# Introducing Pharmacology
## for Nursing and Healthcare

Second edition

Roger McFadden

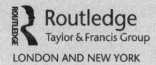
Routledge
Taylor & Francis Group

LONDON AND NEW YORK

First published in 2009
Second edition published 2013 by Pearson Education Limited

Published 2014 by Routledge
2 Park Square, Milton Park, Abingdon, Oxon OX14 4RN
711 Third Avenue, New York, NY, 10017, USA

*Routledge is an imprint of the Taylor & Francis Group, an informa business*

**British Library Cataloguing-in-Publication Data**
A catalogue record for the print edition is available from the British Library

**Library of Congress Cataloging-in-Publication Data**
A catalog record for the print edition is available from the Library of Congress

ISBN-13: 978-1-447-92775-4 (pbk)

Print edition typeset in 9.5/13pt Interstate Light by 35

# Brief contents

# Contents

# Preface to second edition

In the three years since the first edition of *Introducing Pharmacology* was published there have been changes in the world of medicine and medication. Naturally there have been new drugs licensed and old drugs discontinued but there have also been changes in the guidelines and protocols for the treatment of conditions such as hypertension. These changes have been incorporated into this new edition.

Writing the second edition of *Introducing Pharmacology* has also given me the opportunity to extend coverage of the pharmacopoeia with a completely new chapter on anti-cancer drugs. It has also enabled me to fill in some gaps in the first edition with several new sections, including general anaesthetics, hay fever and prescribing for special groups such as children, pregnant women and the elderly.

It's always a pleasure to receive feedback from my students and many have commented positively on the user-friendly style of *Introducing Pharmacology*. So, while the second edition is certainly more comprehensive, I hope students find it retains the readability of the first edition.

*Roger McFadden*
*July 2012*

# Introduction

Welcome, reader, to the fascinating world of pharmacology.

You are probably reading this book because you have enrolled on a course of studies leading to a recognised clinical qualification such as Registered Nurse (RN) or Registered Midwife (RM). Alternatively, you may already be a registered practitioner but are returning to study in order to gain additional qualifications such as Nurse Independent Prescriber or Specialist Practitioner. Whatever your reason for studying the subject, you will find an understanding of pharmacology to be invaluable in your clinical practice. Therapeutic drugs are widely prescribed to patients in most branches of medicine and it is unlikely that any clinical practitioner will be working in an area where patients have not been prescribed some form of medication.

If you are going to be looking after patients who have been prescribed drugs, you need to understand the mechanism whereby those drugs work. For the patient, it will be sufficient to know that an analgesic drug relieves their pain or an anxiolytic drug relieves their anxiety but you, as a clinical practitioner, need to understand the action of these drugs at a much deeper level. You may have had the responsibility for the administration of a drug to a patient or perhaps you are looking after a patient who has been administered a drug by a clinical colleague. In either case, it is you who will be responsible for monitoring the patient's response to the drug and not only must you ensure that the drug is working but also (and equally importantly) whether the drug is causing any unwanted side-effects. To do this effectively it is essential that you understand the drug's mechanism of action – how it produces its therapeutic effect. Increasingly, many non-medical practitioners, nurses, midwives, etc., are trained and licensed to prescribe independently and for them a good understanding of pharmacology is absolutely essential.

*Introducing Pharmacology* has been specially written for the reader without a background in physiology, pathology and pharmacology. In its 12 chapters, *Introducing Pharmacology* focuses on the most commonly prescribed drugs and explains their action relative to the physiology and pathology of the system concerned. Naturally, as you progress in your studies you will need to refer to more advanced textbooks and journals but *Introducing Pharmacology* will start you off with a sound understanding of the basics of the subject.

*Introducing Pharmacology* is divided into two parts.
**Part 1** looks at the fundamentals of pharmacology, taking you down among the cells to the protein structures targeted by drugs. We also look at how the body processes and eliminates the drugs that have been administered. This will help you understand why some drugs can be given in tablet form while others must be

injected or delivered via an intravenous line. Drugs can relieve symptoms and cure disease but they can also cause side-effects so we examine this downside of medication. Drugs also have the potential to interact with other drugs and even some foods. Part 1 explores how this happens and the consequences of these interactions.

**Part 2** examines how individual drugs produce their therapeutic (and sometimes unwanted) effects on the body. Each chapter is devoted to a particular organ system – circulatory, respiratory, digestive, etc. The chapters follow a regular format. Firstly, we examine the basic anatomy and physiology of the organ system. Secondly, we look at key pathologies affecting that system, for example asthma in the respiratory system and high blood pressure in the circulatory system. Finally, when you are sure you understand the physiology and pathology, we then examine the key drugs used to treat those pathologies.

As *Introducing Pharmacology* is an introductory book, it covers primarily those drugs that you will encounter regularly in general clinical practice. Some drugs are rarely found outside specialist areas and to keep the book to its remit of *introducing pharmacology*, these drugs have been touched on only lightly or even omitted. However, all drugs have similarities in their modes of action so by reading this book and understanding the basic principles of pharmacology, you should have the knowledge necessary to access more advanced publications dealing with these specialist drugs.

As you read each chapter, you will find a few special features that will help keep you involved in the learning process and also ensure you have understood what you have just read.

### WHERE ARE WE STARTING FROM?

Provides a few short questions for you to test your background knowledge before you start a chapter.

### ONE SMALL QUESTION

This character pops up frequently and asks those awkward questions that keep us on our toes.

### DID YOU KNOW . . . ?

Interesting snippets of information relating to the text that may broaden your understanding of a particular topic.

### IN PRACTICE

Notes that help you apply your understanding of pharmacology to clinical practice.

### KEY FACT

Highlights important concepts or ideas.

**ANOTHER WAY TO PICTURE THIS**

Sometimes pharmacological concepts can be quite difficult to grasp but by using an analogy from everyday experience they can make more sense.

 **CASE STUDY**

These mini case studies appear in Part 2 and relate to the drugs and diseases that you are exploring in each chapter. You are encouraged to think about what you have learned and apply that knowledge to practice.

 **A QUICK RECAP ON . . .**

Highlights the key concepts and ideas that you have been reading about over the previous few pages.

 **TEST YOURSELF**

Now you have finished the chapter, you can test yourself with these mini-quizzes to find out how much you have learned and remembered. Answers are provided at the end of the book.

## Biomedical terminology

There are a lot of technical terms used in the sciences of physiology, pathology and pharmacology and the practitioner needs to be familiar with them because they are used in clinical practice by other clinical professionals. In *Introducing Pharmacology*, biomedical terms such as *presynaptic receptors* and *ulcerative oesophagitis*, when used for the first time, are written in italics and a brief explanation provided in the Glossary (see p. 319). Where an understanding of these terms is essential, an explanation is highlighted within the text.

In *Introducing Pharmacology* you will find plenty of case studies, clinical notes and self-test questions that break up the narrative into manageable sections. When you have finished working through the book you should have a good grasp of the basics of the subject and the key specialist terms used in pharmacology, and be ready to move onto the next stage of applying what you have learned to your clinical practice.

So, find a nice new pad of A4 paper, sharpen your pencil and get ready for some interesting (if occasionally challenging) pharmacology.

## A brief note about the drug names used in this book

The drugs in *Introducing Pharmacology* use the Recommended International Non-proprietary Names (rINN) from the European Pharmacopoeia, which are replacing the British Approved Names (BAN). Some of these might be slightly different to what you currently encounter in clinical practice so, for example, **phenobarbital** replaces **phenobarbitone**, **furosemide** replaces **frusemide** and **lidocaine** replaces **lignocaine**. The rINN names are the names that appear in the British National Formulary (BNF) and are becoming the accepted form in UK practice.

As is standard for most pharmacology books, *Introducing Pharmacology* uses the generic (rINN) names for drugs rather than the proprietary or trade names. The generic names refer to a standardised formula for that particular drug whereas the manufacturer's proprietary or trade name describes the formulation of the drug supplied by that particular manufacturer. So for example, **fluoxetine** is the generic name of Prozac®, which is the name given to **fluoxetine** by its manufacturer – Eli Lilly & Co Ltd. **Salbutamol** is the generic name for Ventolin® produced by GlaxoSmithKline plc. Although some proprietary names may be better known than the generic names, *Introducing Pharmacology* generally uses the generic names. The reason for this is that some drugs, especially those out of copyright, may have many proprietary versions produced by various manufacturers and it would be impossible to use them all or decide which name among them was the best known. In *Introducing Pharmacology*, the generic name is indicated by the name being highlighted in bold letters, for example **verapamil**, **warfarin** and **ibuprofen**.

## A brief note on pharmacology and clinical practice

Whilst you will find the study of pharmacology very useful and relevant to your clinical practice, it is not strictly a clinical subject and *Introducing Pharmacology* will not be imparting clinical advice. Case studies are included in Part 2 of this book solely to demonstrate the relevance of pharmacology to practice. The decision about which drug to administer to which patient at which dose, at which time and by which route is a clinical decision that requires expertise acquired in clinical practice and clinical training.

*Roger McFadden*

# Acknowledgements

I must above all thank Nicola Peterson (the Lady-wife) for her patience and help during the preparation of the second edition of *Introducing Pharmacology*. I would also like to acknowledge the assistance and advice of clinical and academic colleagues – Tracey Cutler, Simon Dobbs, Christine Hirsch, Caroline Rodrick and Meryl Swann.

# Part 1

# Principles of pharmacology

# Chapter 1

# Let's start at basics: cells and how they work

This chapter looks briefly at the structure and function of cells, which are the prime target for most drugs. We then dip our toes into some basic biochemistry because drugs mostly target biochemical processes in cells.

## CONTENTS

## Introduction

Pharmacology can be quite daunting to the student approaching the subject for the first time. One reason for this is that most pharmacological activity takes place at a cellular or biochemical level and relatively few people are really comfortable down among the cells and molecules. This, however, is the level where we need to be, not only to understand the subject of pharmacology but also to understand the literature relating to the subject. This literature consists of not only textbooks on pharmacology but also clinical reference books such as the *British National Formulary* (BNF) that you will find in daily use in every UK hospital ward and GP surgery. The BNF appears in an updated edition at six-monthly intervals and is published jointly by the British Medical Association and the Royal Pharmaceutical Society of Great Britain. Clinical practitioners use this standard reference book on licensed drugs to ensure that the drug they are prescribing is suitable for the patient, that the patient is being prescribed the correct dose and that the drug will not interact with other drugs. However, a look at the contents page of the BNF will quickly convince you that you need to have some understanding of pharmacology just to access and use this publication. Here is a short sample of the section headings relating to various classes of drugs contained in the BNF:

- Calcium channel blockers
- Selective beta-2 agonists
- Angiotensin-converting enzyme inhibitors
- Alpha-adrenoceptor blocking drugs
- Non-steroidal anti-inflammatory drugs
- $H_2$ receptor antagonists
- Selective serotonin re-uptake inhibitors
- Cyclo-oxygenase-2 inhibitors

If these terms are already familiar, you can probably progress fairly quickly to a more advanced pharmacology book. You might however, recognise the drug groups but not understand the biomedical terminology, in which case you will need to learn them – especially if you are going to be involved in prescribing or administering drugs to patients. Nursing staff who administer drugs to patients are responsible for the safe administration of those drugs. This means that those staff must be familiar with those drugs, how they work in the body, how they may cause side-effects and possibly interact with other drugs. The classes of drugs mentioned above are in fact the clinical names of some of the most common drug groups that include antihypertensives, analgesics, bronchodilators, antidepressants and drugs for heartburn.

One of the key aims of *Introducing Pharmacology* is to familiarise you with the language of pharmacology, the names of drugs and the terms that you will find on every packet of drugs and in every publication dealing with the clinical use of those drugs. You will need this language not only to study and understand pharmacology but also to discuss drugs and their effects with patients and fellow professionals.

## 1.1 Levels of organisation: from cells to systems

Drugs are chemicals that are introduced into the human body to treat or prevent disease. Drugs can relieve symptoms such as pain and swelling, resolve problems such as indigestion and anxiety or manage problems such as heart disease. There are hundreds of different types of drugs designed to treat hundreds of disorders and each type of drug works by a unique action of its own. The way that some drugs work is relatively straightforward while others have quite complex actions. Ultimately, however, if we are going to understand how any of these drugs work, we need to transport ourselves to the level at which most drugs work – the cell.

What exactly is a cell . . . ?

Good question – we will examine cells in some detail later in this chapter. At the moment you just need to know that cells are very small structures that form the building blocks of tissues and organs.

Now, although the basic action of most drugs can be explained at a cellular level, they eventually have an effect on organs and systems that can be observed either by the clinical practitioner or by the patient. This means that to really understand the action of drugs you have to be able to connect their action at cellular level with their effect on organs and systems. Let us illustrate this by looking at some common drugs and drug groups with which you are probably familiar (or at least have heard of) – see Table 1.1. All of these drugs act on specific cells of the body but have an effect above cellular level.

The gap between the target cell and the effect the drug has on the body is highlighted in the table by an arrow and this is largely what pharmacology is about – explaining how a drug that targets a particular cell produces its therapeutic effect on the body. To understand this, you need to appreciate that the body has various levels of organisation.

Table 1.1 Some common drugs, their cellular targets and their effects

| Drug | Target cell | Mechanism | Therapeutic effects |
|---|---|---|---|
| Beta-blockers | Heart cells | ⟶ | Prevents an increase in heart rate |
| Local anaesthetics | Nerve cells | ⟶ | Prevents pain in minor surgery |
| Analgesics | Immune cells | ⟶ | Reduces inflammatory pain |
| Antidepressants | Nerve cells | ⟶ | Relieves depression |
| Statins | Liver cells | ⟶ | Reduces blood cholesterol levels |

We divide the human body into levels of organisation for much the same reason as we divide a book into sections and chapters – it breaks the whole into manageable sections and helps us to understand the structure better. Figure 1.1 shows a simplified hierarchy of structures, starting with cell chemistry and moving upwards to the whole body. As an example of this hierarchy we have used the circulatory system, but bear in mind that this simplified diagram does not imply that the heart is made up of only one type of tissue. There may be only one heart but it is made up of several different types of tissue and these tissues are made up of their own specialised types of cells.

Most drugs interact initially with the first two categories, *cell organelles* and their components, the chemicals of which they are made. However, the effects of drugs are generally observed on the body as a whole or the organ systems. For example, the anti-angina drug **glyceryl trinitrate** (GTN) targets the cells of various blood vessels, including those of the heart itself, but the effect observed by the patient is the lessening of his or her chest pain. Another example is the anti-hypertensive drug **nifedipine**, which reduces blood pressure by targeting the cell membrane of blood vessel muscle cells. Here the effect is on the circulatory system where you will observe a fall in blood pressure.

In Part 2 of *Introducing Pharmacology* we will be following the stories of most of our major drug groups from their interaction with cells right through to their therapeutic effect on organ systems. You will see that when we take each stage a step at a time, then pharmacology is actually quite a straightforward subject and is nowhere near as daunting as it may at first seem. But first things first – we

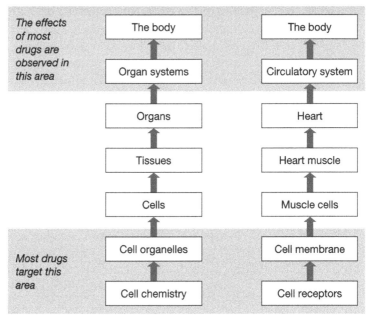

**Figure 1.1** Levels of organisation within the human body. The hierarchy of organisation of the heart and circulatory system is given as an example.

need to familiarise ourselves with cells and some of the basic biochemistry that takes place in those cells.

## 1.2    A brief introduction to cells

Most drugs bind to proteins and most of these proteins are found in and on cells. Those proteins that form the targets for drugs are explored in more detail in Chapter 2, but in the meantime we need to find out a bit more about cells and the proteins they produce.

### Cells and cell components

Cells are the building blocks that make up most tissues and our bodies contain trillions of them. Most cells are specialised to a particular task. For example, muscle cells contract, nerve cells conduct nervous impulses and glandular cells secrete hormones. Drugs interact with these specialised cells and the effects of these interactions will be discussed in detail in Part 2 of *Introducing Pharmacology* when we look at the major drug groups. However, although these cells may look very different on the outside and each may have its own specialised function, inside they are fairly similar. A few cells, such as muscle cells, contain special proteins that enable them to contract, but otherwise cells have many internal features in common. To understand the principles of how drugs work on cells, it is necessary to have a basic understanding of cells, their structure and what goes on inside them. Figure 1.2 is a diagram of a typical cell.

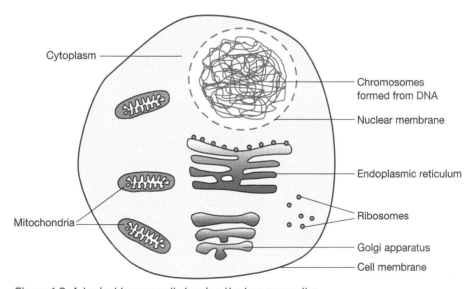

**Figure 1.2** A typical human cell showing the key organelles.

## The components of cells

It is important not to think of cells simply as the building blocks of tissues. In reality they are incredibly complex and dynamic structures, miniature wonderlands of biochemical activity. Every second in every cell there are thousands upon thousands of biochemical reactions taking place to maintain the cell and also to enable it to perform its task as part of a community of cells that makes up our tissues and organs.

## Cell organelles

If you look at a cell through a good-quality, high-powered microscope you can see that cells contain many small structures. These are called the organelles (literally, small organs) and are common to all cells. Each organelle has a specific function.

Several of the organelles work collectively as a team to produce proteins. These are the *nucleus*, the *endoplasmic reticulum*, the *Golgi apparatus* and the *ribosomes*. Tens of thousands of different proteins are made by cells and, as mentioned previously, proteins are the main target for drugs.

*Mitochondria* are small, bean-shaped organelles that produce most of the energy for the cell. They use the energy from fuel such as glucose and lipids to produce *adenosine triphosphate* (ATP), a small packet of energy that powers most of the cell's biochemical processes. You will need to understand more about ATP because some drugs target structures and mechanisms that use ATP. The process whereby our cells make ATP is quite complex but we need to have a basic understanding of the process because some diseases such as angina affect energy production and some drugs such as **glyceryl trinitrate** help to maintain the body's ability to make ATP. This process of cellular energy production is called *cellular respiration* and we will examine it in more detail later in this chapter.

## Cytoplasm

Cytoplasm is a collective term for the contents of the cell. It is composed of the organelles and the cytosol, a semitransparent solution of enzymes, nutrients and electrolytes, necessary for the myriad of processes that take place continuously in each cell.

## Cell membrane

This important structure is a thin membrane that encloses the contents of our cells and separates them from the extracellular fluid outside the cell. The cell membrane regulates what goes into and out of the cell. It is composed mainly of a *phospholipid bilayer* interspersed with cholesterol and it is incredibly thin, around 7 nanometres (1 nanometre is 1000000th of 1 millimetre). The components of the bilayer are arranged as shown in Figure 1.3.

The phosphate heads are hydrophilic (attracted to water) so they happily sit in the watery environment of the *extracellular* fluid outside the cell and the *intracellular* fluid inside the cell. The lipid tails are hydrophobic (repelled by water) and

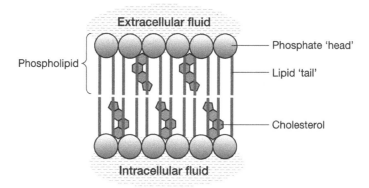

**Figure 1.3** The phospholipid bilayer makes up the cell membrane. Cholesterol molecules within the bilayer help to stabilise it.

form a stable layer in the water-free environment between the outer and inner layer of phosphate heads. Cholesterol molecules give the structure additional stability. There are proteins embedded in the cell membrane that have a variety of roles. These proteins include receptors, ion channels, enzymes and carrier proteins. As mentioned at the beginning of the chapter, proteins are the main targets for therapeutic drugs and these four proteins are our key targets.

*Intracellular* relates to that which is within the cell and *extracellular* is that which is outside the cell.

A section of cell membrane might look like that shown in Figure 1.4.

**KEY FACT**

Many drugs bind to structures in the cell membrane, specifically receptors, ion channels, enzymes and carrier proteins. Not all enzymes are attached to membranes: others may be found inside or outside cells and these also may be the target of drugs.

**Figure 1.4** A section of a cell membrane showing various membrane proteins.

**A QUICK RECAP on our brief introduction to cells**

- Cells form tissues that form organs that form organ systems.
- Cells are complex structures whose organelles are involved in energy production and protein synthesis (among other functions).
- Organelles involved in protein synthesis include the nucleus, the endoplasmic reticulum, the Golgi apparatus and the ribosomes.
- Mitochondria produce most of the cell's energy in the form of ATP.
- The cell membrane controls what enters and leaves the cell.

## 1.3    A brief introduction to (basic) biochemistry

Biochemistry is where biology and chemistry meet; it is basically the chemistry of biological processes. Most people, when they think of chemistry, conjure up images of scientists in white coats doing experiments in laboratories full of strange smells and bubbling test-tubes. Biochemistry labs are very similar except the materials in the test-tubes are of biological origin such as enzymes and lipids. Biochemistry, as with all subjects, can be quite challenging when studied at depth but fortunately, you can learn the essentials, certainly enough for basic clinical pharmacology, without too much chemistry – and not an equation in sight.

*Do we really need to learn this biochemistry?*

Yes, unfortunately you do. Drugs target many biochemical processes that take place in and around cells. For example, most drugs target proteins, so you need to know what proteins are. Some antibacterial drugs target protein synthesis, so you need to understand this process. Statins are a common group of drugs that lower cholesterol, so you need to understand lipids.

### Protein and protein synthesis

Drugs target proteins, but before we look at how the cells make protein, it may be useful to ask ourselves: 'What is protein?' Proteins are an important and probably the most variable class of biological molecules. There are tens of thousands of different proteins in the human body and they perform a wide variety of functions including:

**Structure** – proteins form tendons and ligaments

**Movement** – proteins found in muscles produce muscle contraction

**Communication** – many hormones are proteins

**Defence** – antibodies that attack and destroy bacteria are proteins

**Oxygen transport** – haemoglobin found in red blood cells is a protein.

**Figure 1.5** Chains of amino acids make up a protein. The sequence of the amino acids and the length of the chain largely determine the character of the protein.

As you can see from the above list, the body could not function properly without proteins. Not included in this list are the four protein targets for most of our drugs – ion channels, enzymes, receptors and carrier proteins. These are quite specialised types of protein and are found mainly in and on cells. In Chapter 2 we will explore each of them in some depth.

Proteins are made of chains of amino acids (small nitrogen-containing molecules) – see Figure 1.5. There are 20 different types of amino acid in human protein and we obtain these amino acids from our food. Meat, fish, eggs, nuts and beans are foods that are rich in protein and consequently rich in amino acids. The digestive system breaks down the protein in these foods into its component amino acids, which we absorb into the body for our cells to reassemble into human protein.

The nature of the protein is largely determined by the length of the chain and the order of the amino acids. Another factor characteristic of each individual protein is the way the chain of amino acids folds into its final three-dimensional shape. Some are long and thin such as the structural protein *collagen* found in tendons, and these are called filamentous proteins. Others form a more rounded, globular shape such as the oxygen-carrying protein *haemoglobin*, and these are naturally called globular proteins.

## ANOTHER WAY TO PICTURE THIS

You can think of amino acids rather like letters in the alphabet. There are an infinite number of words that can be formed, each word's individual character being determined by its length and the order of its letters. Similarly, there are an infinite number of proteins that could be made, each protein's individual character being determined by the length of the chain and its sequence of amino acids.

The body's cells all have the ability to make over 20 000 different proteins, the difference determined by the length and sequence of the amino acids in the chain. This means that inside each cell there needs to be a code or instruction to ensure that when the cell makes a particular protein, the amino acids are in the correct sequence and the chain is of the correct length. This code for our proteins is contained within DNA (deoxyribose nucleic acid), an incredibly thin ribbon-like molecule that is found in the nucleus of each cell. There are 46 lengths of DNA in all human cells (except the sperm and egg, which each have 23) and each length of DNA is called a chromosome. Although individual cells do not need to make every kind of protein, each cell contains the codes for every one of our 20 000

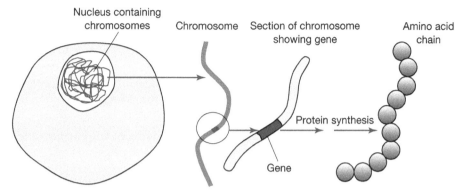

Nucleus containing chromosomes

Chromosome

Section of chromosome showing gene

Amino acid chain

Protein synthesis

Gene

**Figure 1.6** Proteins are produced from information contained in chromosomes. The information coded in each gene is translated into the correct sequence of amino acids by a process called protein synthesis.

or so proteins. How the cell knows which proteins to make and when to make them is not yet fully understood.

The length of DNA that codes for a single chain of amino acids or protein is called a gene (Figure 1.6). There are over 30 000 genes that code for the 20 000-plus proteins that cells make. There are more genes than proteins because some proteins such as haemoglobin are made up of more than one amino acid chain and so need more than one gene to code for each chain.

Some proteins are used within the cell and others are exported from the cell for use in other parts of the body. Many proteins are lodged in the cell membrane such as receptors, ion channels, enzymes or carrier proteins. These are the key drug targets that are examined in Chapter 2. Proteins come in many shapes and sizes and perform many functions. Enzymes are among the most numerous types of protein; they are complex structures that take part in most of the body's biochemical reactions and are also a major target for drugs.

**DID YOU KNOW...** that every cell contains around 2 metres of DNA? There are well over a trillion cells in the human body, so the total length of DNA must be at least 2 billion kilometres, which is more than enough to stretch from the Earth to the Sun over 10 times!!!

## How cells make proteins

When a cell needs to make a protein there follows a complex process that involves finding the correct gene and translating the instructions contained in that gene into a protein with the correct sequence of amino acids, a chain of the appropriate length and folded into the correct shape. The process involves cooperation between several organelles in the cell: the nucleus, obviously, as it contains the chromosomes that carry the code in their genes; the ribosomes that are responsible for the assembly of the amino acids into a chain that will make up the protein, and finally the endoplasmic reticulum and Golgi apparatus that fold the protein into its final shape.

## Lipids

Lipids are an important group of molecules. As well as being a good source of energy and providing insulation from the cold, they are the raw material of some hormones and also form a significant part of cell membranes. As most drugs target proteins in the cell membranes, you will need a basic understanding of lipids in order to understand the nature of the cell membrane and ultimately the action of drugs.

There are many different types of lipid but they can initially be divided into two groups:

- oils – these are liquid at room temperature
- fats – these are solid at room temperature.

Oils are generally obtained from plants and fish whereas fats are mostly obtained from meat such as beef and pork. We can get these fats from the natural foods we eat but a good proportion of our lipid intake is from processed products such as cooking oils, margarine, butter and cheese.

**Triglycerides**, also known as triacylglycerols, are an important group of lipids and most of the lipids that we eat and store in the body are triglycerides. Their structure is relatively simple, just three long fatty acid chains joined to a glycerol molecule (Figure 1.7).

**Figure 1.7** Triglycerides are composed of three fatty acid chains attached to a glycerol molecule.

**Fatty acids** come in various forms and you may have seen their names on the labels of some processed foods. Most of these names refer to the ratio and arrangement of carbon and hydrogen atoms in the fatty acid chains. We will just mention them here so you will understand what they do, but we will not go any deeper into their biochemistry.

- **Saturated fatty acids** – mainly found in animal fats and processed foods.
- **Mono-unsaturated fatty acids** – only vegetable in origin, for example olive oil.
- **Polyunsaturated fatty acids** – only vegetable in origin, for example sunflower oil.

The type and balance of the lipids we consume in our diet has important implications for our health, especially the health of our heart. We are currently recommended to consume less saturated fat and use more mono-unsaturated oils, such as olive oil, in preference.

**Cholesterol** is a sterol lipid that is predominantly made in the liver, but it is also obtained from animal products such as eggs. It is an important substance because it stabilises our cell membranes and is also a component of bile, a digestive product made in the liver and secreted into the digestive tract via the bile duct. Cholesterol is also the raw material for steroid hormones such as oestrogen, testosterone and vitamin D. Cholesterol regulation is important because, if it gets out of balance, it can encourage cardiovascular disease. Various drugs such as statins are widely prescribed to reduce cholesterol levels.

**DID YOU KNOW...** that vitamin D is actually a steroid hormone rather than a vitamin? It is made in the skin when exposed to sunlight but is also obtained in the diet from fatty fish such as sardines and herring. Many foods such as breakfast cereals are fortified with vitamin D. A shortage of vitamin D can cause rickets in children and osteomalacia in adults.

## Carbohydrates and sugars

Just as a car needs fuel to keep it going, the body also needs fuel to provide the energy for the thousands of biochemical reactions that take place every second. Some of these reactions require very little energy; others power processes with a very high energy demand such as muscle contraction. We get the energy primarily from carbohydrates in the form of starches and sugars but lipids also make an important contribution to our energy needs. There are no drugs that have sugars and starches as their prime targets, but these substances play an important role in the body. Drugs such as **insulin** have a direct effect on glucose metabolism so you need a basic familiarity with this important group of molecules.

Carbohydrates can be divided into three groups: monosaccharides, disaccharides and polysaccharides. As 'saccharide' means sugar, these three groups are single sugars, double sugars and multiple sugars respectively.

### Monosaccharides

These are single sugars that include glucose, fructose and galactose. Glucose is one of the most common monosaccharides as it forms the building blocks of polysaccharides such as starch, glycogen and cellulose. Glucose is a key fuel for human metabolism, which is why we need a good supply of carbohydrates for our daily energy requirement. There is very little free glucose in nature and it is mostly found in polysaccharides such as starch. Our digestive systems contain enzymes that break down the polysaccharides into energy-rich monosaccharide glucose molecules. These are transported in the blood to the cells of the body where the glucose is broken down to release its energy to power biochemical processes.

### Disaccharides

These are two monosaccharides joined together. Common disaccharides include maltose, sucrose and lactose. The sugar that we put in our tea and coffee is sucrose, a disaccharide composed of glucose and fructose.

### Polysaccharides

These are long chains of monosaccharides joined together. Common glucose-based polysaccharides include starch, glycogen and cellulose.

**Starch** is a polymer (chain) of glucose molecules that is produced in plants. It is a major source of fuel for humans. Potatoes, wheat and rice contain large amounts of starch and so are important energy-rich foods for us. Starch is broken down into individual glucose molecules by enzymes in the digestive system.

**Glycogen** is a polymer of glucose found in animal cells, stored especially in the liver and skeletal muscle. When the cells require energy, enzymes break down glycogen into glucose molecules. Glucose released by the liver cells can be used to top up the glucose in the blood when circulating levels are low.

**Cellulose** is similar in structure to starch, except for a small biochemical difference that makes it impossible for humans to digest. This is unfortunate because it is a major structural component of plants and the most abundant form of glucose on the planet. Its indigestible nature does confer some benefits because it increases the bulk of our food and provides the fibre necessary for a healthy digestion. Animals such as cows, which get their energy from grass, rely on bacteria in their digestive systems to break down the cellulose into glucose.

**A QUICK RECAP on proteins, lipids and sugars**

- There are many thousands of different proteins in the body.
- Proteins are key targets for drugs.
- DNA in the nucleus of cells codes for our proteins.
- The section of DNA that codes for one protein is called a gene.
- Lipids are an important source of energy and are also components of cell membranes.
- Starch is our main source of energy but needs to be broken down into glucose for use by cells.

## Cellular respiration and the production of ATP

Most of the processes within cells require energy so all cells need energy to function properly. Some cells are especially demanding of energy, for example muscle cells. The heart is primarily made of cardiac muscle cells and beats every second of our lives, increasing its activity when we exercise. Skeletal muscle cells work in groups to contract whole muscles that allow us to engage in sporting activities such as running, tennis and cycling. We can expend a lot of energy when engaged in these sports and this energy comes from the adenosine triphosphate (ATP) produced in every cell of the body. There is a fundamental law of physics that (put simply) says that energy can be transferred but not created; therefore, in the case of cells, there needs to be a source of energy that enables them to produce ATP. This energy is obtained primarily from glucose in energy-rich foods we eat, especially the starchy foods such as rice, potatoes and wheat. Triglycerides from the lipids found in animal and plant products also make a significant contribution to our energy requirements.

**DID YOU KNOW ...** that in some extreme sports, athletes can burn over 30 000 kJ of energy in one day – four times as much as the average person? Someone has calculated that in the Tour de France™ cycle race, where some stages are over 200 km, riders would need to eat 25 cheeseburgers each day to top up their energy!

ATP is produced in every cell of the body because every cell needs energy to perform its numerous biochemical reactions, and the original source of this energy is either glucose or lipids. However, these are large molecules and while they contain plenty of energy, that energy is not in a usable form for most biochemical reactions. As cells need small packets of energy, they break down glucose and lipids by a gradual process into their component parts and during this process energy is released and transferred to ATP.

**KEY FACT**

All cells need energy in the form of ATP. They use the energy from glucose and lipids to make their ATP.

Adenosine triphosphate (ATP) is part of a family of molecules that also includes *adenosine diphosphate* (ADP). If you think of ATP as a small rechargeable battery, it is uncharged in the ADP form and fully charged in the ATP form (Figure 1.8). The biochemical process in the cell that charges ADP into ATP is called cellular respiration.

When ATP has performed its task, perhaps activating an enzyme or moving ions across a membrane, it loses much of its energy and becomes low-energy ADP which must then return to the mitochondria to be recharged into ATP (Figure 1.9).

The process that recharges ADP to ATP is called cellular respiration, which is a fundamental process common to all animals and plants. Cellular respiration is at the heart of our metabolism; it explains why we breathe, why we are warm-blooded animals and why we eat the energy-rich foods we all enjoy. This process takes place in every cell of our body and can be described by a simple word formula:

Carbohydrate/Lipids + Oxygen + ADP $\longrightarrow$ Carbon dioxide + Water + Heat + ATP

**Figure 1.8** Comparing the cell's energy molecule to a rechargeable battery. Cellular respiration charges ADP to its energy-packed form of ATP.

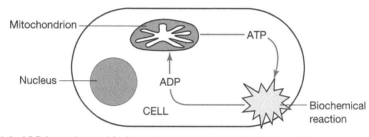

**Figure 1.9** ADP is recharged in the mitochondria to ATP that can then power biochemical reactions in the cell. When it gives up its energy, ATP becomes ADP, which returns to the mitochondria to be recharged again into ATP.

Energy production is all about the ATP that maintains our body's metabolism and therefore life itself. Basically the formula says that in the presence of oxygen the body can use energy-rich foods such as carbohydrate and lipids to energise ADP into ATP. In the process, waste products such as carbon dioxide, water and heat are produced.

The oxygen that is essential for this process is obtained from the air that we breathe and transported in the blood from the lungs to the cells of the body – see Figure 1.10. Carbon dioxide, the waste gas produced in cellular respiration, is transported in the opposite direction, from the cells to the lungs, where it is exhaled into the atmosphere.

The process of cellular respiration involves dozens of enzymes that work in complex pathways to break down carbohydrates and lipids to form ATP. Oxygen is essential for the efficiency of this process and if any disease reduces the supply of oxygen to cells and tissues then the consequences can be very serious indeed: without oxygen, cells cannot produce ATP and without ATP, cells die. This is what happens when someone has a heart attack or stroke – as we will see later in Chapter 4.

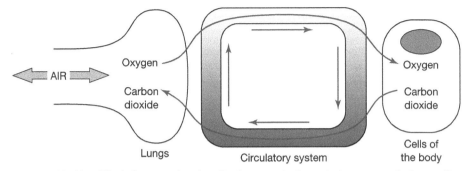

Figure 1.10 Simplified diagram showing the transport of respiratory gases between the lungs and the body's cells. Oxygen carried into the lungs from the air we breathe is transported to the cells via the blood. The waste gas, carbon dioxide, is transported in the opposite direction, from the cells to the lungs, where it is breathed out into the atmosphere.

**IN PRACTICE**

Any disease that affects the lungs can cause problems with gas exchange. Bronchitis and emphysema are very common chronic diseases of the lungs. Shortness of breath, wheezing and cough are common symptoms and lack of oxygen may cause cyanosis (a blue tinge to the lips and fingers).

As for the other waste products in the process of cellular respiration, water simply diffuses into the tissues and mingles with the rest of the water in the body (don't forget we are composed of almost 65 per cent water). The heat produced in cellular respiration helps to keep our body warm with a core temperature steady, around 37°C.

**A QUICK RECAP on cellular respiration**

- Cells need energy for biochemical reactions.
- ATP is the source of energy for these biochemical reactions.
- The energy to produce ATP comes from energy-rich foods.
- The process that produces ATP is called cellular respiration.
- Cellular respiration requires oxygen that is transported from the lungs to the cells of the body.
- Cellular respiration produces carbon dioxide that is transported from the cells of the body to the lungs.

## REFERENCES AND FURTHER RECOMMENDED READING

All recommended websites are open access (but free registration is sometimes required).

Websites

*British National Formulary* (2012) BMJ Group and RPS Publishing.

*British National Formulary* Website – http://www.bnf.org/bnf/

Cells Alive website – www.cellsalive.com

Book

Marieb, E.N. (2011) *Essentials of Human Anatomy and Physiology* (international edn), Pearson.

## Test yourself

Now you have finished reading the first chapter it's time to find out how much you have learned and remembered. If you have not studied in this area before, don't worry if you can't answer all of the questions. Re-read the chapter and make sure that it all makes sense.

*The answers to these questions are at the end of the book (see p. 313).*

1 What is the (outline) function of the following cell organelles?
  (a) Nucleus
  (b) Ribosomes
  (c) Mitochondria
  (d) Cell membrane.

2 Is the cell membrane predominantly made of protein, lipid or carbohydrate?

3 Name the four principal protein targets for drugs.

4 What is the name of the section of DNA that codes for one protein?

5 What are the basic components of proteins?

6 What is the chemical difference between an oil and a fat?

7 What lipid is the raw material for steroid hormones?

8 What kind of polysaccharide is the main food source of energy for humans?

9 What two substances are required for efficient ATP production in humans?

10 What happens to the carbon dioxide produced in the process of cellular respiration?

# Chapter 2

# Protein targets for drugs

This chapter explains why proteins make good targets for drugs, the structure of key protein targets for drugs and what happens when drugs bind to key protein targets.

## CONTENTS

## Introduction

Chapter 1 saw the start of our journey into the interesting if occasionally challenging world of pharmacology. We learned that cells are the prime target for most drugs and that those drugs mostly target biochemical processes in cells. This means that some knowledge of basic cell biology and biochemistry is absolutely essential to an understanding of pharmacology, and in this chapter we will start to apply that knowledge. Chapter 2 is where we start to examine the fundamental principles of pharmacology, where we will focus on the four key protein targets for drugs, namely receptors, ion channels, enzymes and carrier proteins. We will also encounter examples of specific drugs that interact with these protein targets and you should start to gain an insight into the basics of the subject and begin to feel more comfortable with the terminology relating to the cellular and biochemical world where most of our drugs exert their action. In the meantime, make sure that you work through this chapter carefully because the concept of protein targets underpins pharmacology and the terms we use here will appear throughout this book and in clinical manuals such as the *British National Formulary* (BNF), which you will encounter in almost every area of clinical practice.

## 2.1 Why do proteins make good targets for drugs?

As we saw in Chapter 1, most drugs target and bind to proteins, mostly on and in the cell membrane. These protein targets can be divided into four categories . . .

- Receptors
- Enzymes
- Ion channels
- Carrier proteins.

**KEY FACT**

Most drugs bind to proteins, specifically ion channels, enzymes, receptors and carrier proteins.

Chapter 1 introduced us to proteins: what they are, what they do and how they are made. In this chapter we are going to examine the four categories of protein drug targets in some detail and we'll also meet examples of the drugs that target those proteins.

Drugs target and bind to proteins and, via a complex series of consequential events, this produces a therapeutic effect, perhaps reducing inflammation, relieving pain or lowering cholesterol levels etc. How the drugs produce these therapeutic effects will be explained in the second part of this book, where we look at drug groups in more detail. First, however, we must ask ourselves why it is that proteins make such good targets for drugs.

Proteins make good targets for drugs for the three reasons detailed below.

## 1 There are many thousands of different proteins

There are around 20 000 different proteins in the human body and each has its own particular task. This means that there are potentially around 20 000 different targets for drugs – although in reality only a small percentage of proteins are suitable targets. Most proteins are involved in tasks not associated with disease so there is no point targeting those proteins. Others are so crucial to normal cell function that it would be dangerous to target them with drugs. However, if only 1 per cent of those 20 000 proteins are worthwhile targets then that gives us the 200 or so different types of drugs that appear in the pharmacopeia. Naturally there are many more drugs than this on the pharmacy shelves because different drug manufacturers often make their own version of a drug – especially if a particular type of drug is selling successfully.

## 2 Proteins have important roles in physiological processes

Proteins also make good targets because they are key players in every physiological process. Circulation, respiration, nervous activity, digestion, renal function and immunity all depend on proteins. Interfere with a protein by targeting it with a drug and you will interfere with a physiological process. It is important to note, however, that targeting a protein could potentially have an adverse effect on these physiological processes so drug manufacturers need to ensure that the drugs they are developing target specific proteins and produce only therapeutic effects. Very occasionally, drugs have an unforeseen action on a protein and this can result in a manufacturer having to withdraw a drug from the market.

## 3 Each organ and tissue has some protein distinctive to that organ and tissue

If we can identify a protein specific to a particular organ or tissue, it may be possible to design a drug to target that specific protein and exert an effect specifically on that particular organ or tissue. This is very important because we want our drugs to produce predictable results in tissues and organs where there are problems that need to be remedied. If an individual patient has a heart problem, we need a drug that targets the heart and only the heart. Because heart tissue has proteins found only in the heart, we can target those proteins and that specific organ. Similarly, if a patient has a bacterial infection, then we want a drug that kills bacterial cells but does not interfere with human body cells. Because some bacterial protein is substantially different from human protein, we can target that bacterial protein and not interfere with other proteins in the body.

Unfortunately, some proteins that make desirable targets for drugs are found on other organs and tissues, including some that have no involvement in the disease we are attempting to prevent or cure. This can cause problems because drugs can also bind to the proteins in those tissues and produce unwanted side-effects. We will explore this problem in more detail in Chapter 3.

### A QUICK RECAP on why proteins make good targets for drugs

- There are many different proteins in many different tissues, which gives us plenty of targets for our drugs.

- As proteins play key roles in physiological processes, they are worthwhile targeting with drugs because by doing so we can influence those physiological processes.

- Different tissues express their own unique proteins and drugs can therefore target those proteins and exert their effect specifically on those tissues.

- Some tissues express similar proteins to those being targeted and can become the targets themselves – resulting in side-effects.

## 2.2   Protein targets 1: receptors

Communication within the body is very important to ensure that it functions properly. Physiological processes with their myriad of tiny biochemical reactions must be coordinated to occur in the right place at the right time. One part of the brain needs to communicate with other parts of the brain and also with the organs and tissues under its control. Glands such as the pituitary and pancreas need to communicate with cells and tissues to ensure that the body's internal environment is kept stable – a process called *homeostasis*. Sometimes adjacent cells need to communicate with each other so that they work cooperatively to ensure that tissues function properly. All of this essential communication is brought about by chemical messengers that are released from nerves, glands and a host of other cell types. These chemical messengers bind to receptors in and on other cells in the body to produce an effect in those target cells (Figure 2.1).

> *Homeostasis* is the name given to internal regulatory mechanisms that maintain steady-state physiological functions such as blood pressure, temperature and blood gas levels.

In Chapter 1 we saw that the cell membrane is essentially lipid in structure and this prevents most substances (apart from lipids) from passing through it. This explains why many chemical messengers bind to the extracellular region of receptors

**Figure 2.1** Chemical messengers released by a cell bind to receptors on an adjacent cell and produce an effect in that cell.

embedded in the cell membrane. There are also intracellular receptors, found within the cell, and these are generally targeted by steroid hormones, lipid-based mediators and a few neutrally charged molecules that can pass through the cell membrane. Receptors are also very popular targets for drugs and we will devote the first part of this chapter to exploring how drugs interact with receptors.

Examples of some common drugs that interact with receptors include:

- **Salbutamol** – dilates the airways and relieves the symptoms of asthma
- **Atenolol** – slows the heart and relieves angina pain
- **Morphine** – inhibits pain pathways in the spinal cord to relieve severe pain
- **Candesartan** – dilates peripheral blood vessels and reduces blood pressure.

Before we look in more detail at receptors, let us quickly examine some important chemical messengers that can broadly be divided into three groups – hormones, neurotransmitters and mediators. Many drugs mimic these chemical messengers so it is important to understand their function in order to appreciate how those drugs work.

**Hormones** are chemicals released by glandular tissue into the bloodstream. These chemicals circulate in the bloodstream and from there pass into tissues where they bind to cell receptors and produce an effect in those cells. The effect depends on the type of receptor and the type of cell. For example, when the hormone insulin is released by the pancreas it binds to an insulin receptor on a cell, causing that cell to increase its uptake of glucose from the blood. The stress hormone adrenaline binds to adrenaline receptors on many different tissues and produces various effects, such as widening the bronchioles and increasing the heart rate. Steroid hormones such as oestrogen are lipids derived from cholesterol and so pass through the cell membrane to bind to receptors inside the cell. Most other hormones cannot pass through the cell membrane so bind to extracellular receptors.

**Neurotransmitters** are chemicals released from the terminals of neurons (nerve cells). These chemicals bind to receptors on other cells or neurons and produce various effects. For example, *acetylcholine* released from a motor neuron and binding to an acetylcholine receptor on a muscle cell would cause that cell to contract.

*Noradrenaline* released by a *sympathetic* neuron and binding to a noradrenaline receptor on an arteriole (small artery) would cause the arteriole muscle cells (and the arteriole itself) to contract.

> *Sympathetic neurons* are nerve cells of the sympathetic nervous system. The sympathetic system is counterbalanced by the parasympathetic system and together the two systems make up the autonomic nervous system – which controls homeostasis. Generally the parasympathetic system is dominant when we are at rest while the sympathetic system takes over during activity and stress.

**Mediators** are mostly locally acting chemicals that bind to receptors on adjacent or nearby cells and produce an effect. *Histamine* is an example of a mediator that binds to histamine receptors on the cells that line the stomach, stimulating those cells to release the hydrochloric acid that breaks down food particles in the process of digestion.

These natural chemical messengers are often referred to as *ligands* – from the Latin *ligare*, to bind. They are also sometimes referred to as *endogenous ligands*, meaning they are chemical messengers, produced within the body, that bind to receptors. Drugs that bind to receptors would be called *exogenous* (from outside the body) *ligands*.

> **KEY FACT**
>
> Cells of the body have receptors for chemical messengers (*endogenous ligands*) such as hormones, neurotransmitters and mediators.

## Why do chemical messengers bind to receptors?

Chemical messengers bind to receptors because the receptor is the appropriate shape for the chemical messenger to bind to it, just as the lock on your front door is the appropriate shape for your front door key. The chemical messengers produced by the body are exactly the right shape for their receptor target (Figure 2.2). This

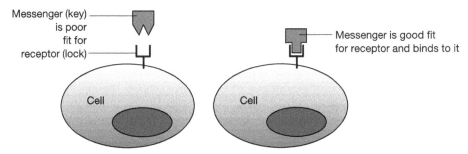

Messenger (key) is poor fit for receptor (lock)

Messenger is good fit for receptor and binds to it

Cell

Cell

**Figure 2.2** Only chemical messengers with a complementary shape to receptors will bind effectively to those receptors.

Keys (hormones)

Locks (receptors)

Figure 2.3 Match the key to its lock. (*Answers on p. 40.*)

correctness of shape is called *specificity* and we will encounter this term later in the chapter when we discuss the interactions between drugs and receptors. The specificity of a chemical messenger for its receptor is predominantly due to shape − like the correct fit of a key to its lock. This binding is enhanced by tiny electrical forces of attraction in the region of the receptor where the chemical messenger docks. These minute forces include *hydrogen bonds* and *van der Waals forces*. However, as this is an introductory book, we will keep things simple and discuss the fit of the chemical messenger for its receptor in terms of shape.

Here is your turn to see whether you can match a chemical messenger to its receptor. The real-life molecular structures of chemical messengers and receptors are rather complex, so we will continue with the analogy of keys and locks. Figure 2.3 shows three keys that may represent three different hormones. The three locks represent three different types of receptor, possibly found on different tissues or organs. Which key best fits into which receptor?

## Why do drugs bind to receptors?

A drug binds to a receptor because the drug's molecular structure gives it a similar shape to that of the natural chemical messenger the body produces to target that receptor.

Here is an example: adrenaline binds to adrenaline receptors in the bronchioles of the lungs and causes bronchodilation (widening of the airways). As the drug **salbutamol** is similar in shape to adrenaline, it also binds to adrenaline receptors and produces the same effect as adrenaline, i.e. bronchodilation. Figure 2.4 shows the molecular structure of the hormone adrenaline and the drug **salbutamol**. You do not need a deep understanding of chemistry to observe the similarities in structure between the two molecules.

Adrenaline          Salbutamol

Figure 2.4 Adrenaline and **salbutamol** have similarities in molecular structure, so they bind to the same receptors.

Why don't we just use the natural chemical messengers as drugs?

Good question. Sometimes we do. For example, adrenaline can be used as a drug in acute anaphylaxis when someone's blood pressure falls rapidly and they go into shock. However, relatively few natural chemical messengers make good drugs. We want drugs that are stable in storage, easy to administer and exert their therapeutic action over several hours or days. Few natural chemical messengers meet these criteria.

## What happens when a chemical messenger binds to a receptor?

The answer to this question depends on the type of chemical messenger, the type of receptor and the type of cell. We have already touched on a few examples, such as insulin causing cells to take up glucose and acetylcholine causing muscle cells to contract. How the binding of these messengers to their receptors produces these effects involves some rather complex intracellular biochemistry and is therefore beyond the scope of this introductory book. From the pharmacological viewpoint, however, the main imperative is to understand the overall effect on the cell or tissue – for example, when the messenger binds to its receptor, does it cause the cell or tissue to contract or relax, increase or decrease its activity, and so on?

## What happens when a drug binds to a receptor?

A drug similar in shape to a natural chemical messenger will bind to the same receptor as that messenger – in fact, competing against the chemical messenger for the receptor site. How successfully it competes depends on the closeness of fit of the drug for the receptor – in other words, its specificity. Once a drug binds to a receptor it can do one of two things: it can either mimic the natural chemical messenger and produce the same effect as that chemical messenger, or bind to and block that receptor and produce no effect.

Drugs that are similar in shape to a natural chemical messenger, bind to its receptor and produce the same effect as the natural chemical messenger are termed *agonists*.

Drugs that are similar in shape to a natural chemical messenger, bind to its receptor but block the receptor without producing a response are called *antagonists*, or sometimes just 'blockers' – as in beta-blockers.

> **KEY FACT**
>
> *Agonist* drugs bind to receptors and mimic the effect of natural chemical messengers. *Antagonist* drugs bind to and block receptors from the effects of their natural chemical messengers.

Figure 2.5 shows a section of membrane with identical receptors for a natural chemical messenger which binds and produces an effect in the cell. Adjacent to

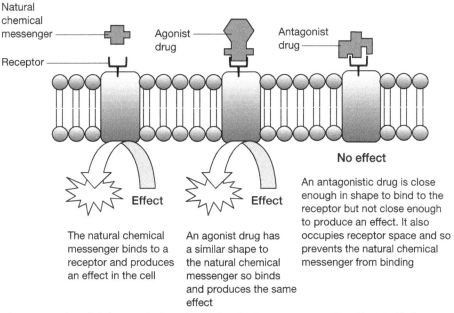

**Figure 2.5** Agonist drugs mimic natural chemical messengers. They bind to their receptors and produce the same effect. Antagonist drugs bind to and block receptors, preventing the natural chemical messengers from binding.

it is an agonist drug that is similar in shape to the natural chemical messenger and so binds to the receptor and produces the same effect. The antagonist drug has enough similarities in shape to the natural chemical messenger to bind to the receptor and block it but not enough to produce a response in the cell.

What's the point of a drug that blocks a receptor but produces no effect?

Good question. It may seem pointless to target a receptor without producing an effect but sometimes we want to prevent the effect that the natural chemical messenger produces. For example, adrenaline increases heart rate so by blocking adrenaline receptors with a beta-blocker we can keep heart rate down – very useful for angina sufferers.

Most drugs that bind to receptors have either an agonist or an antagonist action. We will come across many of these drugs in Part 2 of *Introducing Pharmacology*. Two drugs in common use that you may be familiar with are the bronchodilator **salbutamol** and the anti-angina beta-blocker **atenolol**.

- **Salbutamol** – an agonist for adrenaline receptors in the lungs, mimics the action of adrenaline, stimulates adrenaline receptors and causes bronchodilation (opening of the airways). This helps ease breathing during asthma attacks.
- **Atenolol** – an antagonist for adrenaline receptors on the heart, blocks the receptors from the stimulating activity of adrenaline. This reduces the workload of the heart, which is useful for those suffering from angina.

Both **salbutamol** and **atenolol** have similarities in structure to adrenaline, but whereas **salbutamol** binds to adrenaline receptors and mimics the effect of adrenaline, **atenolol** binds and blocks the receptors without producing any effect in its own right.

## Classes and sub-classes of receptor as drug targets

The observant reader may have noticed from the above account of **salbutamol** and **atenolol** that these two drugs act on different tissues – despite the fact that they both target adrenaline receptors. The reason for this is that the heart's adrenaline receptors and the bronchioles' adrenaline receptors are of different types. On the heart we find beta-1 adrenaline receptors that are targeted by **atenolol** and in the lungs we find beta-2 adrenaline receptors targeted by **salbutamol**.

Receptors that respond to adrenaline (a hormone) or its close relative, nor-adrenaline (a neurotransmitter) are called *adrenergic receptors,* often shortened to *adrenoceptors.* The two classes of adrenergic receptor are often identified simply by their Greek letters, $\alpha$ (alpha) and $\beta$ (beta). These two classes are further divided into sub-classes of receptor. Alpha receptors are divided into alpha-1 ($\alpha_1$) and alpha-2 ($\alpha_2$). Beta receptors are divided into beta-1 ($\beta_1$) and beta-2 ($\beta_2$). There are other sub-classes of adrenergic receptor but these are the only ones of current pharmacological interest.

Different tissues may have different sub-classes of adrenergic receptor; for example, $\alpha_1$ receptors on the arterioles, $\beta_1$ receptors on the heart and $\beta_2$ receptors in the lungs. The fact that there are different types of adrenergic receptor is very important in pharmacology because drugs can be designed to target specific sub-classes of receptor and therefore target specific tissues.

> **KEY FACT**
>
> Drugs can be targeted at the specific sub-classes of receptors that are found on specific tissues.

Other natural chemical messengers have various receptor classes further divided into sub-classes and these are shown in Table 2.1. Don't worry if you do not recognise all of the drug names; the key fact here is that the effect of the natural chemical messenger binding to its receptor depends on the sub-class and location of the receptor. Adrenaline binding to $\beta_1$ receptors on the heart increases the heart rate and force of contraction, but adrenaline binding to $\beta_2$ receptors in the bronchioles causes bronchodilation. This is very important in pharmacology because it means that drugs can be developed that target one specific sub-class of receptor. Thus a drug such as **salbutamol** is a $\beta_2$ adrenergic receptor agonist and will bind preferentially to $\beta_2$ receptors in the lungs rather than any other sub-class of adrenergic receptor. This is why we can have drugs that target specific

Table 2.1 Some common natural messengers, sub-classes of their receptors and examples of agonist and antagonist drugs that target those receptors

| Natural messenger | Class of receptor | Sub-class of receptor | Key locations | Example of agonist drug | Example of antagonist drug |
|---|---|---|---|---|---|
| Adrenaline/ noradrenaline | Adrenergic | Alpha-1 | Arterioles | Phenylephrine | Doxazosin |
| | | Beta-1 | Heart | Dobutamine | Atenolol |
| | | Beta-2 | Bronchioles | Salbutamol | None |
| Acetylcholine | Cholinergic | Muscarinic | Bronchioles | None | Ipratropium |
| | | Nicotinic | Muscles | Suxamethonium | Pancuronium |
| Histamine | Histamine | H-1 | Inner ear | None | Cyclizine |
| | | H-2 | Stomach | None | Cimetidine |
| Opioid-like peptides | Opioid | Mu | Central nervous system | Morphine | Naloxone |
| | | Kappa | | Nalbuphine | None |
| | | Delta | | Pentazocine | None |

organs or tissues such as the heart, lungs, digestive system, nervous system, etc. We also have the option of stimulating the receptor with an agonist or blocking it with an antagonist, whichever is appropriate. Table 2.1 shows that some receptors are targeted by both agonist and antagonist drugs. The key point here is that these different sub-classes of receptors provide useful pharmacological targets.

There is unfortunately a downside to the body having classes of structurally similar receptors. It is useful in that we can target a drug at a particular sub-class of receptor, expressed on a particular tissue to produce a therapeutic effect, but almost inevitably the drug may bind to another receptor of that class, producing an unwanted effect; in other words, a side-effect. This can be a major problem with some drugs and the subject of side-effects is explored more fully in Chapter 3.

**KEY FACT**

Drugs can be targeted at specific sub-classes of receptors but may accidentally bind to other receptors of that class, resulting in unwanted side-effects.

Drugs that bind to types of receptors with either agonist or antagonist actions have been given specific names that you may come across in the pharmacological literature. These terms are *sympathomimetic* and *cholinergic* (both agonist), and *anticholinergic* (antagonist).

A sympathomimetic drug such as **salbutamol** is one that mimics the action of adrenaline or noradrenaline released during sympathetic nervous activity. The bronchodilator **ipratropium bromide** is an antagonist for acetylcholine receptors on the bronchioles of the lungs, and therefore is anticholinergic. There are no direct agonists of acetylcholine in clinical use but **neostigmine**, a drug used to reverse muscle relaxation after surgery, is effectively cholinergic in action.

**A QUICK RECAP on receptors**

- Receptors are proteins found on the cell membrane and also inside cells.
- Receptors are targets for chemical messengers such as hormones, neuro-transmitters and mediators.
- When a chemical messenger binds to a receptor it produces an effect in that cell.
- Drugs are of similar shape to natural chemical messengers and so bind to the same receptors.
- Agonist drugs bind to receptors and produce the same effect as the natural chemical messengers.
- Antagonist drugs bind to receptors and block them from the effects of the natural chemical messengers.
- There are sub-classes of receptors expressed on specific tissues that allow drugs to target those tissues.

## 2.3 Protein targets 2: ion channels

Every major physiological process in the body in some way depends on ions moving across cell membranes, either passively through ion channels or actively through carrier proteins. The rhythmic beating of the heart depends on ions moving across cell membranes, as does the swift movement of nervous impulses along the neurons of the nervous system, the absorption of nutrients by the digestive system and the filtering of waste by the kidneys. It would indeed be difficult to identify a physiological process where the movement of ions across cell membranes did not play a significant part. It is hardly surprising, therefore, that the proteins that facilitate the passage of ions across cell membranes are targets of many of the drugs currently used in clinical practice.

### What are ions?

What, therefore, are ions and why is their transport across cell membranes so crucial to the efficient functioning of the body? Ions are atoms that carry a tiny charge (although ions can also be small molecules). Some common examples of ions found in the body are listed in Table 2.2 and, as you can see from the table, some carry a positive charge and are called *cations* and some carry a negative charge and are called *anions*. Elements such as sodium, calcium and chlorine can exist in non-ionic forms but they are unstable and very reactive and you will not find them in living organisms. The ions that we find in the body are stable and are charged. Most carry either a single positive or single negative charge – although some such as calcium, magnesium and phosphate have a double or even triple charge (hence the $^{2+}$ or $^{3-}$ in superscript after their chemical symbol).

**KEY FACT**

Ions are charged and ions are stable.

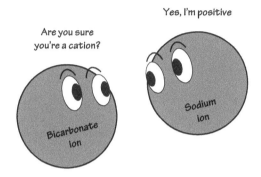

There are many other types of ion found in the human body but those listed in Table 2.2 are the ones that you are most likely to encounter in physiological processes related to pharmacology.

Examples of some common drugs that interact with ion channels include:

- **Lidocaine** – local anaesthetic used in dentistry
- **Diazepam** – anxiolytic (relieves anxiety)
- **Digoxin** – maintains the contractility of the heart
- **Verapamil** – reduces hypertension (high blood pressure).

Table 2.2 Common ions found in the body

| Name of ion | Chemical symbol | Cation or anion |
| --- | --- | --- |
| Sodium | $Na^+$ | Cation |
| Potassium | $K^+$ | Cation |
| Calcium | $Ca^{2+}$ | Cation |
| Chloride | $Cl^-$ | Anion |
| Hydrogen | $H^+$ | Cation |
| Magnesium | $Mg^{2+}$ | Cation |
| Phosphate | $PO_4^{3-}$ | Anion |
| Bicarbonate | $HCO_3^-$ | Anion |

The roles that ions play in physiological processes are discussed in more detail when we examine the various body systems in Part 2 of *Introducing Pharmacology*, along with the drugs that target those systems. Here we will just look at the basic principles of how drugs interact with ion channels.

**IN PRACTICE**

You will often hear the term U & Es used in clinical practice. It stands for urea and electrolytes and must be one of the most common blood tests performed in hospitals. The key electrolytes are $Na^+$ and $K^+$ and deviations from the normal range could indicate various problems such as dehydration. Urea, a waste product, is eliminated in the urine, so high levels in the blood may indicate that the kidneys are not functioning normally.

There are various types of ion channels that perform different tasks in different tissues but essentially they all regulate the passage of ions across the cell membrane. Some ion channels open and close as the electrical activity surrounding the membrane changes. These are called *voltage-controlled ion channels* and are found on cells involved in the transmission of nervous impulses such as neurons and conduction tissue in the heart (Figure 2.6).

Some ion channels are complexed with receptors. These are found in various locations but especially at the junctions between neurons. As the neurotransmitter released by one neuron binds to a receptor on another neuron, this causes the associated ion channel to open (Figure 2.7).

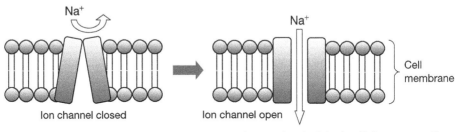

**Figure 2.6** Ion channels open in response to changes in electrical activity surrounding the membrane. In this case a sodium channel opens.

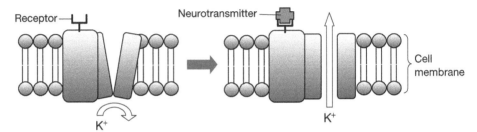

**Figure 2.7** An ion channel opens in response to a neurotransmitter binding to an associated receptor protein. In this case a potassium channel opens.

So how do drugs interact with ion channels? Some drugs simply block the ion channel by inserting themselves into the channel itself and preventing the passage of ions from one side of the membrane to the other. An example of a drug that has this action is the local anaesthetic **lidocaine**.

## Example of an ion channel-blocking drug: lidocaine

**Lidocaine** is a synthetic relation of cocaine and is commonly used as a local anaesthetic to prevent patients experiencing pain during minor operations such as dentistry. As you lie back in the dentist's chair for a filling and the dentist approaches with a syringe, the last thought in your mind is probably about the way that **lidocaine** will make the whole process relatively pain free. However, without **lidocaine**, fillings would be a lot more painful, so read on to find out how this most useful of drugs works.

Figure 2.8 shows a section of the cell membrane of a pain neuron that transmits unpleasant sensations from the site of damage into the central nervous system. Pain impulses, in fact all nervous impulses, depend on $Na^+$ ions entering the neuron through voltage-controlled sodium ion channels. Changes in the electrical activity around the neuron membrane stimulate sodium channels to open, and $Na^+$ ions enter the neuron, causing a change in the electrical activity around the membrane that causes adjacent sodium channels to open – and so on along the neuron. This is the nervous impulse, or *action potential* as it is more correctly called, sending a ripple of ionic activity along the neuron, rather like a Mexican wave at a football match. Naturally there is more to it than this brief explanation and other ions such as potassium are involved, but for this brief example of a channel-blocking drug, you just need to know that pain impulses depend on the opening of sodium channels in pain neurons.

**Lidocaine** and other related local anaesthetics are blockers of sodium channels in pain neurons. They bind to and block sodium channels so that sodium ions cannot enter the neuron and this prevents the progression of the nervous impulse along the pain neuron. Since the perception of pain depends on the brain receiving pain signals from pain neurons, local anaesthetics effectively sever communications between the site of injury and the brain. **Lidocaine** will act preferentially on pain

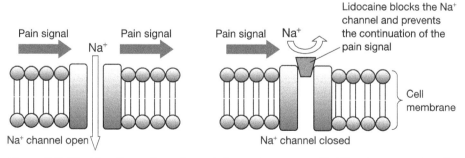

**Figure 2.8** Blocking the sodium channels in a pain neuron with **lidocaine** prevents pain signals from progressing along the neuron and reaching the brain.

neurons but can also affect the motor neurons that control muscles and prevent their proper functioning – as anyone who has had a dental filling and afterwards tried to speak normally will confirm.

Other drugs affect ion channels differently and these are called *modulators*. Two such examples are the anti-anxiety drug **diazepam** and the antihypertensive drug **verapamil**. Modulators change the way that ion channels behave, either enhancing or inhibiting their action. **Diazepam** interacts with chloride channels in neurons of the central nervous system and enhances their opening, so encouraging the movement of chloride ions out of the neuron. **Verapamil** inhibits the opening of calcium channels in the heart and reduces the amount of $Ca^{2+}$ entering certain heart cells. This has the effect of slowing the heart. Despite the fact that it is a modulator, you will find that **verapamil** and other drugs in this class are nearly always referred to as calcium channel blockers or just CCBs.

## 2.4   Protein targets 3: enzymes

Within each cell there are thousands of tiny biochemical reactions taking place every second, mostly involving enzymes – large, complex proteins that catalyse those reactions. These reactions are not easy to describe in simple terms without delving deeper into biochemistry but basically, enzymes change one substance into another substance – for instance, by removing (or adding) a phosphate, breaking (or making) a bond between two carbon atoms and so on. Each enzyme is responsible for catalysing one particular type of biochemical reaction, which it can do time and time again because the enzyme itself remains unchanged by the reaction. The substance that an enzyme converts into another substance is called the *substrate* of that enzyme.

There are many thousands of different enzymes active inside and outside of cells, and they are responsible for the *catalysis* of the myriad biochemical reactions necessary for life. Few enzymes have memorable names, in fact many have abominably long names, making them nigh on impossible to remember. Table 2.3 shows some key enzymes that are targets for common drugs.

Table 2.3 Some enzyme targets and the drugs that target them

| Enzyme target | Drug group | Use |
| --- | --- | --- |
| Angiotensin-converting enzyme | ACE inhibitors | Antihypertensive |
| Cyclo-oxygenase II | NSAIDs* | Analgesic |
| HMG CoA reductase[†] | Statins | Reduces cholesterol |
| Acetylcholinesterase | Cholinesterase inhibitors | Reverses muscle relaxants |

* Non-steroidal anti-inflammatory drugs
[†] 3-hydroxy-3-methylglutaryl coenzyme A reductase (phew . . . !!!)

## How do drugs interact with enzymes?

Drugs generally inhibit enzymes and prevent them from performing their normal physiological tasks. This inhibition is caused by drugs binding to the *active site* of the enzyme, the area where the enzyme interacts with its substrate. Drugs that inhibit enzymes have a molecular shape similar to the substrate; they bind to the active site and inhibit the action of the enzyme (Figure 2.9).

Many enzyme-blocking drugs are targeted at enzymes in *biochemical pathways* so it is important you understand what this term means. In cells, substances are synthesised, not in one complex manoeuvre but in a series of small stages, each change being carried out by a different enzyme (Figure 2.10).

**ANOTHER WAY TO PICTURE THIS**

Rather like the assembly line in a car factory, each worker (enzyme) has his own small task to perform, adding components such as the engine, exhaust, wheels and windows until at the end of the line a finished car is produced.

In Figure 2.11, a drug has blocked the action of enzyme 2. As a result, the pathway is blocked and neither substrate C nor D is produced. It is invariably the final substance in the biochemical pathway that we are trying to prevent being produced. For example, statins such as **pravastatin** and **atorvastatin** block an enzyme in the pathway that produces cholesterol in the liver. High cholesterol in the blood is a contributory factor to coronary artery disease, so reducing cholesterol synthesis with a statin helps to prevent heart attacks. The action of statins is discussed in more detail in Chapter 4.

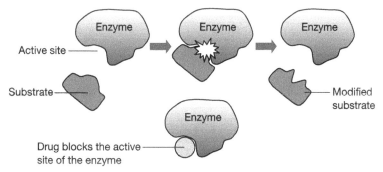

**Figure 2.9** The active site in an enzyme modifies a substrate. A drug with similarities in shape to the substrate occupies the active site and prevents the enzyme from binding to its substrate.

Figure 2.10 A biochemical pathway where substrate A is converted into substrate D via a series of intermediate steps, each catalysed by its own enzyme.

Figure 2.11 A drug binding to the active site of enzyme 2 blocks the pathway by preventing the conversion of substrate B into substrate C.

## 2.5 Protein targets 4: carrier proteins

Of all of the protein drug targets, the carrier proteins form the least coherent group, comprising any membrane protein involved in the active transport of a substance across the cell membrane using ATP as the motive force. For the sake of simplicity we can divide carrier proteins into two broad categories.

### Carrier proteins 1 – ion transporters

The first group of carrier proteins, confusingly perhaps, are those that transport ions across membranes. We have already encountered voltage-controlled ion channels relying on simple diffusion, but some ions are actively transported or pumped across membranes through carrier proteins using ATP. Figure 2.12 shows an ATP-driven carrier protein.

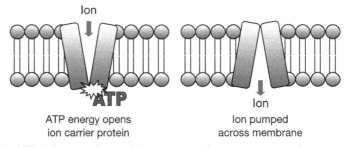

Figure 2.12 ATP-driven carrier protein moves an ion across a membrane.

These ion pumps are found on cell membranes in various parts of the body, but those in the kidneys and lining of the stomach are among the most common targets for drugs. **Furosemide**, a loop diuretic, inhibits an ion carrier in the *loop of Henle*, part of the *nephrons* of the kidney. This interferes with the sodium balance in the kidney, causing it to increase its production of urine. For patients with heart failure, removing fluid from the body can reduce the workload of the heart.

**Lansoprazole**, a proton pump inhibitor (PPI), inhibits the hydrogen ion (proton) pump in the gastric mucosa of the stomach. The pumping of hydrogen ions increases the concentration of hydrochloric acid in the stomach which, in some patients, can cause irritation of the lower oesophagus, a problem known as *gastro-oesophageal reflux* disease (heartburn). Blocking the proton pump with a PPI results in a reduction in the amount of stomach acid which helps to alleviate the symptoms.

## Carrier proteins 2 – neurotransmitter transporters

The second group of carrier proteins targeted by drugs are those found in the junctions between neurons in the complex neural circuits in the brain. These drugs are used in mental health to relieve depression and are dealt with in more detail in Chapter 11. **Fluoxetine** and **paroxetine,** perhaps better known by their proprietary names of Prozac® and Seroxat®, are anxiolytic drugs that block carrier proteins for the neurotransmitter, 5-hydroxytryptamine (serotonin) in neurons in the emotional centres of the brain. How this results in positive changes in mood is complex and by no means fully understood.

**A QUICK RECAP on ion channels, enzymes and carrier proteins**

- Ion channels in the cell membrane allow ions to enter and leave the cell.
- Most physiological processes involve the movement of ions across membranes, especially nervous conduction and heart activity.
- Some drugs simply block ion channels. Other drugs modulate them, which enhances or inhibits the passage of ions across membranes.
- Enzymes are large, complex proteins that act as catalysts in biochemical reactions.
- Enzyme-blocking drugs inhibit the action of enzymes and prevent them binding to their substrate. This often inhibits biochemical pathways.
- Carrier proteins move ions and various other molecules across membranes using ATP as an energy source.
- Drugs acting on carrier proteins generally block the carrier but the effect varies with the type and location of carrier.

**FURTHER RECOMMENDED READING**

McGavock, H (2010) *How Drugs Work: Basic Pharmacology for Healthcare Professionals* (3rd edn). Radcliffe Publishing Ltd.

Rang, HP *et al.* (2011) *Rang and Dale's Pharmacology* (7th edn). Churchill Livingstone.

## Test yourself

Now you have finished reading this chapter you might find it useful to find out how much you have learned and remembered.

*The answers to these questions are at the end of the book (see p. 313).*

1 Approximately how many different proteins are there in the human body?

2 Outline three reasons why proteins make good targets for drugs.

3 Name three types of natural chemical messenger that target receptors.

4 How do natural chemical messengers target their receptors?

5 Why does **salbutamol** bind to adrenergic receptors?

6 Explain the terms *agonist* and *antagonist*.

7 Explain the term *sympathomimetic*.

8 What type of natural chemical messenger would bind to nicotinic and muscarinic receptors?

9 Cations are *negatively/positively* charged ions (delete incorrect option).

10 What type of ion channels open in response to changes in electrical activity across the cell membrane?

11 What is the effect of **lidocaine** blocking $Na^+$ channels in pain neurons?

12 Which part of an enzyme is blocked by enzyme-blocking drugs?

13 What biochemical pathway do statins inhibit?

14 What is the key difference between an ion channel and a carrier protein?

Answers to match the lock and key in Figure 2.3, p. 27.

Lock 1 – Key C
Lock 2 – Key A
Lock 3 – Key B

## Chapter 3

# Side-effects, interactions and pharmacokinetics

This chapter explores the subject of pharmacokinetics – how absorption, metabolism and elimination affect drug levels in the body. It will help you understand how factors such as disease and age can affect metabolism and elimination. It explores the different ways that drugs may cause side-effects and how some drugs may interact with other drugs (and some foods). The factors that determine the correct dosage of drugs are discussed and finally we consider the effects that age, pregnancy and ethnicity can have on drug metabolism.

## CONTENTS

## Introduction

Rather than examining *pharmacodynamics*, the therapeutic effects of drugs on the body, in Chapter 3 we are going to take a step sideways to explore the subject of *pharmacokinetics*. Pharmacokinetics is concerned with what the body does to the drug, how drugs are absorbed into the body, distributed to the tissues of the body, metabolised (usually by the liver) and eventually eliminated. It is an important topic because it explains why some drugs must be delivered directly into the bloodstream while others can be taken orally, in tablet or liquid form. It also explains why some drugs can be given once a day while others need to be administered more frequently. Disease and age can have a profound effect on drug metabolism, which is another area we will touch on briefly.

> *Pharmacodynamics* is what the drug does to the body (principally its therapeutic action) whereas *pharmacokinetics* is what the body does to the drug (mainly absorbs, distributes, metabolises and excretes it).

Chapter 3 also examines the important and problematical subject of side-effects. It may seem slightly odd that after only two chapters and before we have even started to discuss the therapeutic action of drugs, we are about to examine how they cause side-effects. It would be wonderful indeed if drugs always cured diseases and never caused any unwanted effects. However, we are dealing with the human body, an extremely complex machine, and it is inevitable that if we introduce foreign chemicals into that complex machine we will interfere with its normal, efficient running. If you have a *British National Formulary* nearby, open it at any page, choose any drug and check its side-effects. You may (or may not) be surprised to find that every single drug in the BNF produces side-effects – some drugs a few, other drugs many. This does not, of course, mean that everyone who is prescribed a particular drug will experience these side-effects but as a clinical practitioner you need to be aware of the potential side-effects of a drug and also the mechanism whereby it can produce those side-effects. This knowledge will enable you to anticipate potential problems, identify them and respond to them quickly – before they become more serious.

Continuing with Chapter 3, we explore another important area – interactions. Many of your patients will have multiple pathologies and will have been prescribed more than one drug – perhaps many. In this case there is the potential for the drugs to interact; in other words, one drug may change the activity of another. It may increase the other drug's activity to the point where it starts to become toxic or it may reduce that drug's activity to the point where it ceases to have any therapeutic benefit. Surprisingly, common foods such as grapefruit and cabbage can also change the activity of some drugs – as can familiar herbal remedies available from the shelves of health-food shops. The problems of interactions are compounded in elderly patients, many of whom have multiple health problems resulting in them being on a cocktail of drugs, greatly increasing the potential for interactions.

We then examine the factors that determine the dose of a drug that should be administered to a patient. If an insufficient amount is administered, it may not produce the desired therapeutic effect. Conversely, if too much is given, it may produce unacceptable side-effects and even harm the patient. Giving patients the correct dose ensures that the level of drug in the body is appropriate and helps to prevent these potential problems.

Finally in Chapter 3 we consider the use of drugs in special groups of individuals. It is very easy to discuss the use of drugs in general terms, forgetting that in some groups, their age, gender or even race may change the way that their body reacts to the drugs. Also, what happens if the unintentional recipient of the drug is a pregnant woman's baby?

## 3.1 Pharmacokinetics: what the body does to drugs

Have you ever wondered why it is that some drugs are administered orally, perhaps in tablet form, while others can only be given by injection? Why is it that some drugs are given once each day, and others three times each day, while others need continuous administration? The answer to these questions lies in the way that the body absorbs, *metabolises* and eliminates the drugs that we administer to patients.

> *Metabolise* simply means to change by a biochemical reaction. Much of the metabolic activity relating to drugs takes place in the liver.

We must remember that the body is blind to the origin of foreign substances. It does not know that the beneficial chemicals known as drugs have been administered to treat or prevent a disease. To the body, drugs are foreign substances and, like all foreign substances, the body will place barriers to prevent their entry, neutralise those that do gain entry and then dispose of them as quickly as possible. Drug manufacturers have to take these reactions into account when developing a new drug. It is obviously important to ensure that the drug is effective against the disease for which it is being prescribed but it must also survive the body's barriers to entry and subsequent neutralisation by the liver. It must also stay in the circulation long enough to do its job as a therapeutic agent but not so long that it continues to act well after its usefulness to the patient has ended. Pharmacokinetics is important because it explains the reason for the route of delivery, the frequency of administration and also why factors such as age and disease can affect how the drug will act in the body.

We can divide the way that the body deals with drugs into four stages . . .

- The absorption of drugs into the body
- The distribution of drugs to the tissues of the body
- The metabolism of drugs by the body
- The elimination of drugs from the body.

## The absorption of drugs into the body

To act effectively, drugs need to find their way to the site of the disease. We can broadly divide the routes of administration into three main categories:

1 **Topical** – the medication is applied directly to the site of the problem where the drug needs to act. This is usually (but not always) the skin.

2 **Enteral** – the medication is taken orally and absorbed into the bloodstream from the digestive tract. (Note that some drugs may need to remain in the digestive tract if they are to treat digestive tract diseases.)

3 **Parenteral** – the medication is introduced directly into the body usually by intramuscular injection (into a muscle) or intravenously (into a vein).

A pictorial summary of the various routes of administration is given in Figure 3.1.

*Topical administration* Sometimes the problem is localised so near the surface of the body that the drug can be applied directly to the skin. **Hydrocortisone**, a topical corticosteroid used for eczema, is an example of a drug applied directly to the skin. **Ibuprofen** gel can ease superficial aches and pains. Inhaled bronchodilators such as **salbutamol** and **ipratropium bromide** probably fit best in this category as they are delivered into and act directly on lung tissue.

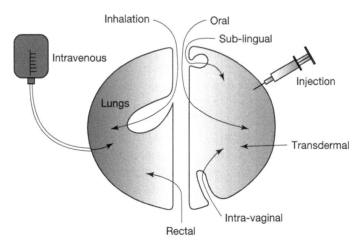

**Figure 3.1** There are many ways to introduce drugs into the body. The route chosen depends on various factors, including the nature of the drug, the pathology, the state of the patient and the required response time.

*Enteral administration* The oral administration of drugs is perhaps the most acceptable method to the conscious and cooperative patient because, given the choice, most people prefer to take a couple of tablets than have a hypodermic needle stuck into them! Drugs taken orally must be sufficiently robust to withstand the rigours of the digestive system such as stomach acid and digestive enzymes. If the drug has survived its passage through the stomach and duodenum into the absorptive section of the small intestine it will start to be absorbed into the circulatory system and here we encounter the first of the body's defences against foreign substances – the liver. This organ plays a major role in drug metabolism and we will shortly discuss it in more detail.

*Parenteral administration* This really covers any drug that is not administered orally, and while the term is generally applied to injections and intravenous (IV) lines, it can also cover other routes. Injection is an effective way of introducing a drug quickly into a subcutaneous (under the skin) area. Sometimes the drug stays in the area of injection such as the dental anaesthetic **lidocaine**. Other drugs such as **insulin** diffuse from the site of injection into the bloodstream for distribution around the body. **Insulin** is an example of a drug that cannot survive the passage through the digestive tract. As a protein, it would be quickly denatured by digestive enzymes and unlikely to reach the bloodstream. Drugs administered directly into a vein have an almost immediate effect as there is little of the transport delay that occurs between the gut and the blood as in the case of oral administration. This type of delivery is very suitable where the amount of drug in the bloodstream must be carefully controlled. For example, **morphine** used to control severe pain is often delivered IV by a dispenser controlled by the patient. As the pain levels increase, the patient is able to obtain almost immediate relief by increasing the rate of delivery of the **morphine**. This is called patient-controlled analgesia or PCA for short.

There are some drugs that fall between categories. These are drugs that have a systemic action but are not delivered orally or by injection or IV. These are drugs that pass through one of the body's membranes to be absorbed into the bloodstream. Various membranes can be used to absorb drugs, for example the sub-lingual (under-the-tongue) route can be useful for drugs that cannot survive the trip through the stomach to the bloodstream such as the anti-angina drug **glyceryl trinitrate**. Rectal delivery by incorporating the drug into *suppositories* can be useful for those unable to take medication by mouth, for example analgesia for patients who are recovering from an operation. The absorption of drugs transdermally (through the skin) is generally poor but lipid-soluble drugs such as anti-inflammatory corticosteroids and the hormone oestrogen can be delivered successfully by this route. Inhaled general anaesthetics such as **sevoflurane** and **nitrous oxide** quickly pass from the lungs into the bloodstream and thence to the brain.

> **IN PRACTICE**
>
> It is very important that drugs are administered by the correct route because often the doses can vary between routes. Generally IV doses are much smaller than oral doses because of drug metabolism in the liver situated between the gut and the circulatory system. There have been several cases of fatalities where drugs have been delivered by the wrong route.

## The distribution of drugs to the tissues of the body

Drugs are distributed around the body in the blood but relatively few drugs exert their pharmacological action in the blood itself. Anticoagulants and anti-platelet drugs are obvious examples, interacting with clotting proteins and platelets in the blood. Most other drugs need to move from the blood into the interstitial fluid to interact with their target proteins in and on cells. How much of a drug will move out of the bloodstream and into another area of the body depends to a large extent on the chemical nature of the drug. Some drugs need to move into the central nervous system (CNS) and the *blood–brain barrier* represents a significant obstruction. Sometimes this can be quite useful if a peripherally-acting drug would cause neurological side-effects were it to enter the CNS. Conversely this impermeability can be a problem such when an antibacterial drug needs to cross the blood–brain barrier to treat bacterial *meningitis*. This may require the drug to be injected directly into the *cerebrospinal fluid* that surrounds the brain and spinal cord.

Many drugs do not travel freely dissolved in the blood but are bound to plasma proteins – especially albumins. Drugs bind to and unbind from plasma proteins but it is only the free, dissociated drug that can exert its therapeutic effect. Conditions such as burns or malnutrition that reduce levels of plasma albumin provide less binding sites for drugs and so leave more free drug in the blood. Depending on the drug, this may result in more pronounced side-effects.

## The metabolism of drugs by the body

Once the drug has survived its passage through the stomach and the duodenum and into the small intestine it will start to be absorbed into the circulatory system. Here we encounter the first of the body's defences against foreign substances – the liver.

We need to start by learning a bit of anatomy relating to the circulatory and digestive system. Most tissues and organs have conventional vascular plumbing consisting of an artery that supplies oxygenated blood and a vein that removes deoxygenated blood, returning it to the general circulation. The digestive system, however, has a slight variation on this theme for although it has a conventional blood supply via the *mesenteric artery*, the blood is returned by a vein that feeds

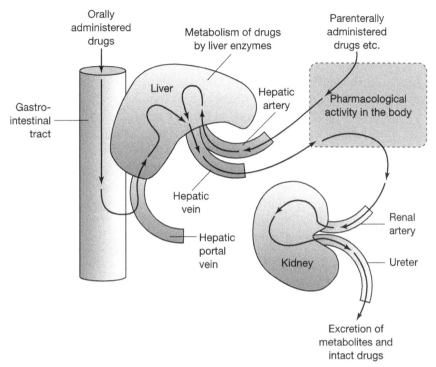

**Figure 3.2** Summary of drug metabolism in the body. Drugs in the digestive system travel through the liver before being released into the general circulatory system.

directly into the liver – rather than into the general circulation. This vein is called the *hepatic portal vein* and ensures that all of the nutrients and other substances that we absorb from the gut first pass through the liver (Figure 3.2).

Why do all the nutrients and miscellaneous substances absorbed from the digestive system have to first pass through the liver? Well, imagine you have just been out for a birthday meal with your pals and as a special treat you have a double helping of sticky toffee pudding and custard (it is your birthday, after all). Very nice indeed, but imagine the effect on your blood glucose levels if all the sugar from that pudding emptied directly into your circulation from your intestine! Fortunately, the sugar initially feeds into the liver via the hepatic portal vein where much of it is stored as glycogen. This means that the blood leaving the liver through the *hepatic vein* will not be excessively high in glucose.

The liver not only acts as a *buffer* to nutrients absorbed from the digestive system, it also acts as a barrier to unwanted substances and potential toxins. These substances appear naturally in our food and include numerous plant chemicals, most of which are not particularly toxic but still need to be processed before they enter the bloodstream. The liver also acts as the body's main 'detox' organ, metabolising and neutralising substances that have been produced in metabolic reactions in the cells and tissues. These include hormones and other substances that have fulfilled their purpose and need to be removed from the system.

A *buffer* is a structure, substance or process that resists or helps to prevent change. In this case, the liver acts to prevent major changes in blood nutrients after a meal.

The mechanism whereby the liver performs this valuable task involves a large family of *cytochrome P450* enzymes that metabolise unwanted substances into a form that is easier for the kidneys to excrete in urine. These liver enzymes originally evolved to respond to the many unwanted substances that occurred naturally in the leaves, nuts, roots and fruits that formed a significant part of our diet. These plant substances included many hydrophobic (water-hating) alkaloids and the liver's P450 enzymes evolved to change these hydrophobic alkaloids into hydrophilic substances. These dissolve more easily in the blood and can be disposed of by the kidneys in the process that produces urine. The P450 reactions are divided into two main types . . .

- **Phase I reactions** change lipophilic substances into hydrophilic metabolites, mainly by oxidation.
- **Phase II reactions**, also called 'conjugation' reactions, attach a molecule such as a sugar to the unwanted substance, making it more water-soluble and easier for the kidneys to excrete.

Although originally evolved to deal with unwanted substances from plants, these days the P450 enzymes also have to metabolise drugs. This has important implications for drug delivery and, as we shall see later in this chapter, drug interactions.

Drugs that are absorbed from the digestive tract all pass through the liver and to a greater or lesser extent will be metabolised by the P450 enzymes before they enter into the circulatory system. This is called *first-pass metabolism* and the extent of the metabolism will determine the amount of a drug that appears in the circulation to perform its therapeutic task – sometimes referred to as its *bioavailability*. Some drugs are almost completely metabolised by the liver, resulting in such low bioavailability that the drug is therapeutically ineffective. The anti-angina drug **glyceryl trinitrate** is an example of a drug subject to almost complete first-pass metabolism, which is why it is generally delivered by sub-lingual spray. From under the tongue, GTN will be absorbed directly into the bloodstream and will have just enough time to exert its therapeutic effect before being inactivated by the liver.

**KEY FACT**

P450 enzymes in the liver play a key role in drug metabolism. They metabolise both drugs absorbed from the digestive tract and those already in the system.

If you return to Figure 3.2, you will see that parenteral drugs, introduced directly into the circulation by IV line, etc., will eventually pass through the liver where they come into contact with P450 metabolising enzymes. As the blood circulates around the body, drugs carried in the blood are subject to hepatic metabolism each time they pass through the liver. How long a drug remains in the circulation depends on various factors, including how quickly it is metabolised by the P450 enzymes. However, enough of the drug needs to remain in the circulation to diffuse from the blood into the tissues and perform its therapeutic task. Not all drugs are inactivated by the liver; some need to be metabolised before they become active. These are called *pro-drugs* and include **enalapril** (an antihypertensive ACE inhibitor), the anti-clotting drugs **aspirin** and **clopidogrel** and the anti-inflammatory drug **prednisolone**.

*Bioavailability* is a commonly used but rather imprecise term that refers to the amount of an orally administered drug that reaches the circulation after first-pass metabolism.

## The elimination of drugs from the body

As we have just discussed, most drugs are metabolised by the liver into metabolites. This usually involves an oxidation reaction or adding a sugar molecule to the drug in order for it to become more soluble in blood. This makes it easier for the kidneys to remove it from the body. The kidneys are the main excretion organs of the body, acting as complex filter beds; they remove unwanted materials from the blood while conserving the useful materials such as glucose, salts and amino acids. In this manner drugs and their metabolites eventually find their way to the kidneys where they are filtered out of the blood and appear in the urine. Some drugs, especially those of large molecular weight, such as **vincristine**, **rifampicin**, **doxorubicin**, **vecuronium** and **amiodarone**, are eliminated by the liver in the bile. Bile is a mixture of cholesterol, acids and pigments that plays an important part in fat digestion. Drugs eliminated in bile are transported to the digestive system via the bile duct and eliminated in faeces.

**DID YOU KNOW ...** that urine tests in sport are searching for tell-tale traces of metabolites that indicate the athlete concerned has been using performance-enhancing drugs? Some athletes try to evade detection by using substances naturally produced in the body such as testosterone and erythropoietin. Others use diuretics to remove the tell-tale metabolites more quickly.

**IN PRACTICE**

Any disease that affects the liver or kidneys can have an effect on the bio-availability of drugs. Cirrhosis of the liver reduces its ability to metabolise drugs, which means that circulating drug levels are elevated. Renal failure means that drugs and their metabolites are excreted more slowly, again elevating levels in the circulation.

## 3.2    How drugs can cause side-effects

There is a popular saying among pharmacologists that goes . . .

*'A drug that does not cause side-effects is a drug that does not work.'*

No one is quite sure who first said this but, unlike most popular sayings, this one is invariably true. All drugs have the potential to cause side-effects and a quick glance at the *British National Formulary* will confirm this. Some drugs may cause relatively few side-effects while the list of side-effects for other drugs is so long that one wonders why anyone would ever prescribe them.

Firstly, some patients will experience few, if any, side-effects and if those side-effects are relatively minor then the therapeutic benefit of a drug will generally outweigh any problems. For example, a slight feeling of nausea may be acceptable if an antibacterial drug rids us of a painful infection.

Secondly, the condition of the patient may be so serious that even quite unpleasant side-effects may be tolerated if it ensures the patient's recovery. For example, drugs used to treat cancer can have very unpleasant side-effects but if they save the individual's life, then that will be a price worth paying.

Patients vary in the side-effects they experience. Give the same drug to two patients, matched for age, gender, weight, etc., and if they do experience side-effects, those side-effects are quite often different for each patient. This is a common phenomenon but precisely why it happens is not always easy to determine. Everyone is physiologically different and these differences can be observed in people's height, weight, hair colour, facial features, body shape, etc. There are also differences within the body, in particular the way that our bodies deal with drugs. Most of these differences manifest themselves at a cellular level, which is where drugs interact with the body. Drugs target specific proteins and variation in these proteins between individuals can mean that the body's response to drugs can vary, in respect of therapeutic effects and side-effects. The way that our bodies absorb, metabolise and eliminate drugs also varies between individuals, perhaps because of age or disease, and this can result in variations in the amount of drug circulating in the blood. This can affect both therapeutic effects and side-effects – as we will see later in this chapter.

There are also differences between drugs in their tendency to cause side-effects. Some drugs cause many side-effects while others cause fewer problems. Some drugs regularly cause minor inconveniences such as nausea or constipation but rarely cause any serious problems. Other drugs quite regularly cause unpleasant side-effects and need monitoring carefully. The message is that every drug is different and it will behave differently in each individual patient. This is not, of course, to imply that there is a complete lack of predictability with the drugs that we administer but, because of individual differences, there will inevitably be some variation between patients both with regard to their therapeutic response and their susceptibility to side-effects.

> **KEY FACT**
> Patients will differ in their response to drugs, especially with the side-effects they may experience.

## How drugs can cause side-effects 1: tipping the balance too far

Individuals react differently to drugs and their response can vary with factors such as age, disease and simply the normal genetic variability between people. Manufacturers are aware of this and during the testing process they decide the appropriate dosage that will provide the optimum therapeutic effect with the minimum of side-effects. Sometimes, however, variability in response to a drug means that the drug delivers a more pronounced therapeutic effect than originally intended. Now you might think that this is a good thing because a patient who experiences an enhanced therapeutic effect will automatically be better off, but this is not always the case. If the drug is attempting to return a physiological factor such as high blood pressure to normal, a super-efficient drug action can actually tip the patient too far to the other side of normal – into hypotension (low blood pressure).

### ANOTHER WAY TO PICTURE THIS

Think of your central heating system at home that is controlled by a thermostat that allows you to set the temperature of your house. If the house is too cold you turn up the thermostat, but if you turn it up too far, an hour later you are sweating. This is like a drug that has a greater effect than intended and tips the balance the other way.

Clotting is another example where the balance can be tipped too far. The anti-clotting drugs **warfarin** and **heparin** need to be used carefully or they can tip the balance of blood coagulation too far in the other direction and cause haemorrhage (unwanted bleeding). Stimulant laxatives such as **senna** can prove to be too effective and cause diarrhoea. **Codeine phosphate** used for acute diarrhoea can work too well and cause constipation.

Most examples of drugs tipping the balance too far are dependent on the dose, therefore we say that the effect is *dose-related*. The greater the dose, the more pronounced is the action of the drug and the greater is the side-effect produced.

## How drugs can cause side-effects 2: hitting the wrong target

We saw in Chapters 1 and 2 that most drugs bind to protein targets such as receptors, enzymes, ion channels and carrier proteins and they bind because their shape is compatible with specific regions of those proteins. These protein targets seldom exist as solitary individuals, but are mostly members of a larger group of similar proteins. Each family of proteins will have core similarities in molecular structure that define their group. This means that drugs targeting one member of the family are quite likely to bind to other members of that family because of these similarities in molecular structure. This principle applies to all of our target proteins – receptors, enzymes, ion channels and carrier proteins, most of which are part of families whose members can become unintended targets for drugs. When a drug binds to these unintentional targets then unintended things happen in the form of side-effects.

> **KEY FACT**
> Many side-effects are caused by drugs accidentally binding to unintended targets and producing unwanted effects.

## Hitting the wrong target 1: Receptors

Drugs that bind to receptors do so because they are of a similar shape to the natural chemical messengers of the body and so bind to the messengers' target receptors – either stimulating or blocking those receptors. We compared this action to a key fitting into a lock, the drug being similar to the key and the receptor to the lock. We saw in Chapter 2 that there are several families of receptors – adrenergic, cholinergic, dopaminergic, opioid and histamine, etc. Within these families are classes and sub-classes of receptor but as these receptors are all related, they have key similarities in structure. Generally, each tissue or organ will express a particular sub-class of receptor and respond in a way specific to the messenger and receptor. For example, adrenaline binding to $\beta_1$ adrenergic receptors on the heart causes tachycardia (excessively fast heart rate) while adrenaline binding to $\beta_2$ adrenergic receptors on the lungs causes bronchodilation (Figure 3.3).

### ANOTHER WAY TO PICTURE THIS

Think of the key to your car as a hormone. It can produce two different effects depending on which lock (receptor) it goes into. The key will fit into your car door

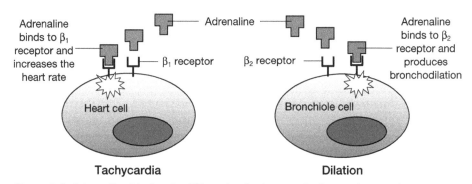

**Figure 3.3** Adrenaline binding to different sub-classes of adrenergic receptor produces diverse effects in different tissues.

lock and open the door and also fit into your ignition lock and start your engine. One key, two locks and two different effects.

Drugs will target specific receptors to produce specific therapeutic effects. Using the above beta-adrenergic receptors as an example, the anti-angina beta-blocker **atenolol** targets $\beta_1$ adrenergic receptors on the heart and, being an antagonist (blocker), causes a slowing of the heart rate. The anti-asthmatic drug **salbutamol** targets $\beta_2$ adrenergic receptors on the lungs and, being an agonist (mimic of adrenaline), causes bronchodilation.

This specificity is what is required from drugs because we want heart drugs to target the heart, lung drugs to target the lungs and so on. However, in order for **atenolol** to bind to $\beta_1$ adrenergic receptors on the heart and **salbutamol** to bind to $\beta_2$ adrenergic receptors on the lungs, both drugs have to have a structural similarity to adrenaline. This means there is a strong likelihood that **atenolol** might bind to $\beta_2$ adrenergic receptors on the lungs and that **salbutamol** might bind to $\beta_1$ adrenergic receptors on the heart. If this happens then **atenolol** could block the $\beta_2$ adrenergic receptors on the lungs, causing bronchoconstriction and, even worse, preventing **salbutamol** from binding to its $\beta_2$ adrenergic receptors when asthma sufferers use their inhalers (Figure 3.4).

There is also the distinct possibility that if the asthma sufferer uses his or her inhaler then **salbutamol** could bind to $\beta_1$ adrenergic receptors on the heart and cause tachycardia (Figure 3.5).

A quick check on the side-effects of these two drugs confirms this. **Atenolol** can cause bronchoconstriction and block the action of bronchodilators. This latter action could be very serious in asthmatics and so beta-blockers such as **atenolol** are *contra-indicated* in patients with asthma. As well as an example of a side-effect (bronchoconstriction) this is also an example of a mechanism of interaction where the two drugs compete for the same receptor. **Salbutamol** has various side-effects including tachycardia and palpitations, both caused by the drug binding to $\beta_1$ adrenergic receptors on the heart.

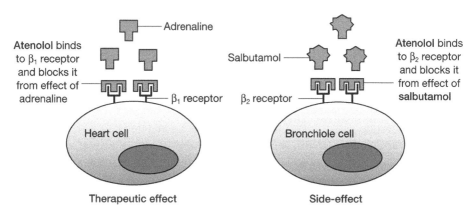

**Figure 3.4** Beta-blockers can cause bronchospasm by binding to $\beta_2$ receptors on the bronchioles and blocking them from the bronchodilatory action of **salbutamol**.

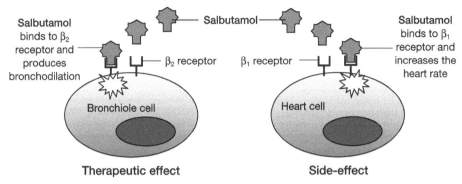

**Figure 3.5 Salbutamol** produces the side-effect of tachycardia by binding to $\beta_1$ receptors on the heart as well as its target $\beta_2$ receptors.

From this example of how drugs can cause side-effects it is fairly obvious that the more specific a drug is for its targeted receptor, the less likely it will bind to an unintended receptor – and cause unwanted effects. Some beta-blockers, for example **atenolol** and **bisoprolol**, are relatively cardioselective; in other words they are more specific for the heart's $\beta_1$ adrenergic receptors so their main action will be on the heart. Other beta-blockers such as **carvedilol** are non-cardioselective but their ability to bind to alpha adrenergic receptors on arterioles makes them useful in treating hypertension.

> **KEY FACT**
>
> The more specific a drug is for its intended target, the fewer side-effects it is likely to produce.

### Hitting the wrong target 2: enzymes

Many of our most common drugs such as ACE inhibitors, NSAIDs and statins bind to the active site of key enzymes and block their action. This produces beneficial results such as lowering blood pressure, relieving inflammatory pain and reducing blood cholesterol. However, these enzymes are often members of families of enzymes and drugs can stray off target, bind to other members of the family and cause side-effects.

ACE inhibitors such as **captopril, enalapril** and **ramipril** are widely prescribed antihypertensive drugs. As we shall see in Chapter 5, these drugs bind to an enzyme called angiotensin converting enzyme (ACE) and inhibit its action of converting angiotensin I to angiotensin II. By interfering with various processes such as sodium balance, this reduces blood pressure. However, in the lungs there are *kininases*, enzymes similar to ACE, and these metabolise a chemical called *bradykinin* into its metabolites. Unfortunately ACE inhibitors also have an affinity for these enzymes and can inhibit its action, resulting in the build-up of bradykinin, which has an irritant action on the lining of the lungs. This is what causes the dry cough that prevents some people from using ACE inhibitors (Figure 3.6).

**Figure 3.6** ACE inhibitors block kininases that break down bradykinin which accumulates, irritates the bronchioles and causes a dry cough.

## Hitting the wrong target 3: ion channels

As we saw in Chapter 2, ion channels are popular targets for drugs. Because ion channels are present in every cell, tissue and organ of the body, a drug that not only binds to its intended target but blocks ion channels elsewhere in the body, will inevitably result in side-effects.

**Verapamil** is used both for hypertension and also for arrhythmias. It works by inhibiting the opening of calcium channels in various cells of the heart and preventing $Ca^{2+}$ entering those cells. This has the effect of slowing the heart and maintaining a steady rhythm. However, calcium channels are widely distributed around the body, as well as on the heart. The smooth muscle cells that surround all of the hollow organs of the body, such as the blood vessels and the gut, contract in response to calcium entering those cells. This means that if the calcium channels on those cells are blocked with a $Ca^{2+}$ blocking drug such as **verapamil**, this interferes with contraction and promotes dilation. Other classes of calcium channel blockers such as **amlodipine** exploit this action by causing dilation of the peripheral arterioles and reducing blood pressure – as we will see in Chapter 5. Unfortunately, blocking contraction of smooth muscle in the gut has less beneficial results because it inhibits peristalsis (the rhythmic muscular contraction that pushes food and partially digested material from one end of the digestive system to the other). It is little wonder, therefore, that **verapamil** and other $Ca^{2+}$ blocking drugs have constipation as one of their side-effects (Figure 3.7).

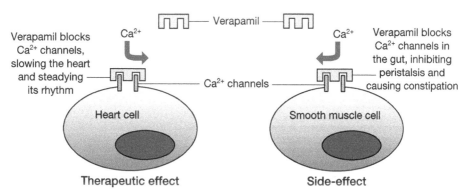

**Figure 3.7** **Verapamil** blocks calcium channels in the gut, inhibiting peristalsis and causing constipation.

## Hitting the wrong target 4: carrier proteins

This diverse group of protein drug targets includes many drugs used in the treatment of mental health problems. Any drug acting on such a complex organ has the potential for unwanted interactions with other carrier proteins in other parts of the brain. **Amitriptyline**, now mainly used for neuropathic pain, targets noradrenaline and serotonin carrier proteins in the emotional centres of the brain. It is also profligate in its binding with unintended proteins, in the brain and other parts of the body. Side-effects are many, including sleep defects, dizziness and agitation as well as anti-muscarinic effects such as dry mouth and constipation. In the heart, **amitryptyline** can interfere with ion channels, causing life-threatening arrhythmias, especially in overdose.

**A QUICK RECAP on side-effects caused by drugs hitting the wrong target**

- Drugs bind mainly to proteins, mainly by shape, like a key fits a lock.

- Some proteins are members of families of similarly shaped proteins and drugs can bind to other members of the protein family, as well as their intended target.

- When drugs bind to an unintended target they can cause unwanted side-effects.

- Adrenaline has many sub-classes of receptor so drugs have the potential to bind to unintended adrenaline receptors and produce unwanted side-effects.

- Salbutamol targets $\beta_2$ adrenergic receptors in the lungs, but can also bind to $\beta_1$ receptors on the heart and cause tachycardia.

- Atenolol targets $\beta_1$ adrenergic receptors on the heart but can also bind to $\beta_2$ receptors on the lungs, blocking them from the action of salbutamol.

- Drugs can inadvertently block an unintended enzyme. For example, ACE inhibitors can inhibit bradykinin-degrading enzymes in the lungs, resulting in a dry cough.

- Drugs can inadvertently block an unintended ion channel. For example, **verapamil** can block calcium channels in the wall of the digestive system resulting in a reduction in peristalsis, thus causing constipation.

## How drugs can cause side-effects 3: drugs that are intrinsically hazardous

Some drugs, especially those used to treat cancers, work by inflicting damage on rapidly dividing cells. They do this by a variety of means, including sticking together the DNA strands, fragmenting DNA, blocking enzymes essential to DNA synthesis and paralysing the cells' microtubules (fine tubes that form a sort of cellular skeleton). Although this damage is targeted at rapidly dividing cancerous cells, inevitably other cells receive unwanted attention from these quite unpleasant drugs – especially those that are dividing legitimately such as *epithelial* cells and white blood cells. This explains some of the common side-effects such as dry mouth, hair loss, gastro-intestinal disturbance and neutropaenia (low levels of circulating neutrophils). In addition to interfering with normal cell division, many of the anti-cancer drugs are intrinsically toxic and need careful monitoring as they can cause damage to the heart, nervous tissue, lungs and kidneys. Nausea and vomiting are frequent side-effects of anti-cancer treatment and are very distressing to patients. Some drugs, such as **cisplatin** and **cyclophosphamide**, are notorious for this problem.

Why would anyone want to use such dangerous drugs?

Cancer is a very serious, life-threatening disease and some of the drugs used to treat it have a fairly brutal mechanism of action on the body, so it is not surprising that their side-effects are among the most unpleasant of all drug groups. However, as they can be life-saving or at least life-prolonging, their benefit generally outweighs the disagreeable side-effects they may cause.

> *Epithelial cells* are those that line the parts of the body exposed to the external environment, including the skin, lungs and digestive tract. Lining cells inside the body such as those that line blood vessels are called endothelial cells.

## 3.3   Drug interactions

Many patients, especially the elderly, have multiple health problems that require a combination of drugs. Patients may be suffering from diabetes, rheumatic pains, hypertension, fluid retention and digestive problems so inevitably different drugs will be prescribed for each of these disorders. Multiple prescribing, or *polypharmacy* as it is sometimes called, can cause some of the drugs to interact with one another and this can cause additional side-effects for the patient. Drug interactions are not rare and a glance at Appendix 1 of the current *British National Formulary* will show the extent of the problem, with around 90 pages listing how one drug can interact with another.

Interactions between drugs will either increase or decrease the activity of one of those drugs. However, to be worthy of interest, an interaction must be of clinical significance. For example, drug A may marginally decrease the activity of drug B but if this does not produce any measurable change in the therapeutic effectiveness of drug B or change its side-effects profile then the interaction is of little or no clinical relevance. Those drugs where a small change in concentration can have severe consequences are more likely to have serious interactions. These drugs include some of the anticoagulants (anticlotting drugs) and anti-arrhythmics (drugs to restore normal heart rhythm).

> *Polypharmacy* literally means 'many drugs' and is a term used when a patient has been prescribed several different drugs. This is especially a problem for the elderly who often have multiple problems, each requiring its own range of drugs.

## Interactions involving hepatic P450 enzymes

Cytochrome P450 enzymes in the liver specialise in metabolising unwanted substances – including many drugs – making them more soluble and easier for the kidneys to excrete. When an unwanted substance, which might be a potential toxin, is present in the blood, the liver will respond by increasing the production of P450 enzymes specific to that substance. This is the basis for P450 inter-actions. Some drugs can induce an increase in enzyme activity that results in other substances being metabolised more quickly, and these substances can include other drugs. This means that when the activity of certain P450 enzymes is increased, those drugs that are substrates for those enzymes are metabolised more quickly and this decreases their bioavailability (Figure 3.8).

Like most other enzymes, P450 hepatic enzymes can be inhibited by drugs and other substances. When a particular P450 enzyme is inhibited, drugs that are substrates for that enzyme are metabolised more slowly. Clearance is reduced, which increases circulating levels of those drugs (Figure 3.9).

Examples of drugs that inhibit P450 enzymes are given in Table 3.2, together with some of the drugs whose circulating levels are increased as a consequence.

Examples of drugs that induce P450 enzyme activity are given in Table 3.3, together with some of the drugs whose circulating levels are reduced as a consequence.

**Figure 3.8** The effect of drug B inducing the production of additional P450 enzymes is to increase the overall rate of metabolism and so decrease levels of drug A.

**Figure 3.9** Drug A is metabolised into its metabolites by a P450 enzyme. The effect of drug B inhibiting that enzyme is to increase levels of drug A.

Table 3.2 Examples of drugs that inhibit P450 enzymes and so increase the circulating levels of other drugs

| Drugs that inhibit P450 drug metabolising enzymes | Drugs affected by inhibition (circulating levels are increased) |
|---|---|
| Cimetidine (reduces stomach acid) | Amiodarone (anti-arrhythmic)<br>Pethidine (pain reliever)<br>Warfarin (anticoagulant) |
| Corticosteroids (anti-inflammatory) | Amitriptyline (antidepressant) |
| Ciprofloxacin (antibacterial) | Theophylline (asthma reliever) |
| Phenelzine (antidepressant) | Pethidine (pain reliever) |

Table 3.3 Examples of drugs that induce P450 enzyme activity and so decrease the circulating levels of other drugs

| Drugs that increase the activity of P450 drug metabolising enzymes | Drugs affected by induction (circulating levels are reduced) |
|---|---|
| Phenobarbital (anti-epileptic) | Warfarin (anticoagulant)<br>Oral contraceptives<br>Corticosteroids (anti-inflammatory)<br>Ciclosporin (immunosuppressant) |
| Rifampicin (antibacterial) | |
| Griseofulvin (antifungal) | |
| Phenytoin (anti-epileptic) | |
| Ethanol (alcoholic drinks) | |
| Carbamazepine (anti-epileptic) | |

DID YOU KNOW... that many other substances can cause interactions besides drugs? The herbal remedy St John's Wort (*Hypericum perforatum*) is a strong inducer of P450 enzymes while grapefruit juice acts as an inhibitor and increases levels of various drugs, including the cholesterol-lowering drugs **simvastatin** and **atorvastatin** plus the anti-arrhythmic, **amiodarone.**

## Other mechanisms of drug interactions

There are many other mechanisms whereby drugs interact. As we saw earlier in this chapter, beta-blockers such as **atenolol** can compete with **salbutamol** for $\beta_2$ adrenergic receptors in the lungs. This means that for any asthmatic who suffers an asthma attack, their **salbutamol** inhaler will be rendered ineffective because their $\beta_2$ adrenergic receptors are blocked by beta-blockers.

The anticoagulant drug **warfarin** is susceptible to interactions with both antibiotics and common foods. **Warfarin** competes with vitamin K for the active site

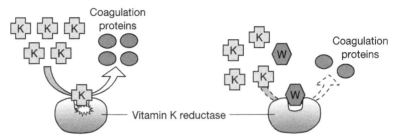

**Figure 3.10** Vitamin K (K) and **warfarin** (W) compete for the active site of the enzyme vitamin K reductase. Fluctuating levels of vitamin K affect the ability of **warfarin** to compete for the active site.

of *vitamin K reductase*, a key enzyme in the production of various circulating coagulation proteins, and the effectiveness of **warfarin** largely depends on levels of vitamin K (Figure 3.10).

Antibacterial drugs such as **rifampicin**, used to treat digestive infections, also reduce the population of friendly bacteria in the large intestine. Normally, these friendly bacteria produce vitamin K so, if levels of this vitamin fall due to **rifampicin**, the effectiveness of **warfarin** is enhanced. Fewer coagulation proteins are produced, so increasing the chance of haemorrhage. Conversely, a rise in vitamin K levels has the opposite effect, decreasing the effectiveness of **warfarin** and promoting coagulation. In fact **phytomenadione** (vitamin K) is used to counteract the effects of excess **warfarin**. This also explains why patients on **warfarin** are warned against suddenly consuming large amounts of vitamin K-rich leafy green vegetables such as cabbage, broccoli and kale.

Drugs with a similar therapeutic activity can cause problems if administered together. This is called additive or summative action and an example would be the co-administration of the anticoagulants **warfarin** and **aspirin**. Although their mechanisms of action are different, when given together they can result in an increased risk of haemorrhage and can be especially problematical if the patient develops a peptic ulcer, which can cause bleeding into the stomach. Another herbal remedy worth mentioning here is the maidenhair tree, *Ginkgo biloba*, which is reputed to improve cerebral circulation. As the *ginkgolides* contained in its leaves have an anticoagulant action, it would be inadvisable to use this herb with either **aspirin** or **warfarin** because of the potential additive effect causing unwanted bleeding.

**A QUICK RECAP on how drugs interact**

- P450 enzymes in the liver metabolise drugs.

- Some drugs can either increase or decrease P450 activity.

- If P450 enzyme activity is increased, some drugs are metabolised more quickly and this reduces those drugs' bioavailability.

- If P450 enzymes are inhibited, some drugs are metabolised more slowly and this increases those drugs' bioavailability.

- Some drugs interact by competing for the same receptor, e.g. **salbutamol** and **atenolol.**
- Drugs that have a similar effect can produce an additive effect if taken together.
- Herbal remedies and even common foodstuffs, such as grapefruit juice and cabbage, can interact with drugs.

## 3.4    Factors that determine the correct dosage of drugs

A key objective in the administration of a drug is to produce a therapeutically appropriate level of that drug in the blood and tissues. There are two key factors that affect the blood concentration: the rate of administration and the rate of elimination. Ideally, where treatment is to last several days or weeks, the rate of administration should match the rate of elimination so that the amount of drug in the body remains fairly constant.

**ANOTHER WAY TO PICTURE THIS**

Getting the right levels of drug in the patient is rather like running a bath with the plug missing. Water is coming in via the taps (drug administration) and water is leaving via the plughole (drug elimination). The only way to keep the level constant is to ensure that water is going in at the same rate as it is leaving the bath.

Generally, for each individual drug, the rate of elimination is reasonably constant as it is continuously metabolised by the liver and excreted by the kidneys. Administration, on the other hand, tends to be periodic, either by regular injections or by ingestion. Parenteral administration resolves this problem with continuous delivery. Patient-controlled analgesia (PCA), where the patient has control of the rate of delivery of pain-relieving drugs, is designed to achieve a reasonably steady state or a level appropriate for effective pain relief.

Once the rate of elimination has been determined, it is possible to calculate the dose required to reach therapeutic levels. This level of drug in the body is important because if levels are too low, the drug will be ineffective and if levels are too high, the drug may produce toxic effects. There are two terms used to describe these levels . . .

1  **Minimum effective concentration** (MEC). This is the minimum amount of drug that will produce the desired therapeutic effect.

2  **Maximum safe concentration** (MSC). This is the maximum amount of drug that can be tolerated before it starts to produce toxic effects.

Correct drug administration should ensure that the level of circulating drug is maintained between these two values for the period determined to be required

**Figure 3.11** A correctly administered drug maintains levels between the minimum effective concentration and the maximum safe concentration.

for the course of treatment. Figure 3.11 shows a correctly administered enteral drug whose concentration in the blood always remains between the MEC and the MSC. After each dose, levels rise and then fall as the drug is metabolised and eliminated from the body. However, before the level of drug falls below the MEC, another dose is administered to top up the level.

The difference between the MEC and MSC is sometimes called the *therapeutic window* and the calculated ratio of MEC to MSC defines the *therapeutic index* (TI) by the following formula:

$$\text{Therapeutic index (TI)} = \frac{\text{MSC}}{\text{MEC}}$$

This usually means that if a drug has a wide therapeutic index, there is less likelihood of adverse reactions or toxicity if the normal dose is exceeded for any reason. However, it cannot be stressed strongly enough that there is no room for any error in the administration of drugs – even when a drug has a wide therapeutic index. Drugs that have a very narrow therapeutic index, such as **digoxin, heparin, theophylline** and **warfarin**, need very careful monitoring indeed to ensure that levels are kept tightly controlled within the therapeutic index.

Establishing the therapeutic index of a drug does not tell us how frequently it needs to be administered because the TI does not measure the rate of elimination. The rate at which a drug is eliminated is quantified by its *half-life* ($T\frac{1}{2}$), the time it takes for the concentration of a drug to decrease by half, from (say) 100 micrograms per litre to 50 micrograms per litre. The longer the half-life, the longer the drug will remain in the circulation and vice versa. The shorter the half-life, the more frequently a drug needs to be administered and vice versa. Look at the two drugs in Figure 3.12.

It can be seen from Figure 3.12 that the time taken for drug A and drug B to fall from a plasma concentration of 100 micrograms per litre to 50 micrograms per litre (i.e. by half) is different. $T\frac{1}{2}$ for drug A is around 6 hours while $T\frac{1}{2}$ for drug

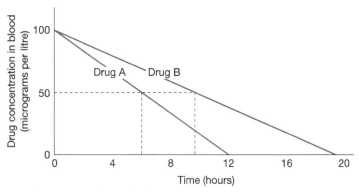

Figure 3.12 Differences in the rate of metabolism or elimination give drugs A and B different half-lives.

B is around 10 hours. Drugs with short half-lives such as **morphine** may need to be administered fairly frequently in order to maintain therapeutic levels but because **morphine** has a relatively narrow therapeutic window it cannot be given in larger doses at less frequent intervals. Modified-release formulations of **morphine** may be administered less frequently, providing a slower rate of absorption that keeps levels within the therapeutic window. For drugs with a wider therapeutic index, a larger dose may be appropriate and safely given at less frequent intervals. Fortunately for those who administer drugs, these calculations are done in the development process by the drug manufacturers and it is then the responsibility of clinical staff to ensure that they administer the correct dosage of the drug in accordance with current recommendations.

A QUICK RECAP on factors that determine the correct dosage of drugs

- For drugs that are to be prescribed over a period of days or weeks, the delivery of the drug needs to match the rate of metabolism and elimination.
- The level of drugs in the body needs to be kept above the minimum effective concentration (MEC) and below the maximum safe concentration (MSC).
- The difference between the MEC and the MSC is called the therapeutic window and its calculated ratio is the therapeutic index (TI).
- The half-life of a drug ($T\frac{1}{2}$) is the time it takes for the concentration of a drug to fall by one half.

## 3.5 Drugs and special groups

It is very easy to generalise about the way drugs interact with the body, forgetting that there may be considerable physiological and genetical variation between individuals. Pharmacokinetic variation can affect the way individuals absorb, metabolise, distribute or eliminate drugs, either increasing or decreasing circulating levels. Pharmacodynamic variation can result in significant differences in the way that people respond to drugs, either increasing or decreasing the individual's response. Given this potential for pharmacokinetic and pharmacodynamic variation, those prescribing or administering drugs need to be aware of the possible problems, particularly in special groups – as we shall learn . . .

## Drugs and the elderly patient

There is probably more variation between elderly patients than any other group; after all, they have had seventy or so years to diverge from one another. Some old people age well while others seem to have developed every conceivable ailment and be taking half the drugs listed in the BNF (we shall return to the problem of polypharmacy shortly). You can probably recall examples from your own experience of healthy and unhealthy old age. Reasons for this diversity are legion but predominantly involve lifestyle, diet, smoking and social class as well as a degree of genetic serendipity. If you desire a healthy old age then exercise regularly, eat wisely, don't smoke – and choose your parents carefully . . . ! Given this variation, we still need to make a few generalisations about older people in order to prepare ourselves for potential pharmacological problems.

The two organs that most affect circulating drug levels are the liver and the kidneys and the effectiveness of both declines with age. Both the mass of the liver and its blood flow decreases as we get older. In addition, there may be a decline in activity of various P450 enzymes, affecting the clearance of some drugs. Renal function gradually declines with age so we frequently have a situation where drugs are both metabolised and excreted more slowly. These changes generally increase circulating levels for a standard dose but the clinical relevance can depend on the individual and the drug. In some cases it can result in toxicity – especially for drugs with a narrow therapeutic window such as anti-arrhythmics, benzodiazepines, opioids and **warfarin**. An increase in the severity of side effects may also be expected as levels become elevated. This is why for many drugs, lower than standard doses may be prescribed for the elderly patient. If the drug is well tolerated then the dose may be increased in steps to achieve the desired therapeutic effect.

> **KEY FACT**
> Levels of circulating drug are most likely to increase in old age, possibly resulting in more side-effects or, for some drugs, toxicity.

Polypharmacy is the prescribing of many drugs to one individual. This is a particular problem in the elderly because many diseases such as rheumatism, angina, hypertension, diabetes, arthritis, osteoporosis, etc., are chronic diseases that develop as a person ages. Add to these co-morbidities the almost ubiquitous gastro-intestinal problems of heartburn and constipation and it is understandable why many elderly people will be on a cocktail of drugs. Obviously, the potential for interactions increases with the number of drugs being taken. Add to this changes in metabolism and elimination and the prescribing of drugs to the elderly person with many co-morbidities can become a real problem.

With polypharmacy, the number of potential side-effects increases and these may either be mistaken for normal signs of ageing or, worse still, treated with still more drugs. Adding to the problem is the fact that many elderly people suffer from confusion and poor eyesight and concordance (adhering to the prescribed medication regime) may be less than optimal.

## Drugs and the young patient

Ideally, children should be given medicines only when necessary and the prescribing of medicines for children needs to be done in consultation with both the child and their parents or carer. All medicines have potential risks and these need to be balanced against the benefits. When discussing medication, the potential side-effects need to be explained and distinguished from symptoms of the medical condition for which the drugs are being prescribed. The simplest medication regime is often preferable, making it easier for children to be involved in the responsibility for taking their medication and so improving concordance. The prescribing and administration of drugs to children is a complex and sensitive area and it is recommended you refer to specialist publications such as the BNF's companion guide, *BNF for Children*.

Children are not an homogeneous group, ranging from the pre-term neonate to the adolescent. Generally, there is not a huge amount of physiological variation between children of the same age group and gender so the pharmacokinetic or pharmacodynamic variations are also likely to be of marginal clinical significance. Within an age group, some children will no doubt be bigger and some smaller but this will be allowed for by adjusting the dose to the size of the individual child. In children's medicine, many drugs have their dose determined by the weight of the child or in some cases, the child's surface area. Obesity can complicate these calculations and where children are significantly overweight, the average weight for their age will often be used.

So far we have been considering the typical 'normal' child but some children have diseases that can significantly affect the way their bodies handle drugs. For example, children who have renal impairment will need adjustments to their dosage to allow for reduced drug clearance. Again, you are recommended to refer to specialist publications.

Younger children differ from adults in the rate that they metabolise and eliminate drugs. You might think that because children have smaller livers and smaller kidneys that they metabolise and eliminate drugs more slowly. For some drugs this rule applies but for other drugs, the immature liver metabolises more quickly – in other words, it is not possible to generalise on the rate of drug metabolism in young children.

Neonates, usually defined as children under four weeks old, need special consideration because their liver and kidneys are immature and, for a pre-term infant (any child born before 37 weeks gestation), their organs will be even less mature. Liver enzymes in the neonate are significantly underactive compared to the adult, which means that they take much longer to metabolise drugs. Kidneys are also immature at birth so the renal elimination of drugs is reduced but these organs mature fairly rapidly. Taken together, liver and renal immaturity can significantly increase the half-life of drugs in the neonate compared to the adult. This has obvious implications for the prescribing and administration of drugs.

Categories are often created for the convenience of the professional and may not reflect a physiological reality. Neonates may technically become children four weeks after birth but their livers do not suddenly mature overnight. Effectively, drug metabolism and clearance can be affected in the very young child, well beyond the neonatal stage.

## Drugs and the pregnant and breast-feeding patient

Sound, pharmacological evidence relating to the effects of drugs in pregnancy is rather thin. For obvious reasons, it is considered unethical to use pregnant women in clinical trials so evidence in this area is often based on animal studies. Drugs prescribed to a pregnant woman may well reach her unborn child but there is variation between drugs in their ability to cross the placenta. Lipophilic drugs will cross much more easily than hydrophilic drugs but once a drug has reached the foetal circulation, elimination is slow.

Advice regarding prescribing in pregnancy tends to err on the side of caution. Unless absolutely necessary, it is recommended that drugs should not be taken during pregnancy, especially during the first trimester (three months). This is because many drugs are teratogenic (cause malformation of the developing foetus), especially those used for the treatment of cancers. These drugs are extremely teratogenic and often will not be prescribed until it is confirmed that a woman is not pregnant. During the second and third trimesters drugs are less likely to be teratogenic but may affect the baby's growth and development. Some drugs such as opioids and antidepressants may cause withdrawal symptoms in the newborn baby so should be used with caution. Given the paucity of evidence, it is usually recommended that if medicines are prescribed during pregnancy they should preferably be drugs that have been extensively used and found to be safe during this period.

As you are (I hope) aware, it takes two people to make a baby and men are not immune from the effects of drugs. Some drugs, especially the anti-cancer drugs, can damage sperm and lead to malformation or developmental problems if the child is conceived while the man is taking medication.

When a woman is breast-feeding there is a possibility that any drug she has taken will appear in her milk and be transferred to her baby. Ideally, babies, especially neonates, should not be exposed to drugs or their metabolites but the amounts transferred in the milk are generally so small as to produce no discernible effect in the baby. Pre-term babies and those with infant jaundice are most at risk but evidence is poor and, erring on the side of caution, nursing mothers are advised not to take medicines unless absolutely necessary.

> **DID YOU KNOW ...** the majority of drugs are not licensed for use in children even though they appear in the *BNF for Children* ... ? To get a product licence, manufacturers have to provide evidence, usually from clinical trials, but for ethical reasons it is very difficult to recruit children as trial subjects. These drugs are regularly prescribed 'off-licence' to children but on the basis of clinical expertise and evidence obtained from adult trials.

## Drugs and ethnicity

There is genetic diversity between racial groups but there is also genetic diversity within groups and this makes it difficult to predict with certainty how an individual of any race may react to a particular drug. Much of the genetic diversity of pharmacological interest manifests itself in P450 polymorphisms that influence the rate that drugs are metabolised, especially in the liver. Unfortunately, it is not always easy to determine the clinical relevance of P450 and other biochemical polymorphisms and currently in the UK we have only one class of drug whose prescribing is according to guidelines based on a patient's ethnic origin. ACE inhibitors such as **captopril**, **enalapril** and **ramipril** are not recommended as first-line antihypertensive treatment for people of Afro-Caribbean origin. These drugs act on the renin-angiotensin system and are less effective in Afro-Caribbeans because circulating renin levels are naturally lower in this ethnic group. In the USA a combination of **isosorbide dinitrate** and **hydralazine** for congestive heart failure in African Americans became the first drug to be licensed for a specific ethnic group. The future holds the prospect of drug regimes tailored to an individual's genetic profile but whether more race-specific drugs will be introduced remains to be seen.

**A QUICK RECAP on drugs and special groups**

- Elderly people tend to metabolise and eliminate drugs more slowly so for standard doses, circulating levels may be higher, resulting in more pronounced side-effects.
- This problem is compounded by polypharmacy, increasing the potential for drug–drug interactions.
- Prescribing drugs for children needs great care and doses need to be adjusted to the individual child.
- Neonates have very immature livers and kidneys so metabolise and eliminate drugs more slowly.

- Pregnant women should ideally not take medicines, especially in the first trimester, as they may cause deformities in the unborn child.
- Breast-feeding mothers should ideally not take medicines unless absolutely necessary.
- There is variation in the way that different races respond to drugs but currently in the UK only ACE inhibitors are prescribed according to the ethnic origin of the patient.

## REFERENCES AND FURTHER RECOMMENDED READING

Books

Barrett, T.G., Lander, A. and Diwakar, V. (Eds) (2002) *A Paediatric Vade-Mecum*. Hodder Arnold.

*British National Formulary* (2012) BMJ Group and RPS Publishing.

*BNF for Children* (2012) BMJ Group and RPS Publishing.

Coleman, M. (2010) *Drug Metabolism*. Wiley-Blackwell.

Websites

All recommended websites are open access (but free registration is sometimes required).

British National Formulary (and BNF for Children): http://www.bnf.org/bnf/

UK Teratology Information Service (UKTIS): http://www.uktis.org/html/maternal_exposure.html

## Test yourself

Now you have finished reading the chapter it's time to find out how much you have learned. Side-effects, drug metabolism and interactions are important aspects of pharmacology so it's essential that you understand these topics.

*The answers to these questions are at the end of the book (see p. 313).*

1 Name a drug or group of drugs that can cause unwanted effects by tipping the balance too far as they try to restore homeoostasis.

2 What is the effect of adrenaline binding to a $\beta_1$ receptor on the heart?

3 Why may salbutamol, a $\beta_2$ receptor agonist, cause tachycardia?

4 ACE inhibitors such as **captopril** can accidently bind to and block kininase enzymes in the bronchioles – how might this cause the side-effect of dry cough?

5 How may calcium channel blockers such as **verapamil** cause constipation?

6 Name the three major routes of drug administration.

7 Describe the passage of drugs from the digestive system to the circulation.

8 Why can **insulin** not be administered orally?

9 Why can **glyceryl trinitrate** (GTN) not be administered orally?

10 What is first-pass metabolism?

11 If P450 enzymes are inhibited by a drug is it more likely that other drugs will be increased or decreased in their bioavailability?

12 What is the most likely effect of an increase in vitamin K on a patient taking **warfarin** – thrombosis or haemorrhage?

13 What is the therapeutic window?

14 What is the half-life of a drug?

15 Why are circulating drug levels likely to be higher in the elderly patient?

# Part 2

# The major drug groups

# Chapter 4

# The cardiovascular system (1): drugs used in the management of coronary artery disease

Chapter 4 is the first of two devoted to the cardiovascular system. This first chapter starts by examining the basic anatomy and physiology of the circulatory system. We then discuss the all-too-common pathology of coronary artery disease and its consequences. Finally, we apply this knowledge as we explore the pharmacological action of the major drug groups used to prevent and to treat coronary artery disease. Chapter 5, the second on the circulatory system, is devoted to the problem of hypertension (high blood pressure) and the drugs used in its treatment.

## CONTENTS

The chapter contains some brief case studies and finishes off with some self-test questions, so you can make sure that you have understood the physiology, pathology and pharmacology of this important area.

### IN PRACTICE

You will find that coronary artery disease is depressingly common, especially among the elderly and particularly those from poorer, underprivileged backgrounds. The disease itself can take many forms from mild angina through to congestive heart failure and it is often associated with other chronic diseases such as diabetes and hypertension. In any branch of adult medicine you will undoubtedly encounter patients with heart problems, so you need to understand the nature of the disease and also the many different types of drugs used in its treatment.

## Introduction

Let's start off with a less than cheerful statistic: according to the UK Office for National Statistics, coronary artery disease (CAD) is the cause of more deaths in the UK than any other disease. This is a sad (but true) fact and it's almost certain that most of us will know a relative or acquaintance who has had a heart attack. Fortunately, the chances of surviving a heart attack have been greatly improved in recent years and many people are alive today thanks to the excellent standard of treatment by paramedics and emergency care teams, not to mention advances in drug therapy. You can see, therefore, how important it is for all clinical practitioners to have a basic knowledge of the circulatory system, the nature of coronary artery disease and also familiarity with the common drugs used in its prevention and treatment.

This chapter follows a format that will become familiar to you as you read the subsequent chapters in Part 2. Firstly, we make sure that you understand the basic anatomy and physiology of the circulatory system. Secondly, we help you to understand something about the pathology of coronary artery disease, its causes and its consequences. Finally, we put this knowledge to good use when we explore how the main groups of anticoagulant, anti-anginal and lipid-lowering drugs work to help to prevent and treat this disease. We also include a brief section of some common but fairly specialised drugs used to treat abnormal heart rhythms.

In this and the next chapter you will find that several drugs have more than one indication; in other words, they are used for more than one type of cardiovascular disease. For example, some of the beta-blockers such as **propranolol**, **atenolol**, **bisoprolol**, etc., are used to alleviate angina, lower high blood pressure, help with heart failure and prevent *arrhythmias* (abnormal heart beat) – not to mention relieving various symptoms associated with anxiety. To save repetition, we will just explain the action of each drug once rather than repeat its action for each type of cardiovascular problem.

*Arrhythmias* such as palpitations can be annoying but not life-threatening whereas others, especially after a heart attack, can be very serious indeed. The term *arrhythmia* can refer to an irregular heart beat or one that is abnormally slow or fast.

## WHERE ARE WE STARTING FROM?

In the next two chapters we shall look at the circulatory system and its associated pathologies in some detail – as well as the drugs that are used to treat those pathologies. *Introducing Pharmacology* is primarily (as the title implies) a book about pharmacology so we cannot explain all the anatomy, physiology and pathologies of the circulatory system in great detail. We will, however, cover enough of the basics of these topics in Chapters 4 and 5 to enable you to understand the action of the main drugs used to treat cardiovascular disease. The general physiology and pathophysiology books in your college or university library will help you to explore the subject in more depth. Some suggestions for recommended reading are provided at the end of this chapter.

Do we really need two chapters just devoted to the circulatory system?

Yes, indeed we do. An understanding of the circulatory system is essential to anyone training or working in clinical practice. Think how often nurses and doctors take their patients' blood pressure or pulse. Also, if you do not understand the basic physiology of the circulatory system you will never understand the action of the drugs used to treat cardiovascular diseases.

You might care to try this short quiz to find out how much you know before beginning the chapter:

1 Point to your heart – is it on the left or right side of your chest?

_____

2 Do arteries carry blood to or from the heart?

_____

3 How many chambers are there in the heart?

_____

4 Starting from the heart, arrange these blood vessels in the order that the blood flows – capillaries, arteries and veins.

_____

5 What is the name of the arteries that supply the heart muscle with blood?

_____

*Answers are at the end of the chapter on p. 108.*

How did you do? If you think you might need to brush up on the anatomy and physiology of the circulatory system, this topic is covered in the first section of this chapter.

## 4.1 The physiology of the cardiovascular system

The circulatory system is made up of the heart, the blood vessels and blood and can be thought of as the body's internal transport system, carrying messages and materials from one part of the body to another. The circulatory system is also central to maintaining the stability of the internal environment, those processes that control nutrient levels and waste disposal as well as water and temperature regulation. The need for an internal transport system arose hundreds of millions of years ago when single-celled organisms started to aggregate into larger, multicellular organisms. Their increase in size then became limited by the rate at which nutrients and gases could be obtained from the environment by simple diffusion. The development of a simple circulation meant that nutrients and gases could be collected by specialist organs such as the gut and gills* and then transported to all of the cells of the body. We might speculate that without the development of the circulatory system, animal life as we know it today would not exist – including perhaps ourselves!

### Overview of the circulatory system

The circulatory system is the main transport system of the body, carrying nutrients, respiratory gases, wastes, hormones, immune cells and clotting proteins around the body in the blood. It also has other functions, such as temperature control and acidity regulation, that are essential for the well-being of the individual. In the context of pharmacology, it is also the system that transports most of our drugs around the body, from the site of administration to the tissues targeted by those drugs.

The circulatory system is divided into two parts, the *pulmonary system* supplying the lungs and the *systemic system* supplying the rest of the body (Figure 4.1). At the centre of both systems is the heart, a large, muscular pump that beats 70 or so times each minute from a few weeks after conception to the last minute of the individual's life. A simple calculation indicates that by the age of 70, the heart

---

* The move from single-celled to multicellular animals probably happened in the sea, so these primitive animals would have had gills rather than lungs to collect oxygen.

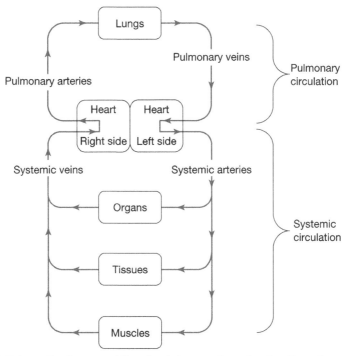

**Figure 4.1** Schematic diagram of the circulatory system showing the pulmonary and systemic systems.

has beat over 2.5 billion times. Although it is a single organ, the heart is not a single pump but, rather, two separate pumps joined together and beating in unison. The right-hand pump sends blood to the pulmonary circulation, around the lungs from where it returns to the left-hand heart pump. From the left-hand pump the blood is sent around the systemic circulation to the tissues and organs of the body. The blood then returns to the right-hand pump from where it is again sent around the pulmonary circulation.

## Blood vessels

Blood vessels are the body's plumbing system, carrying blood from one part of the circulatory system to another. These vessels can be divided broadly into three types: arteries, veins and capillaries, each having a different structure and function.

- **Arteries.** These thick-walled, muscular tubes carry high-pressure blood away from the heart, supplying blood to organs and muscles where they branch into smaller arteries called *arterioles*. The body can adjust the diameter of the arterioles to control blood pressure – as discussed in more detail in Chapter 5.
- **Veins.** These have thinner walls than arteries and carry low-pressure blood back to the heart. Small one-way valves help to keep the blood moving in one

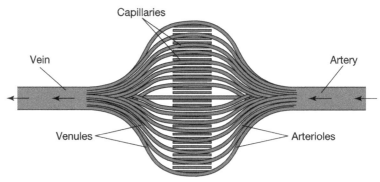

**Figure 4.2** Relationship between the blood vessels of the arterial and venous system. The arrows indicate the direction of blood flow.

direction. Veins are larger in diameter than their arterial counterparts and over 60 per cent of the body's blood is retained in the veins at any one time. The tiniest of veins, where they emerge from tissues and organs, are called *venules*.

- **Capillaries.** These are the smallest of the blood vessels, being only one cell thick, and they permeate nearly every cubic millimetre of every tissue of the body. The walls of arteries and veins are too thick to allow gases and nutrients to cross their walls, so it is in the capillaries where the exchange of materials between the blood and the body's cells takes place.

**CASE STUDY**

Harry is admitted to A & E complaining of severe chest pains and difficulty breathing but an *electrocardiogram* (ECG) confirms that he has not suffered a heart attack. Further tests indicate a pulmonary thromboembolism – a blood clot in the lungs. The consultant diagnoses that the problem originated with a deep vein thrombosis (DVT) in Harry's leg. Explain how a DVT in the leg might cause problems in the lungs.

*Comment on case study* A blood clot that forms in the veins of the leg (deep vein thrombosis) can often cause a pulmonary thromboembolism – a blood clot in the lungs. The blood clot travels in the ever-widening veins to the right side of the heart where it enters the pulmonary circulation and soon blocks one of the ever-narrowing pulmonary arteries, causing chest pain and difficulty in breathing.

## The circulatory system and gas exchange

As we saw in Chapter 1, glucose and fatty acids are broken down in the body's cells to produce adenosine triphosphate (ATP) and this requires a good supply of oxygen. Carbon dioxide is a waste produced during cellular energy production and needs to be removed from the cells, otherwise its accumulation could inhibit metabolic activity. The transport of oxygen to the tissues and the removal of carbon dioxide is a very important function of the circulatory system and must be maintained constantly throughout the life of the individual. Any disease or trauma that interferes with the transport of gases, especially oxygen, quickly results in problems, the death of cells and even the demise of the individual.

If you refer to Figure 4.1 (p. 77) you will see that blood constantly flows between the pulmonary and systemic circulation. In the pulmonary circulation, the blood collects oxygen then travels via the systemic circulation to the muscles, organs and tissues where the oxygen is released to the cells in order that they may produce energy. During the process of energy production, carbon dioxide, which is produced in the cells, is collected by the blood and transported to the pulmonary system, where it is disposed of into the atmosphere via the lungs.

## The heart

Ask most people where their heart is situated and they will point vaguely to the left side of their chest. The heart is in fact situated in the centre of the chest, directly under the sternum (breastbone) but on a slightly tilted axis so that the lower pointed part or apex is on the left-hand side. This means that when the heart is beating strongly, the heart beat can be heard more clearly on the left-hand side, where you can also feel it by placing your fingers just to the left of the sternum.

### The structure of the heart

The heart consists of four chambers – two atria and two ventricles. Blood arriving at the heart from the vena cava and the pulmonary veins first enters the atria, from where it passes into the ventricles, which are the main pumping chambers of the heart. When the left and right ventricles contract, blood is forced into the aorta and pulmonary arteries respectively. Separating the atria and the ventricles are one-way valves, collectively known as the atrioventricular valves. Another set of valves called the semilunar valves separate the ventricles from the arteries. Figure 4.3 shows the general structure of the heart and Figure 4.4 shows the route by which the blood flows through it. Most of the force that pumps the blood out of the heart comes from contraction of the thick muscular wall of the heart – the *myocardium*. The myocardium consists almost entirely of cardiac muscle cells which are unique to the heart, being found in no other part of the body. As might be expected in a muscle mass that may beat continuously for over 70 years, energy supply is of prime importance and the cardiac muscle cells are rich in ATP-producing mitochondria.

The pumping cycle of the heart can be divided into two stages: *diastole* (pronounced *die-ass-toe-lee*), when the heart is relaxed and filling with blood, and *systole* (pronounced *sis-toe-lee*), when the heart is contracting and pumping blood into the arteries. We will learn more about systole and diastole in Chapter 5 when we examine the control of the heart and how the body regulates blood pressure.

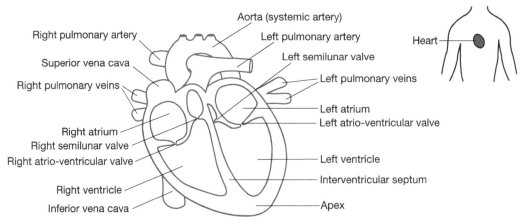

Figure 4.3 Front view of the heart in section. The small diagram to the right shows the position of the heart in the thoracic cavity.

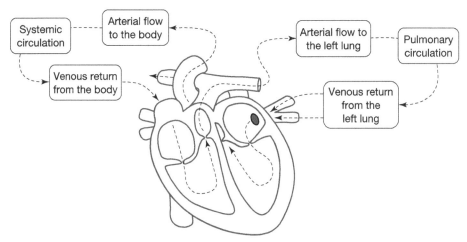

Figure 4.4 Simplified diagram of blood flow through the heart, the systemic circulation and the pulmonary circulation. Left pulmonary blood flow only is shown for clarity.

*Myocardium* is the middle layer of the heart wall and comprises cardiac muscle cells. As the cells contract, a wave of contraction in the myocardium pumps blood out of the heart into the arteries.

## The blood supply to the myocardium

Most people would assume that the heart obtains its oxygen and nutrients from the blood that is constantly being pumped through the atria and ventricles. However, if you look back at Figure 4.3 you will see that the myocardium, the muscular wall of the heart, is quite thick, too thick in fact to obtain its nutrients and oxygen by simple diffusion. To resolve this problem, the heart has its own blood supply via its own blood vessels and this is called the coronary circulation

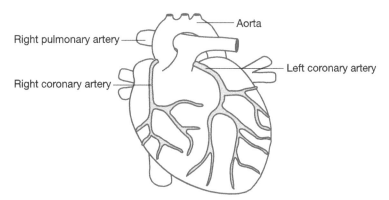

Figure 4.5 The coronary circulation. Blood vessels emerging from the aorta supply the heart muscle with blood, nutrients and oxygen.

(Figure 4.5). The blood supply for the coronary circulation comes from the two coronary arteries which emerge from the base of the aorta. These coronary arteries wrap themselves around the heart, the right coronary artery supplying the right atrium and right ventricle and the left coronary artery supplying the left atrium and left ventricle. The arteries are initially visible on the surface of the heart but then dive into the heart muscle and divide into arterioles and capillaries.

DID YOU KNOW ... why the arteries of the heart are called coronary arteries? It is because they are vaguely shaped like a crown worn by the Monarch. The words *coronation* and *coroner* derive from this root. Turn Figure 4.6 upside-down and you will see. You might well be forgiven for thinking the inverted arteries look more like reindeer antlers than a crown ...

A QUICK RECAP on the circulatory system

- The main function of the circulatory system is the transport of materials around the body. Of special importance is the transport of oxygen from the lungs to the cells of the tissues.

- There are two parts of the circulatory system – the pulmonary circulation and the systemic circulation.

- There are three main types of blood vessels – arteries, veins and capillaries. All of these vessels transport blood but it is in the capillaries that exchange takes place between the blood and the cells.

- The heart is the double driving pump of the circulatory system – the left half pumps blood through the systemic circulation and the right half pumps blood through the pulmonary circulation.

- The heart has its own blood vessels – the coronary arteries, which supply blood to the heart muscle, the myocardium.

## 4.2    The pathology of coronary artery disease

Atherosclerosis in the coronary arteries is the principal cause of angina, myocardial infarction (heart attack) and heart failure. In the carotid arteries that supply the brain, atherosclerosis can result in stroke.

Cardiovascular disease is undoubtedly the principal cause of death in the UK and the cost of treating this problem places an enormous drain on the resources of the National Health Service. Hundreds of thousands of people are afflicted with this disease; many are unable to enjoy normal activities as their lives are blighted by a pathology that is largely avoidable.

Early in the life of some individuals, the first recognisable event in the development of atherosclerosis is the formation of fatty streaks in the walls of the arteries. White blood cells called *macrophages* containing fat droplets of cholesterol migrate from the blood to the area just under the inner lining of the arteries called the subendothelium. Generally, in the healthy individual these fatty streaks remain inconspicuous but in some people they develop into *atheromata* (singular, atheroma) (Figures 4.6a to 4.6d).

Smooth muscle cells in the area are prompted to multiply in a disorganised and haphazard fashion and the fatty streaks enlarge into cholesterol-rich structures called atherosclerotic *plaques* that can become inflamed and unstable. In this

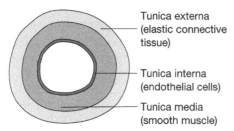

(a) Structure of a healthy coronary artery

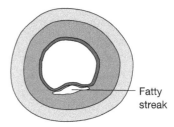

(b) Fatty streak develops in the subendothelium

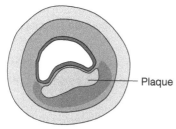

(c) Fatty streak enlarges, muscle cells divide and the area becomes inflamed. It is now is termed an atherosclerotic plaque

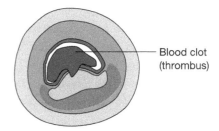

(d) Damage to plaque from inflammation, trauma, exercise etc. results in a thrombus forming. This may completely block the artery

**Figures 4.6** (a)–(d) show the development of an atherosclerotic plaque and the formation of a thrombus.

state, the plaques can partially block the coronary arteries, resulting in angina. Even worse, the plaque can rupture and a *thrombus* (blood clot) can form, blocking the coronary artery and causing a myocardial infarction, commonly known as a heart attack.

> *Macrophage* literally translated means 'big eater'. Macrophages are important members of the white blood-cell family of immune cells with many functions, including the destruction of bacteria.

Apart from a few people who inherit a genetic defect in lipid regulation, most atherosclerosis is due to the lifestyle adopted by the individual. The key risk factors for cardiovascular disease are smoking, lack of exercise, eating too much saturated fat and not eating enough fruit and vegetables. Add to these risk factors obesity and diabetes and you can almost guarantee that an individual will have heart problems. How these factors increase the risk of cardiovascular disease is quite complex but the epidemiological evidence that they do is well established.

**CASE STUDY**

Jim is 58, works as a truck driver and is complaining about feeling out of breath when he climbs the stairs. He is overweight, smokes and eats most of his meals in transport cafes. Given what you know about the causes of cardiovascular disease, what would you advise for Jim?

*Comment on case study* Jim is at risk of developing cardiovascular disease and his breathlessness definitely needs to be discussed this with his GP. The best advice to improve his health would obviously be to give up smoking and change his diet by reducing his intake of saturated fats and eating plenty of fresh fruit and vegetables. He should also start to take regular exercise. This advice would, however, require a radical change in Jim's lifestyle and it may be more productive to tackle the problem in stages, with smoking cessation the first priority.

## Angina pectoris

The gradual blockage of the coronary arteries by atherosclerotic plaques can result in insufficient blood and oxygen being delivered to the myocardium during exercise. Remember, whatever group of muscles you are exercising, the heart has to respond by beating faster to increase its output of blood. However, when heart muscle cells cannot get sufficient oxygen they do some clever biochemistry and switch on metabolic pathways that keep energy production going despite the shortage of oxygen. Unfortunately, this switch in pathways results in the production of lactic acid that stimulates pain neurons and this produces the pain associated with angina. In chronic stable angina, the arteries occluded (obstructed) by plaques produce a predictable, exercise-associated pain. Unstable angina is defined as new-onset angina, angina at rest or angina after a heart attack. The cause of unstable angina needs investigating as it may signal a thrombosis in the coronary arteries.

## Heart attack or myocardial infarction

When a plaque ruptures it can result in a blood clot forming around the site of rupture and this can partially or completely block the coronary artery. The section of heart muscle supplied by the artery is deprived of sufficient blood and oxygen and is said to be ischaemic. If the blood supply is not restored quickly, the myocardial muscle cells die, forming an infarct (area of dead tissue). This is a heart attack or myocardial infarction (MI). Damaged heart muscle can severely incapacitate the heart's ability to pump blood and eventually this may lead to heart failure and possibly death. The extent of the damage to the heart depends on the size and location of the artery that has been occluded. A large clot can block a large artery, which cuts off blood to a significant section of the heart muscle, causing a major heart attack. A clot forming in a small terminal artery may affect only a relatively small area of muscle and the damage is potentially less serious (Figure 4.7). Sometimes the ischaemic tissue can be rescued by *collateral circulation*, the blood supply from adjacent, unaffected arteries, keeping the tissue alive until the paramedics arrive.

> **IN PRACTICE**
>
> The pain experienced in a heart attack is often felt in the arm and neck as well as the chest because the pain neurons that originate in these areas all feed into the spinal cord at the same point. The brain is unable to identify the precise source of the problem so that pain is perceived as emanating from a different area to the source. This is called *referred pain*.

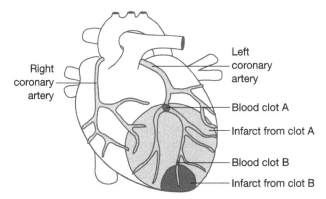

**Figure 4.7** Two blood clots form in the coronary arteries. Blood clot A is large and blocks two branches of the descending left coronary artery, depriving a large area of heart muscle of blood and oxygen and severely affecting the heart's ability to pump blood. Blood clot B is smaller, blocks a minor artery and affects a smaller area of tissue.

## Heart failure

The consequences of a heart attack can vary depending on the location of the thrombus, the area of heart tissue affected and, most importantly, the time it takes for the paramedics to arrive. If the patient's life is saved but a significant area of the myocardium is irreparably damaged, this can eventually lead to heart failure. This is a complex process where the heart becomes more and more weakened as it attempts to maintain blood pressure and eventually becomes irreparably damaged, leading to complete failure and death.

# Surgical interventions in coronary artery disease

Many people with severe coronary artery disease will be admitted to hospital for surgery to improve the supply of blood to the heart muscle. There are two common procedures, usually abbreviated to CABG (pronounced 'cabbage') and PCI. As these surgical procedures are common, it is worth outlining them to contextualise the drugs we shall shortly be describing. In coronary artery bypass grafts (CABG), the heart is exposed and a healthy vein or artery is removed from elsewhere in the patient and transplanted so that it bypasses the damaged coronary artery. Percutaneous coronary intervention (PCI) is performed using radiographic imaging (x-rays) to insert a long, thin wire called a catheter into the arterial system and directing it into the blocked coronary artery. Here, a small balloon on the end of the catheter is expanded to open up the blocked artery. A small metal cage called a stent is often attached to the end of the catheter and as the balloon expands so does the stent, holding open the artery and allowing blood to flow freely.

While CABG and PCI can undoubtedly prolong and improve the quality of life for those with coronary artery disease, most of these patients will continue to be maintained on a regime of anticlotting drugs that we will discuss later in the chapter.

**IN PRACTICE**

Could you explain to a patient or relative the difference between a coronary artery bypass graft and a percutaneous coronary intervention?

**A QUICK RECAP on coronary artery disease**

- Atheromata are fatty growths that form in the wall of the coronary arteries.
- Atheromata can partially block the coronary arteries resulting in stable angina – reversible heart pain brought on by exercise.
- Atheromata can rupture, causing a thrombus (blood clot) to form in the arteries.
- The thrombus can block a coronary artery, cutting off the oxygen supply to areas of heart muscle – ischaemia.
- The continued lack of blood and oxygen can cause an infarct – death of heart muscle; this is a myocardial infarction (MI) or heart attack.

## 4.3 Drugs used in the treatment of coronary artery disease

### Anti-angina drugs

#### What are we trying to do with these drugs?

The principal purpose of anti-angina drugs is to relieve the pain associated with the disease rather than treating the disease itself. This is not to say we can't help the sufferer of stable angina but the drugs used to relieve the pain do little, if anything, to resolve the cause of the problem, which is primarily the formation of atherosclerotic plaques in the coronary arteries. The PCI procedure described above is often performed to give relief from pain to angina sufferers.

The full treatment regime for anyone suffering from stable angina will include lifestyle changes such as giving up smoking, taking controlled exercise and eating a healthy diet that includes more fruit and vegetables and less saturated fat. To reduce the rate at which atherosclerosis develops, statins such as **atorvastatin** may be prescribed to lower cholesterol levels in the blood. Angina sufferers also run the risk of clots forming in the coronary arteries, so **aspirin** may be pre-scribed on a long-term basis to prevent this. The action of statins and **aspirin** will be discussed later in the chapter.

A variety of drugs are available to reduce angina pain and these include nitrates, beta-blockers and calcium channel blockers. The general aim of these drugs is to reduce the workload of the heart or dilate the coronary arteries, so delivering more oxygenated blood to the heart muscle. In this section of the chapter we will concentrate on the action of nitrates and beta-blockers and leave any detailed discussion of the calcium channel blockers until Chapter 5, when we examine their role as antihypertensive drugs.

> **KEY FACT**
>
> Anti-angina drugs relieve angina pain by reducing the workload of the heart or by increasing the blood supply to the heart muscle.

#### Anti-angina drugs group 1: glyceryl trinitrate and related drugs

**Glyceryl trinitrate** (GTN) is regularly prescribed as first-line treatment in stable angina. It is available as tablets or as a spray, both of which are used under the tongue, from where the drug speedily enters the bloodstream and quickly relieves angina pain. Transdermal patches are also available to deliver **GTN** over a longer period.

The action of nitrates on cells is complex but their main effect is to release nitric oxide, a potent vasodilator that causes relaxation of the smooth muscle

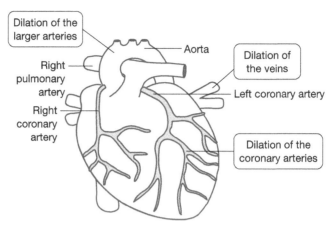

**Figure 4.8** Summary of the effects of nitrates on the heart.

cells surrounding blood vessels and so produces vasodilation. Nitrates have various effects on different blood vessels (Figure 4.8).

● **Venodilation** (dilation of the veins) reduces pressure in the veins, which in turn reduces the amount of blood returning to the heart. Less blood in the ventricles when they are contracting reduces the workload of the heart.

● **Vasodilation of coronary arteries** increases blood flow to the heart muscle, bringing with it more oxygen. This reduces lactic acid production and thus pain.

● **Vasodilation of larger arterioles** lowers blood pressure and reduces the amount of effort needed by the heart to pump blood out of the ventricles.

**IN PRACTICE**

A **GTN** tablet or spray dissolves under the tongue rather than being swallowed because **GTN** is almost completely metabolised by the liver on its way from the digestive system to the general circulation. Dissolved under the tongue, **GTN** passes straight into the bloodstream. Other formulations are available that can survive passage through the liver.

GTN itself has a very short life in the circulation of around five minutes, so other formulations such as **isosorbide dinitrate** and **isosorbide mononitrate** have been developed to provide longer-term relief from angina. Nitrate tolerance can be a problem with these drugs as their effectiveness diminishes with long-term use.

*Side-effects* A drug group that causes general vasodilation can cause hypotension (low blood pressure) in some patients. Throbbing headache is another common side-effect of nitrates.

**CASE STUDY**

John has been suffering from angina for nearly one year. He has been using a **GTN** sub-lingual spray which seems to ease the pain that he experiences when he climbs the stairs. Recently his chest pain has returned despite the **GTN**. What may be the cause?

*Comment on case study* There are several possible causes but it could be that he is becoming tolerant to **GTN** and his medication needs reviewing. Another explanation could be that John's coronary arteries are becoming more occluded by the atheromata so further tests are required.

**DID YOU KNOW . . .** that glyceryl trinitrate is the same substance as nitroglycerin, the explosive component of dynamite invented by Alfred Nobel in the nineteenth century? Modern formulations of **GTN** do not carry the risk of explosion but one wonders if early pharmacists had a few close shaves with this potentially dangerous substance! **GTN** is also one of the oldest drugs still in use – its first appearance in the pharmacopoeia was in the 1880s.

## Anti-angina drugs group 2: beta-blockers

This group of drugs is more correctly called beta-adrenoceptor antagonists in that they antagonistically block adrenergic (adrenaline) receptors. They have been in the pharmacopoeia for over 30 years and earned their inventor, Sir James Black, the Nobel Prize for Medicine in 1989 for the synthesis of **propranolol.**

Examples of this group used in the treatment of angina include **acebutolol, atenolol, bisoprolol, carvedilol, labetalol, metoprolol, nadolol, oxprenolol, pindolol, propranolol** and **timolol.** Selected members of this group of drugs are also used for hypertension and arrhythmias and heart failure.

The sympathetic neurons release the neurotransmitter noradrenaline and this stimulates $\beta_1$ adrenoceptors on the heart pacemaker cells and the heart muscle. This increases both the heart rate and contractility which in turn increases the workload of the heart and so the probability of angina-induced pain. Beta-blockers bind to and block $\beta_1$ receptors on the heart and this reduces its responsiveness to sympathetic activity (Figure 4.9). This lowers the heart's workload to a level where the oxygen demand of the heart muscle can be met, even by the narrowed coronary arteries.

Beta-blockers also reduce blood pressure by a complex mechanism that is by no means fully understood (see Chapter 5). When blood pressure (BP) is reduced in the aorta, this means that the heart has to beat less forcefully to push blood into the arterial system. This also helps to reduce the heart's workload and so prevents angina pain.

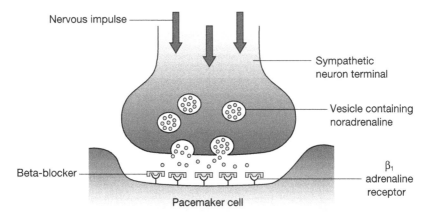

Figure 4.9 At the synapse between a sympathetic neuron and a pacemaker cell, noradrenaline is prevented from binding to its receptors by beta-blockers which lower the heart rate.

**IN PRACTICE**

Beta-blockers should not be prescribed to anyone suffering from asthma. This is because these drugs can block $\beta_2$ adrenaline receptors in the bronchioles of the lungs and these receptors are the targets for bronchodilators such as **salbutamol**. If they are blocked by beta-blockers, then **salbutamol** cannot bind and activate its receptors, which could be potentially very serious for anyone having an asthma attack.

## Anti-angina drugs group 3: calcium channel blockers

Examples of calcium channel blockers (CCBs) include **amlodipine**, **diltiazem**, **felodipine**, **nicardipine**, **nifedipine** and **verapamil**. CCBs are a diverse group of drugs and exert their effects by different mechanisms. CCBs are a popular group of drugs that are also used in the treatment of hypertension. We will meet them again in Chapter 5 when we discuss antihypertensive drugs, and we will examine in more detail how they reduce blood pressure.

Calcium channel blockers act on calcium ion channels in the muscle cells of the heart, the conduction system of the heart and the smooth muscle cells of blood vessels. These diverse targets all result in a reduction in the pain associated with angina but by a variety of mechanisms:

1 **Reduction in heart rate.** Slowing the heart rate reduces the workload of the heart and helps to ease angina pain.

2 **Reduction in the force of contraction.** This again reduces the workload of the heart and helps to ease angina pain.

3 **Reduction in blood pressure.** Vasodilation dilates the blood vessels and this reduces blood pressure. The heart has to pump less forcefully to push blood into the arteries.

*Side-effects* These are many, including hypotension, flushing, oedema, headaches and constipation (especially with **verapamil**).

### Miscellaneous anti-angina drugs: potassium channel openers – nicorandil

**Nicorandil** acts on smooth muscle cells of blood vessels where it opens $K^+$ channels in the cell membrane, making the muscle cells more resistant to contraction. **Nicorandil** also dilates the coronary arteries, thus increasing blood and oxygen supply to the myocardium. In addition to its action as a $K^+$ channel opener, **nicorandil** (nicotinamide nitrate) also has a nitrate-like action, acting in a similar manner to GTN.

### Miscellaneous anti-angina drugs: funny channel blockers – ivabradine

This is not a joke – **ivabradine** really does block a mixed $Na^+/K^+$ ion channel on the heart's pacemaker called the funny channel (who says scientists don't have a sense of humour?). This lowers the heart rate which, in turn, reduces oxygen demand by the heart muscle. This means that even with partially blocked coronary arteries, sufficient oxygenated blood can be supplied to the myocardium to prevent the muscle cells from producing the lactic acid that causes angina pain.

Ivabradine blocks funny channels in the heart.

### Miscellaneous anti-angina drugs: ranolazine

Used as an adjunct to other anti-angina drugs, **ranolazine** appears to reduce workload in the heart by interfering with $Na^+$ and $Ca^{2+}$ balance in the heart's muscle cells. The drug may also shift energy production in the heart away from lipids towards more efficient carbohydrate metabolism.

**A QUICK RECAP on anti-angina drugs**

- Nitrates such as **glyceryl trinitrate** reduce angina pain by general vasodilation. This reduces pressure in the arteries and ventricles and so reduces the workload of the heart. The coronary arteries are also dilated, supplying more blood and oxygen to the heart muscle.
- Beta-blockers such as **atenolol** block the heart from the effects of sympathetic stimulation, and this helps to reduce the heart's workload.
- Calcium channel blockers such as **diltiazem** vasodilate arterioles, slow the heart rate and reduce the force of contraction. All of these actions result in a reduction in the heart's workload.
- Miscellaneous anti-angina drugs include potassium channel openers such as **nicorandil**, funny channel blockers such as **ivabradine** and drugs that affect $Na^+$ and $Ca^{2+}$ balance such as **ranolazine.**

## Lipid-regulating drugs

### The regulation of lipid metabolism

Cholesterol is a major constituent of the atherosclerotic plaques that develop in the coronary arteries. It is a lipid that is obtained from animal fats in the diet but can also be synthesised in the liver. The body needs a regular supply of cholesterol as it is important for the structural stability of cell membranes and forms the raw material for the manufacture of steroid hormones and vitamin D. It is also a component of *bile* produced by the liver.

*Bile* is the alkaline, detergent-like substance produced by the liver and secreted into the duodenum via the bile duct. Its main function is the emulsification of lipids that enables their digestion.

Cholesterol is transported in the blood in small water-soluble spheres called *lipoproteins*. Being a lipid, cholesterol will not mix readily with blood, which is watery in nature. In the centre of a lipoprotein sphere, however, the cholesterol is isolated from the blood by the phospholipid shell. This clever arrangement allows the lipoprotein sphere to dissolve in blood (Figure 4.10).

There are two clinically relevant types of lipoprotein – *high-density lipoprotein* (HDL) and *low-density lipoprotein* (LDL). The density of the two lipoproteins refers to the relative amounts of protein in the spheres but essentially it is the different roles that interest us. HDL scavenges cholesterol from tissues, removing it to the liver where it is stored, metabolised or incorporated into bile. LDL has a different role, including the transport of cholesterol from the liver to the tissues. Most importantly, it is LDL that is chemically modified and taken into developing atheromata by macrophages. Here it forms part of the developing atherosclerotic plaques.

**Figure 4.10** A lipoprotein sphere consisting of a phospholipid and protein shell isolating triglycerides and cholesterol from the watery environment of the blood.

The ratio between HDL and LDL is important. Generally, high levels of HDL and low levels of LDL are best for cardiovascular health. Lifestyle factors such as lack of exercise, high cholesterol diet and smoking can adversely affect the HDL:LDL ratio, decreasing HDL or increasing LDL levels.

> **KEY FACT**
>
> To help prevent coronary artery disease it is important to reduce LDL and maximise HDL cholesterol.

Ideally, cholesterol levels should be controlled by diet, exercise and abstinence from harmful habits such as smoking and drinking too much alcohol. In reality, patients are often reluctant to change their lifestyle and for those at high risk of cardiovascular disease, pharmacological intervention can help to regulate cholesterol levels. Typical recommended UK values for serum cholesterol and triglycerides are as follows:

**Typical UK recommended cholesterol and triglyceride values**

| | |
|---|---|
| Total cholesterol | 5.2 mmol/L* or lower |
| LDL (bad) cholesterol | 3.5 mmol/L or lower |
| HDL (good) cholesterol | 1.0 mmol/L or higher (men) 1.2 mmol/L or higher (women) |
| Triglycerides | 1.7 mmol/L or lower |

* millimoles per litre (see below)

## A BRIEF EXPLANATION of moles and molarity

Chemists measure quantities in moles, and 1 mole of a substance is about $6 \times 10^{23}$ atoms. Molarity is the number of moles per litre of solution and 1 mole of a substance dissolved in 1 litre of water would be a 1 molar solution. The mole represents rather a lot of atoms so in biological chemistry you will generally find the millimole

One mole

One millimole?

(mmol) rather than the mole. One millimole is one thousandth of a mole. Put simply, the greater the molarity, the more of a substance there is in a solution.

## Drugs used to lower lipids: statins

The most commonly prescribed drugs used to lower serum cholesterol for the prevention and management of cardiovascular disease are statins. There are a few other drugs such as anion-exchange resins and fibrates but statins are by far the most popular. Examples of this group include **atorvastatin, fluvastatin, pravastatin, rosuvastatin** and **simvastatin**.

You might think that simply cutting down on fats in the diet would reduce cholesterol levels sufficiently but unfortunately, when cholesterol intake is reduced, the body can respond by manufacturing cholesterol in the liver. This can result in elevated serum cholesterol despite a reduction in dietary intake. Remember that cholesterol is a useful substance as well as a potentially harmful one so when levels fall then the body responds by making more of it.

> **KEY FACT**
>
> Reducing dietary cholesterol intake may not be enough to control levels because the liver sometimes responds by synthesising more cholesterol.

Statins are inhibitors of the enzyme 3-hydroxy-3-methylglutaryl-Coenzyme A reductase, usually shortened to HMG CoA reductase. This enzyme takes part in a reaction in the pathway that produces cholesterol in the hepatocytes (liver cells) (Figures 4.11a and 4.11b). Because the liver needs cholesterol to make bile, when production is blocked by a statin, the hepatocytes pull more LDL cholesterol from the blood and this reduces circulating LDL and so reduces the risk of cardiovascular disease. Naturally, statins need to be used in conjunction with a reduction in dietary

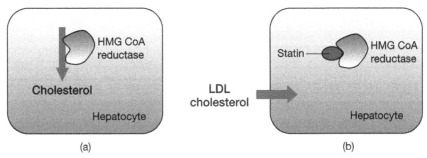

(a)                                                (b)

**Figure 4.11** (a) The hepatic enzyme HMG CoA reductase is involved in the production of cholesterol; (b) Statins block the action of HMG CoA reductase, inhibiting the production of cholesterol, so hepatocytes import LDL cholesterol from the blood.

intake of cholesterol, together with changes in lifestyle to ensure a healthy HDL:LDL ratio.

*Side-effects* Apart from the usual GI disturbances, statins can occasionally cause muscle pain and inflammation.

> **IN PRACTICE**
> Statins are generally taken in the evening because the liver is most active in the production of cholesterol at night.

**A QUICK RECAP on lipid-regulating drugs – statins**

- Cholesterol is a lipid that is essential for the proper functioning of the body but it is also a key component of atherosclerotic plaques.
- We obtain cholesterol from our diet but it can also be synthesised by the liver.
- Cholesterol is transported in the blood in lipoprotein spheres. Two types are clinically important – high-density lipoprotein (HDL) and low-density lipoprotein (LDL).
- Ideally, LDL levels should be minimised and HDL levels maximised for good cardiovascular health.
- A healthy diet, not smoking and taking plenty of exercise helps regulate cholesterol levels.
- Statins inhibit HMG CoA reductase, a liver enzyme involved in the synthesis of cholesterol. A reduction in intracellular cholesterol also stimulates the hepatocytes to absorb LDL cholesterol from the blood.

## Anticoagulant drugs

### Let's start with the basics: what is clotting?

When someone gets injured it is important that blood loss is minimised, otherwise they may eventually lose so much blood that they go into shock, a state where blood pressure falls to the point where tissues are not supplied with sufficient oxygen. Animals have therefore evolved a mechanism that responds to injury involving damage to blood vessels by converting the blood in the area of damage from its normal fluid form into a solid clot. This staunches the flow of blood and prevents further blood loss. Having dealt with the immediate emergency, further mechanisms are then initiated by the body to make more permanent repairs to the injured area in a process called wound resolution.

In most situations, clotting is a desirable process that prevents a loss of blood from a wound but in the case of the coronary arteries the formation of a clot on a ruptured plaque can be disastrous because it can cut off the blood supply to the

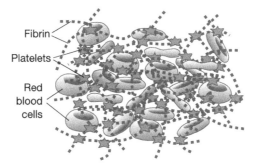

Fibrin

Platelets

Red blood cells

**Figure 4.12** Blood clot showing the platelets, fibrin and red blood cells.

heart muscle, which could then die from lack of oxygen. In this chapter we will examine the process more closely and find out what drugs are available to keep the blood flowing in the coronary arteries.

**DID YOU KNOW ...** that there's a sound reason for sucking your finger when you have a small cut? Saliva contains an enzyme called lysozyme that attacks and destroys bacteria and so prevents your injury becoming infected.

## What is a clot?

The blood clot itself is composed of three elements – platelets, fibrin and red blood cells. The platelets are small cell fragments that have the ability to bind to fibrin, a filament-like protein which forms a web-like structure that traps red blood cells and forms a clot. You can think of it as a fishing net, the platelets being the knots that tie the fibrin strands together (Figure 4.12).

## Overview of clotting

Clotting, like most things in the body, is quite complex but can be understood more easily if we divide it into two key processes:

- **Activation of platelets** – these small cell-like structures are key players in the formation of a blood clot. Without them a clot will not form (a fact exploited by the many antiplatelet drugs).
- **Conversion of fibrinogen into fibrin** – fibrin is a thread-like protein that, together with platelets, forms a web that traps red blood cells. This is another process targeted by anticlotting drugs.

## Part 1 of the clotting process: the activation of platelets

Platelets (also called thrombocytes) circulate in the blood and are key players in the clotting process. Produced primarily in the bone marrow, they are disc-shaped cell fragments without a nucleus and 3–4 μm diameter. Around 300 million are found in each millilitre of blood, with an average life of around ten days. Platelets

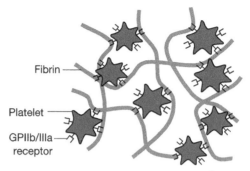

**Figure 4.13** Activated platelets bind to fibrin by their GPIIb/IIIa receptors.

are generally inactive as they circulate in the blood until they come into contact with proteins such as collagen in the wall of a damaged blood vessel. This activates the platelets, which change their shape from smooth to spiky and they also produce receptors on their cell membrane. These receptors, designated GPIIb/IIIa receptors, bind to circulating fibrin, making the web that entraps red blood cells and forms the clot (Figure 4.13).

The mechanisms involved in the activation of platelets needs to be explained briefly in order that you can understand the action of our antiplatelet drugs, **aspirin**, **clopidogrel**, **prasugrel** and **ticagrelor**. In response to tissue damage, platelets become activated and produce two chemicals, *thromboxane A2* (TXA$_2$) and adenosine diphosphate (ADP), that cause the platelets to increase the production of GPIIb/IIIa receptors and display them on their cell surface where they can bind to fibrin.

### ANOTHER WAY TO PICTURE THIS

Imagine the platelets as children in a cold playground so they have their hands (GPIIb/IIIa receptors) in their pockets. On the floor are lots of skipping ropes (fibrin) and when the teacher blows a whistle all the children take their hands out of their pockets and grab hold of any two skipping ropes, forming a kind of net. Hold on to this scene as we will return to it later when discussing antiplatelet drugs.

### Part 2 of the clotting process: the conversion of fibrinogen into fibrin

We have seen how the platelets are activated and now we will look at the second important process in the formation of a blood clot, the conversion of fibrinogen into fibrin. In the blood, fibrin circulates as an inactive soluble protein called fibrinogen. Because it is soluble when dissolved in the blood, fibrinogen will not interact with the platelets because the GPIIb/IIIa receptors cannot bind to it. Imagine trying to grab hold of jelly – that's like platelets trying to bind to fibrinogen. However, when fibrinogen is converted into fibrin it becomes insoluble and visible and can be seen through a high-powered electron microscope as tiny, cotton-like threads. In this form, the platelet GPIIb/IIIa receptors bind eagerly to fibrin and form the web-like structure that traps the red blood cells and forms the blood clot.

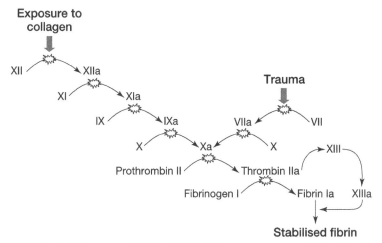

**Figure 4.14** The clotting cascade (simplified). Injury or exposure of the blood to the connective tissue collagen causes a series of reactions in the blood that result in the formation of stabilised fibrin, a key component of blood clots.

The clotting process looks pretty complex

Yes, it is quite complex but you really need to know how the clotting process works in order to understand the action of common anti-clotting drugs such as **aspirin**, **clopidogrel**, **heparin** and **warfarin**.

Circulating in the blood are a family of clotting proteins (also known as clotting factors), most of which are identified simply by Roman numerals. Fibrinogen itself is one of these proteins and is designated Factor I. Fibrinogen is converted into fibrin (Factor Ia) as the result of a cascade of enzymic reactions involving these clotting factors.

The clotting cascade is triggered by either blood coming into contact with damaged tissue or exposed collagen. This causes the activation of clotting factors VIII or XII, each of which activates another clotting factor in the cascade and this activates the next factor and so on. In Figure 4.14 you will note that the factors when activated take the suffix 'a' ('a' stands for activated). Eventually an enzyme called prothrombin (Factor II) is converted to its active form of thrombin (Factor IIa). Thrombin is of key importance because it converts soluble fibrinogen into stabilised insoluble fibrin with the help of Factor VIIIa. In its stable, insoluble form, fibrin and platelets together form the web-like structure that traps blood cells and makes the blood clot.

## Drugs used to prevent clotting

Individuals who have coronary artery disease are at greater risk of clots forming and blocking their coronary arteries, resulting in ischaemia and infarction. The aim of anticoagulant therapy therefore is to interfere with the clotting process and so reduce the chances of clots forming, especially in the coronary arteries. As we have seen, there are two key processes involved in the clotting process –

the activation of platelets and the conversion of fibrinogen into fibrin. Drugs used to inhibit clotting can also be broadly divided into two groups: antiplatelet drugs and drugs targeting the clotting cascade.

> **KEY FACT**
> Anticlotting drugs work either by inhibiting the activity of platelets or by inhibiting the clotting cascade that converts fibrinogen into fibrin.

### Anticoagulant drugs group 1: antiplatelet drugs

There are many drugs used to inhibit the activation of platelets but those that you are most likely to encounter are **aspirin** and **clopidogrel** plus the more recently introduced **ticagrelor** and **prasugrel**, prescribed either singly or together after a heart attack or a surgical revascularisation procedure. All of these drugs act on platelets and prevent them from expressing the GPIIb/IIIa receptors that bind to fibrin, producing the web-like structure that traps red blood cells and forms a blood clot. Other antiplatelet drugs such as **dipyridamole**, **tirofiban**, **eptifibatide** and **abciximab** tend to be used more in specialist cardiology units for patients at high risk of myocardial infarction or undergoing surgical procedures such as percutaneous coronary intervention (see Section 4.2 towards the beginning of this chapter).

   **Aspirin** is one of our oldest non-steroidal anti-inflammatory drugs (NSAIDs) and, although used less often these days as an analgesic for pain relief, it has found a new role as an antiplatelet drug for the prevention of myocardial infarction. It is also used to prevent a *stroke*, which involves a similar pathology to coronary artery disease but in this case the atherosclerotic plaques form in the carotid arteries that supply the brain with oxygen. Rupture of a plaque in these arteries can cause a clot to develop that cuts off blood to the brain, sometimes causing permanent damage.

> *Stroke* is a serious disturbance in the blood supply to the brain caused by the formation of a blood clot or haemorrhage in the arteries that supply the brain.

**Figure 4.15** Aspirin blocks the action of cyclo-oxygenase 1 (COX-1), reducing the production of thromboxane A2, a mediator in platelet activation.

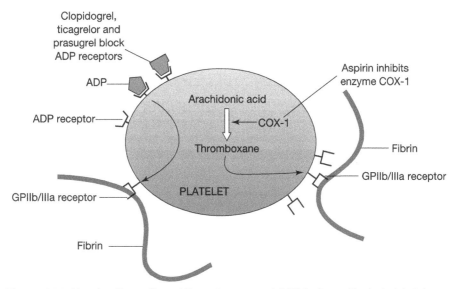

**Figure 4.16** Showing the action of thromboxane and ADP in the activated platelet. Both mediators increase the expression of GPIIb/IIIa receptors and so promote the clotting process. **Aspirin** inhibits thromboxane production. **Clopidogrel, ticagrelor** and **prasugrel** block ADP receptors.

**Aspirin** or acetylsalicylic acid works by inhibiting the production of a chemical called thromboxane A2 ($TXA_2$), a member of the prostaglandin family. Some of the prostaglandins are associated with inflammation and we will meet them again in Chapter 7. Activated platelets produce thromboxane, which increases the production of GPIIb/IIIa receptors that bind to fibrin and form the blood clot as described earlier. $TXA_2$ is produced from *arachidonic acid* by an enzyme called *cyclo-oxygenase-1* (COX-1). **Aspirin** irreversibly binds to COX-1, inhibiting its action and so preventing platelets from making thromboxane (Figure 4.15). As thromboxane levels fall, platelets are less able to express their receptors and without receptors, platelets cannot bind to fibrin and so clotting is inhibited (Figure 4.16).

As the inhibition of COX-1 is irreversible it means that the platelet cannot produce any more GPIIb/IIIa receptors. However, platelets only have a life of around ten days so the clotting function is restored as new platelets are produced.

> **DID YOU KNOW ...** that **aspirin** was originally obtained from willow bark? Willow is *Salix* in Latin and its name can still be traced in the chemical name of **aspirin** – acetylsalicylic acid.

**Clopidogrel, ticagrelor** and **prasugrel** also work by inhibiting the production of GPIIb/IIIa receptors on platelets, but by a different mechanism to **aspirin**. Adenosine diphosphate (ADP) is a mediator released by platelets during activation that stimulates the production of GPIIb/IIIa receptors by binding to ADP receptors on the surface of adjacent platelets. **Clopidogrel**, **ticagrelor** and **prasugrel** are all ADP antagonists that block ADP receptors, preventing ADP binding and so inhibiting the expression of GPIIb/IIIa receptors (Figure 4.16).

### ANOTHER WAY TO PICTURE THIS

Remember that we compared platelets to children in a playground? As it's cold, they have their hands (GPIIb/IIIa receptors) in their pockets. Antiplatelet drugs induce the children to keep their hands firmly in their pockets to prevent them grasping the skipping ropes (fibrin) that forms the web-like net (clot).

*Side-effects* **Aspirin** can cause gastro-intestinal haemorrhage. Prostaglandins have a protective effect on the gastric mucosa and their production is inhibited by **aspirin**. **Aspirin** (and other NSAIDs) can also induce asthma (see 'In practice' below). **Clopidogrel**, **ticagrelor** and **prasugrel** can cause the usual gastric upsets and may also cause haemorrhage.

### IN PRACTICE

It is estimated that around 10 per cent of asthma sufferers are sensitive to **aspirin** and other non-steroidal anti-inflammatory drugs (NSAIDs). They can induce an asthma attack, often accompanied by symptoms of runny nose, sneezing and facial flushing. The mechanism is uncertain but NSAIDs may increase the production of *leukotrienes*, mediators implicated in asthma.

### Anticoagulant drugs group 2: drugs acting on the clotting cascade

*Parenteral anticoagulants* This group of drugs includes **heparins** and **warfarin** as well as some of the less well-known anticoagulants such as **bivalirudin**, **lepirudin** and **fondaparinux**. As these last three are unlikely to be encountered outside of specialist surgical settings, we will only note them in passing.

**Heparins** are mainly used in hospitals and are prescribed primarily to prevent venous thromboembolism and pulmonary embolism in patients undergoing surgery. They are also used extensively in coronary care for patients with unstable angina and to prevent clots forming after cardiac interventions. There are two forms of **heparin** in current use, **unfractionated heparin** and **low molecular weight heparin** (LMW heparin), the latter often being preferred these days as it has a longer duration of action so needs less frequent administration. Examples of LMW heparins include **bemiparin**, **dalteparin**, **enoxaparin** and **tinzaparin**. Heparins inhibit clotting by activating a protein called *antithrombin*, part of the body's own anticlotting mechanism. Antithrombin, as the name implies, inactivates thrombin but also inhibits various other clotting factors (Figure 4.17). Unfractionated **heparin** and **LMW heparin** effectively do the same task in activating antithrombin, but there are small differences in which of the other clotting factors they inhibit.

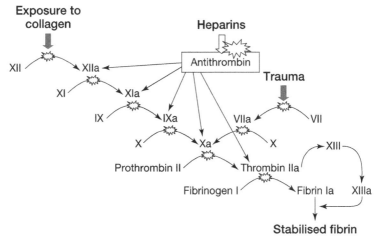

**Figure 4.17** Heparins activate the natural anticlotting protein antithrombin that in turn deactivates various clotting factors as shown in the diagram. The clotting cascade is halted, preventing the formation of stabilised fibrin, a key component of blood clots.

**IN PRACTICE**

The clots that form in the veins are subtly different from those that form in the arteries. Arterial clots generally form in response to vascular injury and this activates platelets so these clots are said to be platelet rich. Venous thrombi, on the other hand, more often form due to inadequate blood flow and so are fibrin rich and platelet poor. This is why drugs such as **heparin** and **warfarin** rather than antiplatelet drugs are used to prevent deep vein thrombosis.

*Side-effects* As with all anticoagulants, **heparin** and **LMW heparin** can both cause unwanted bleeding but there is a lower risk of heparin-induced *thrombocytopenia* (low platelet levels) with **LMW heparin**.

**CASE STUDY**

Betty has been admitted for a hip replacement and with the prospect of her remaining immobile for several weeks there is the risk of DVT developing. Apart from a suspected peptic ulcer, Betty is otherwise in reasonable health. Would you advise **aspirin** to prevent DVT – or perhaps some other anticlotting drug?

*Comment on case study* **Aspirin** should not be given to anyone with a peptic ulcer, as there is a strong risk of causing a gastro-intestinal (GI) bleed. All anticoagulant drugs have the potential to cause problems in patients at risk from bleeding. Non-pharmacological solutions such as thromboembolism deterrent (TED) stockings may be a better option.

**Figure 4.18** Being similar in structure, **warfarin** competes with vitamin K for the active site on vitamin K reductase, a key enzyme in the production of clotting factors II, VII, IX and X. Note that the structures of **warfarin**, vitamin K and the pathway are simplified for clarity.

*Oral anticoagulants* **Warfarin** is an oral anticoagulant used for prevention of deep vein thrombosis (DVT), pulmonary embolism, atrial fibrillation and after the surgical insertion of prosthetic heart valves. **Acenocoumarol** and **phenindione** are anticoagulants with similar properties to **warfarin**.

**Dabigatran etexilate**, **apixaban** and **rivaroxaban** are three recently introduced drugs that have somewhat confused the previously neat categories of oral and parenteral anticoagulants. These three are all administered orally (like **warfarin**) but act directly on the clotting cascade (like **heparin**).

**Warfarin** acts in the liver to prevent the production of clotting factors II, VII, IX and X. Being similar in structure to vitamin K, it competes for the active site on vitamin K reductase, a key enzyme in the production of clotting factors (Figure 4.18). Inhibition of the enzyme by **warfarin** reduces circulating clotting factors and compromises the body's ability to form sufficient fibrin to make structurally stable clots.

*Side-effects* The most common side-effect with **warfarin** is unwanted bleeding. This may be countered by the administration of **phytomenadione** (vitamin $K_1$). This tips the balance of competition for the active site of vitamin K reductase towards vitamin K and promotes the production of clotting factors.

*Interactions* **Warfarin** is matched only by **carbamazepine** for its number of interactions. Many of these interactions involve the induction or inhibition of hepatic P450 enzymes. The anticoagulant effect of **warfarin** is enhanced by **amiodarone**, **trimethoprim** and cranberry juice and reduced by (no surprise) **carbamazepine** and the herbal remedy, St John's Wort. Plus many, many more interactions . . .

**IN PRACTICE**

The anticoagulant effects of **warfarin** take 48–72 hours to develop fully. This is because **warfarin** inhibits the synthesis of new clotting factors but does not affect those already in circulation.

Dabigatran etexilate, apixaban and rivaroxaban are all licensed for the prevention of thromboembolism after hip or knee replacement. Recently introduced (2012) guidelines from the National Institute of Health and Clinical Excellence (NICE) have also recommended **dabigatran** and **rivaroxaban** for use in the prevention of thromboembolism in atrial fibrillation (AF) in high risk groups.

**Dabigatran** directly inhibits the enzyme thrombin and has a rapid onset of action. **Apixaban** and **rivaroxaban** inhibit activated factor X. All of these drugs can cause haemorrhage and patients need to be monitored for bleeding.

> **DID YOU KNOW . . .** that the evocative smell of newly-mown hay is the same aromatic compound that produces **warfarin**? These chemicals, known as coumarins, sometimes undergo fermentation in silage and can cause a disease responsible for haemorrhage in cattle.

## Anticoagulant drugs group 3: fibrinolytic drugs

So far we have seen how both groups of anticlotting drugs, antiplatelet and coagulation cascade inhibitors can prevent clots from forming in the arteries and veins. We will now examine drugs that can be used in emergency situations where a patient is experiencing a myocardial infarction caused by a blood clot that has formed in the coronary arteries. We now need powerful drugs that will break down and disperse a blood clot, thus restoring blood and life-giving oxygen to heart tissue. These drugs are called fibrinolytic or thrombolytic drugs because they lyse (break down) fibrin and consequently the structural integrity of the thrombus collapses. These drugs include **alteplase**, **reteplase**, **streptokinase** and **tenecteplase**.

All of these drugs act by stimulating **plasmin**, the body's own clot-busting enzyme that breaks down fibrin. Plasmin is formed from its inactive form **plasminogen**, which becomes incorporated into the clot as it forms. The body needs to ensure that when a wound has healed the clot will dissolve as part of the repair process. Plasminogen is eventually converted into plasmin by a protein called *tissue plasminogen activator* (t-PA) (Figure 4.19). Fibrinolytic drugs are similar in structure to t-PA and so produce activated plasmin that breaks down fibrin and dissolves the clot.

**Streptokinase** is a bacterial enzyme derived from *β-haemolytic streptococci*. As a foreign, bacterial protein it can trigger an immunological reaction and is therefore not used beyond four days after its first use. After that period, *antibodies* produced in response to the initial administration will attack and neutralise the drug.

**Figure 4.19** Showing how plasminogen is converted into its clot-destroying form of plasmin by tissue plasmin activator (t-PA).

Alteplase, tenecteplase and reteplase are recombinant tissue plasminogen activators (rt-PA) that act by the same mechanism as streptokinase but are more specific for clot-bound plasminogen and also, being non-bacterial in origin, do not elicit the same immune response as streptokinase. Recombinant technology involves genetic manipulation, removing a gene from one organism and splicing it into another, generally a bacterium or yeast, in order to produce significant quantities of a protein – in this case, tissue plasminogen activator.

> *Antibodies*, or immunoglobulins, are potent immune proteins produced by B-lymphocytes in the lymph nodes. Released into the bloodstream, they attach themselves to invading *pathogens* and mark them for destruction by white blood cells.

Tranexamic acid is a drug that has the opposite effect of the fibrinolytic drugs in that it promotes clotting in emergency situations involving severe haemorrhage. The drug inhibits the conversion of plasminogen into plasmin, which helps prevent fibrin dissolution.

### CASE STUDY

Sam, an agricultural worker, collapses at work, complaining of shortness of breath and severe 'indigestion' like pain that is spreading up his left side. An ambulance arrives within 20 minutes and the paramedics perform an electrocardiogram (ECG) on Sam. After consulting with the hospital they decide to administer 10000 units of tenecteplase by intravenous (IV) injection. What is happening to Sam?

*Comment on case study* Sam has the classic symptoms of a myocardial infarction or heart attack. The ECG would show subtle changes in the heart's electrical activity that are signs of a MI. Because Sam works in the countryside he may be some distance from a hospital, therefore to restore the blood supply to his heart muscle, thrombolysis will be performed by the paramedics. Sam's prospects for survival and recovery are better with early treatment.

### A QUICK RECAP on drugs used to prevent clotting

- Clotting is the body's emergency repair system which prevents excessive blood loss after injury.
- Clots consist of fibrin strands cross-linked by platelets. This forms a mesh-like structure that traps red blood cells.
- Anticlotting drugs can be divided into two types – drugs that prevent the activation of platelets and drugs that inhibit the coagulation cascade and the formation of fibrin.
- Antiplatelet drugs such as aspirin and clopidogrel inhibit platelets from expressing GPIIb/IIIa receptors so they cannot bind to fibrin.

- Parenteral anticoagulants such as **heparin** interfere with the clotting cascade and so prevent fibrinogen being converted into fibrin.

- Oral anticoagulants such as **warfarin** that act on the coagulation cascade inhibit an enzyme in the liver responsible for producing circulating clotting factors. As circulating levels of these factors diminish, so does the blood's ability to form clots.

- **Dabigatran etexilate** and **rivaroxaban** are oral anticoagulants that interfere with the clotting cascade.

- In emergencies, such as a heart attack, thrombolytic drugs such as **streptokinase** convert plasminogen into plasmin – an enzyme that breaks down blood clots.

- In emergencies involving excess bleeding, **tranexamic acid** promotes clotting.

## Arrhythmias and anti-arrhythmic drugs

The use of drugs to control arrhythmias (abnormal heart rhythms) is a very specialised area and it is beyond the scope of this introductory book to explain the action of these drugs in any great detail. However, some anti-arrhythmic drugs such as **amiodarone**, **verapamil**, **digoxin** and beta-blockers are regularly prescribed to people with heart problems, so it is worth discussing them briefly to ensure that you are at least familiar with their names.

If you place your fingers half way down your rib cage, just to the left of your sternum (breast bone), you should feel the steady, rhythmic beating of your heart. This is called *sinus rhythm* and is set by the heart's main pacemaker, the *sino-atrial (SA) node*, located in the front wall of the right atrium. The SA node generates a regular impulse that spreads across the heart muscle causing it to contract and force blood out of the atria and ventricles respectively. The SA node rate is governed by nerves from the parasympathetic and sympathetic divisions of the autonomic system. Normally the parasympathetic division dominates at rest, keeping the heart rate at its resting level, typically between 65 and 75 beats per minute. During exercise or stress, the sympathetic division becomes dominant and the rate increases, causing the heart to pump more oxygenated blood around the body.

There are many types and many causes of cardiac arrhythmias that require specialist diagnosis, usually with the aid of an electrocardiogram (ECG), a device that measures electrical activity in the heart and displays that activity as a series of traces on a graph. This enables clinicians to determine the location and nature of any abnormalities in heart function.

Some arrhythmias are defined by an abnormal heart rate – either tachycardia (excessively fast rate) or bradycardia (excessively slow rate). Tachycardia may be caused by pain, stress, fever, shock or by drugs such as **salbutamol**. Hypothermia can cause bradycardia, as can drugs such as **digoxin** and beta-blockers. Some arrhythmias are the result of damage to the heart's internal conduction system, often caused by heart attacks that can result in cells outside the SA node starting to act as pacemakers and sending abnormal signals across the myocardium. Sometimes, the impulse that spreads across the heart muscle in one direction then turns back on itself and becomes a circular *re-entrant rhythm*. Whatever the cause of the arrhythmia, it will affect the normal pumping of the heart and clinical intervention is often needed to restore a normal rhythm.

## Anti-arrhythmic drugs

**Amiodarone** is a drug commonly used to prevent arrhythmias, although its mechanism of action is not fully understood. It is believed to block some of the $K^+$ and $Na^+$ (and possibly $Ca^{2+}$ channels) on the heart's conduction tissue and muscle cells. This slows the wave of contraction with each heart beat, helping to produce a more stable rhythm. This drug has a propensity to cause many side-effects and with an average half-life of over 30 days, these side-effects are not always easily reversible.

*Side-effects* Unusually, **amiodarone** contains iodine and, having structural similarities to the thyroid hormone thyroxine, this can affect iodine metabolism, sometimes resulting in hypothyroidism (low levels of thyroxine) and, less frequently, in hyperthyroidism (high levels of thyroxine). Deposits in the cornea of the eye are common with long-term use, as is the tendency for **amiodarone** to cause the skin to turn blue-grey when exposed to sunlight.

 **Verapamil**, discussed earlier in this chapter in its role as an anti-anginal drug, helps to prevent arrhythmias by blocking $Ca^{2+}$ channels especially in the heart's conduction tissue, thus slowing the heart and helping in the treatment of tachycardias.

 **Digoxin** is a cardiac glycoside, originally extracted from the purple foxglove *Digitalis purpurea* (now mostly from *Digitalis lanata*). It has a complex action that increases $Ca^{2+}$ concentration in the myocytes which, in turn, increases the force of contraction of the myocardium. It also acts on the central nervous system, reinforcing parasympathetic activity and reducing heart rate.

 **Beta-blockers** are used for several cardiovascular problems including angina, hypertension and heart failure. Those used as anti-arrhythmics include **propranolol**, **atenolol**, **esmolol**, **metoprolol** and **sotalol**. The action of these drugs was discussed earlier in this chapter in the section on anti-anginal drugs, but essentially they block $\beta_1$ receptors on the heart from the effects of adrenaline and noradrenaline and this reduces heart rate and contractility. **Sotalol** appears also to have a broad spectrum of anti-arrhythmic activity similar to that of **amiodarone**.

**A QUICK RECAP on arrhythmias and anti-arrhythmic drugs**

- Arrhythmias (abnormal heart rhythms) can be caused by heart disease or as a side-effect of some drugs.

- The diagnosis and treatment of arrhythmias is complex and requires specialist clinical knowledge.
- Anti-arrhythmic drugs such as **amiodarone**, **verapamil** and beta-blockers work by a variety of mechanisms but they all have an inhibitory action on the heart rate and slow the speed of contraction of the myocardium.
- **Digoxin** slows the heart rate and increases the force of contraction of the myocardium.

## REFERENCES AND FURTHER RECOMMENDED READING

Books

Opie, L. and Gersh, B.J. (2008) *Drugs for the Heart* (7th edn). Saunders.

Websites

All recommended websites are open access (but free registration is sometimes required).

Bandolier: cardiology – http://www.medicine.ox.ac.uk/bandolier/

British Heart Foundation – http://www.bhf.org.uk/

European Medicines agency – http://www.ema.europa.eu/

Medscape: cardiology – http://emedicine.medscape.com/cardiology

NICE Guidelines (2012) – TA249 (dabigatran), TA256 (rivaroxaban) – http://publications.nice.org.uk/

Office for National Statistics – http://www.ons.gov.uk

Student, BMJ cardiology – http://student.bmj.com/student/student-bmj.html

## Test yourself

Now you have finished reading this chapter it is worthwhile finding out how much you have learned and remembered. Cardiovascular disease is extremely common and can be found in most patient groups so it is important that you understand the action of the various associated drugs.

*The answers to these questions are at the end of the book (see p. 314).*

1 List at least six functions of the circulatory system.

2 In which of the blood vessels does exchange between the blood and the cells takes place?

3 What is the name of the blood vessels that supply blood to the myocardium?

4 What is the main lipid found in atherosclerotic plaques?

5 Why may an artery that is partially blocked by a plaque result in angina pain?

6 GTN dilates the coronary arteries – why may this reduce angina pain?

7 What might be the consequence of a plaque rupturing in the coronary arteries?

8 Why would slowing the heart rate with a beta-blocker reduce angina pain?

9 What type of circulating lipoprotein is implicated in the formation of plaques?

10 Why may reducing dietary cholesterol not always result in a fall in blood cholesterol?

11 How does inhibiting HMG CoA reductase with a statin reduce blood cholesterol?

12 What are the three main components of a blood clot?

13 How does aspirin prevent clotting?

14 What is the key difference between the action of **warfarin** and **heparins**?

15 Under what circumstances might a thrombolytic drug be used?

Answers to the questions on p. 75.

1 Neither, it is in the middle of the chest.
2 From the heart.
3 Four chambers – two atria and two ventricles.
4 Arteries, capillaries and veins.
5 The coronary arteries.

# Chapter 5

# The cardiovascular system (2): hypertension and antihypertensive drugs

This chapter explains the anatomy and physiology underpinning the regulation of blood pressure, the pathology of hypertension and its consequences. We then explore the pharmacological action of the antihypertensive drug groups and finally take a quick look at the pharmacological response to hypotension.

## CONTENTS

The chapter contains some brief case studies and finishes off with some self-test questions to enable you to be certain that you have understood the physiology, pathology and pharmacology of this important area.

**IN PRACTICE**

Blood pressure is something that everyone in clinical practice needs to understand because almost everyone in clinical practice will need to measure blood pressure, perhaps the most common of clinical procedures, at some time in their professional career. The maintenance of a healthy blood pressure is essential for the efficient functioning of the body and problems occur if blood pressure deviates significantly from its healthy norm. If blood pressure falls then the patient can go into shock and this is a medical emergency that requires emergency action. A rise in blood pressure tends to be a long-term problem rather than an emergency but the consequences can be quite serious. Regardless of their pathology, it is likely that many of your adult patients will have high blood pressure and will be taking medication to reduce their blood pressure, so it is essential that you understand how both antihypertensive drugs and the body itself work to regulate blood pressure.

## Introduction

Hypertension (high blood pressure) is a very common problem, especially in developed countries such as the UK where, by the age of 50, almost 25 per cent of the population are hypertensive. People with sustained high blood pressure are at greater risk of developing diseases such as diabetes and heart problems so it makes sense for them to take steps to reduce it. Ideally, a reduction in blood pressure should be achieved with changes in diet and exercise, but antihypertensive drugs are an alternative for the many people who find it difficult to change their lifestyle. There are many different drugs with a wide variety of actions and this chapter examines them in detail.

It is only in the last 50 years that high blood pressure has been classified as a serious disease. This is evident from the term 'benign hypertension' which was originally ascribed to high blood pressure that did not appear to be adversely affecting the patient. In a 1931 lecture to the British Medical Association Dr John Hay stated that . . .

> *'There is some truth in the saying that the greatest danger*
> *to a man with high blood pressure lies in its discovery,*
> *because then some fool is likely to try and reduce it.'*

Looking at the antihypertensive drugs available in those days, Dr Hay may have been correct. Later in the lecture he recommended bed rest and doses of calomel, which sounds pleasant enough until you realise the formula for calomel is $Hg_2Cl_2$, i.e. mercurous chloride! In the second half of the twentieth century it was becoming obvious to medical researchers that high blood pressure, while initially without symptoms, could if not treated eventually cause serious cardio-vascular problems. Modern drugs are not without their side-effects but at least do not have the toxicity of earlier mercurial compounds.

This chapter follows a format that will be becoming familiar to you. Firstly, we make sure that we understand the physiology – the nature of blood pressure and how the body maintains that blood pressure. Secondly, we need to understand the pathology of hypertension, what causes it and its consequences. Finally we put this knowledge to good use when we explore the pharmacology, how the main groups of antihypertensive drugs work to lower blood pressure. Case studies and clinical scenarios will help to reinforce your understanding of this subject.

## WHERE ARE WE STARTING FROM?

Before you start this chapter you need to have read through the basics of circula-tory physiology in Chapter 4. Let's see how much you have remembered . . .

1 Which blood vessel carries blood from the heart to major organs such as the kidneys and liver?

 

2 Which side of the heart (left or right) pumps blood to the lungs?

 

3 When blood returns to the heart from the veins, does it first enter the atria or the ventricles?

 

4 Which is the highest pressure in the blood vessels – systole or diastole?

 

5 Do the pulmonary veins carry oxygenated or deoxygenated blood?

 

6 Is the vena cava a vein or an artery?

 

*Answers are at the end of the chapter on p. 137.*

Good, we will assume that you answered all or most of the answers correctly and that you know the basic structures and functions of the circulatory system.

We can now get down to learning about blood pressure, hypertension and the antihypertensive drugs.

## 5.1 The physiology of blood pressure

### Let's start with the basics: what is blood pressure?

When we talk about blood pressure, we are generally referring to the pressure of blood in systemic arteries such as the aorta. As we saw in Chapter 4, the systemic arteries are those that carry blood from the left side of the heart, via the aorta, to the organs and tissues of the body. These organs include the brain, liver, kidneys and digestive system and tissues such as the muscles and skin. Naturally, the blood is also under pressure in the pulmonary arteries carrying blood from the right side of the heart to the lungs, but this pressure is much lower and not as easy to measure because the pulmonary arteries lie deep within the thoracic cavity.

Arterial pressure is important to the well-being of the body because it is this pressure that causes oxygenated blood from the lungs to flow to the cells of the organs and tissues. This pressure pushes the blood through the arteries and into the tiny capillaries of the body where gas exchange takes place between the blood and the cells. These capillaries permeate every cubic millimetre of the body and are essential for the health of our cells. A constant supply of fresh blood is required to supply cells with their oxygen and nutrients and take away waste such as the gas carbon dioxide (Figure 5.1). If pressure falls and the blood moves more slowly through the capillaries, then cells do not get enough oxygen and cannot get rid of their carbon dioxide.

### Understanding arterial blood pressure

Arterial pressure is pulsatile in nature in that it fluctuates between a high pressure and a low pressure. The maximum pressure of blood on the arterial walls is the systolic pressure and the lowest pressure is the diastolic. Some systemic arteries

**Figure 5.1** Capillaries, the smallest of our blood vessels, supply cells with oxygen and remove carbon dioxide.

You will find
your radial
pulse here

Figure 5.2 How to find your radial pulse.

appear near the surface of the body and pressure changes in these arteries can be measured relatively easily with the familiar *sphygmomanometer*, often just called a 'sphyg'. Place the tips of your first and second finger in the groove just below the end of your radius bone and you will experience the systolic expansion of the arteries as a pulse in the radial artery just under the skin (Figure 5.2).

> A *sphygmomanometer* is a device for measuring systemic arterial blood pressure. An inflatable fabric cuff wrapped round the upper arm detects systolic and diastolic pressures. Results are displayed either manually on a dial or digitally in units of millimetres of mercury (mmHg). Mercury-column sphygmomanometers have their adherents and are still in occasional use today.

The heart beats around 70 times each minute and with each beat the ventricles contract and force blood into the arteries. The elastic walls of the arteries stretch as the pressure increases to maximum systolic pressure. Then, when the heart goes into its diastolic phase and relaxes, their elastic walls steadily recoil, continuing to push the blood through the millions of tiny arterioles and capillaries.

Figure 5.3 is a simplified graph of fluctuations in blood pressure in a systemic artery such as the aorta. Note that there is always a minimum pressure in the arteries of (typically) 70–80 mmHg. Because there is always this pressure in the arteries, there is always a constant flow, pushing blood through the arterioles and capillaries.

The rapid rise in pressure seen in Figure 5.3 is caused by the ventricles contracting, forcing blood into the arteries – this is systole. As the heart relaxes to fill with blood again, the pressure in the arteries falls as the blood is pushed through the arterioles and capillaries – this is diastole.

KEY FACT

The blood pressure in the arteries fluctuates with each heart beat between systole (maximum pressure) and diastole (minimum pressure).

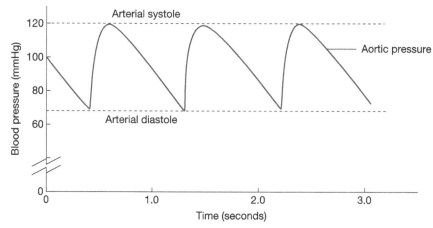

**Figure 5.3** Typical blood pressures in a systemic artery such as the aorta.

## The control of arterial blood pressure

It is very important that systemic arterial blood pressure is maintained sufficiently high to drive the blood through the millions of capillaries to provide nutrient supply, gas exchange and waste removal from the cells of the body's tissues, but not so high that it ruptures the small blood vessels or places undue strain on the heart.

Maintaining blood pressure is very important and is subject to constant monitoring and adjustment by the body to make sure that it never falls so low as to compromise the blood supply to essential organs such as the brain.

Blood pressure is maintained in the short term by the complex interaction of systemic vascular resistance (SVR) and cardiac output (CO). Longer-term regulation also calls for adjustment to blood volume. We are going to look at the long-term and short-term control of blood pressure because we will need to understand them when we later examine the action of antihypertensive drugs.

## The short-term regulation of blood pressure

> **KEY FACT**
>
> The short-term regulation of blood pressure is largely determined by two factors – cardiac output and systemic vascular resistance.

The following facts are very important so we will list them separately:

1  **Cardiac output** (CO) is the amount of blood pumped by the heart each minute.
2  Cardiac output is determined by two factors:
   (a) **Heart rate** (HR) – the rate at which the heart beats
   (b) **Stroke volume** (SV) – the amount of blood pumped by the ventricle in each beat.

3 **Systemic vascular resistance** (SVR) is the resistance to blood flow as determined by peripheral blood vessel diameter in the systemic circulation.

### ANOTHER WAY TO PICTURE THIS

Imagine the arterial system like a long, thin balloon with a small hole in the far end. To maintain pressure in the balloon you have to blow regularly into one end (cardiac output) and restrict the amount of air coming out of the hole at the other end (systemic vascular resistance).

Blood viscosity and the total length of blood vessels also contribute to systemic vascular resistance, but they remain relatively static in the short term so SVR is largely determined by the diameter of the arterioles.

We can best express the relationship of the factors that determine blood pressure by a simple formula:

$$BP = CO \times SVR$$
(Blood pressure = Cardiac output × Systemic vascular resistance)

Cardiac output is expressed by another simple formula:

$$CO = HR \times SV$$
(Cardiac output = Heart rate × Stroke volume)

Do I really need to learn this formula?

**YES** (sorry to shout) – you most certainly do! You don't need to learn many formulae to study basic physiology but this one is very important – if not *the* most important. So it is worth spending a few minutes working through this section to make sure you understand it.

If formulae are a bit of a mystery to you then just substitute some values instead of the words. For example, a typical heart rate might be 70 beats per minute (bpm) and typical stroke volume 70 millilitres (ml) of blood.

Cardiac output = 70 bpm × 70 ml

This gives us a typical cardiac output of 4900 millilitres, nearly 5 litres of blood pumped each minute. Because the formula indicates that the figure on the left side of the equals sign is determined by the product of both figures on the right of the equals sign, this means if you change either of the two figures on the right side then the figure on the left side changes. For example, if the individual started to exercise, then heart rate and stroke volume might both increase as follows:

Cardiac output = 100 bpm × 85 ml

This means that cardiac output increases to 8500 millilitres of blood pumped each minute. Similarly, if either of the two figures on the right side of the formula decrease then the figure on the left side decreases. Perhaps the individual has an accident causing loss of blood which causes a reduction in stroke volume as follows:

$$\text{Cardiac output} = 70 \text{ bpm} \times 50 \text{ ml}$$

In this case, cardiac output falls to 3500 millilitres of blood pumped each minute. Going back to our blood pressure formula . . .

$$BP = CO \times SVR$$

This just indicates that blood pressure (BP) is equal to the product of cardiac output (CO) and systemic vascular resistance (SVR). It also indicates that if either CO or SVR increases, then BP will increase. On the other hand, if either CO or SVR decreases, then BP will decrease. This gives us a clue as to how the body will respond to changes in blood pressure.

**KEY FACT**

If either CO or SVR increases then BP will increase. If either CO or SVR decreases then BP will decrease.

First we need to understand the mechanisms that the body has at its disposal to regulate blood pressure.

### Systemic vascular resistance

Systemic vascular resistance (SVR) is defined as the combined resistance of the peripheral arterioles of the systemic circulation. Arterioles are surrounded by bands of smooth muscle and in vasoconstriction when these collectively contract, the internal diameter of the blood vessel decreases and so resistance increases. In vasodilation the bands of smooth muscle collectively relax, the internal diameter of the blood vessel increases and so resistance decreases.

**ANOTHER WAY TO PICTURE THIS**

Imagine a crowd of football fans leaving through the stadium gates at the end of the game. If the ground staff had left some of the gates partially closed, pressure in the jostling crowd would increase. Vasoconstriction has the same effect, making it harder for the blood to flow through the arterioles and so increasing the pressure in the arteries.

Arterioles are controlled by both the nervous system and chemical messengers released into the blood as a response to changes in blood pressure. Each arteriole is connected to the central nervous system by nerves from the sympathetic division of the autonomic nervous system. The autonomic nervous system is formed from groups of nerves originating in the central nervous system that maintain homeostasis – the steady state of the internal environment. When blood pressure drops, the sympathetic division is activated to restore pressure to within normal values. Sympathetic nerves connected to arterioles cause each arteriole to contract, resulting in an increase in systemic vascular resistance (Figure 5.4).

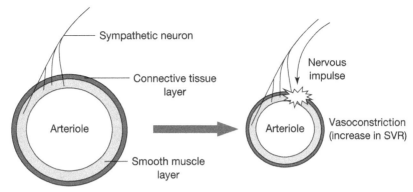

**Figure 5.4** Sympathetic nerves cause vasoconstriction that increases systemic vascular resistance (SVR).

The maintenance of blood pressure is critical to organs such as the brain while tissues such as the skin are less susceptible to fluctuations in pressure. This is why, when blood pressure falls, it is primarily the arterioles of the skin that vasoconstrict, increasing SVR and shunting blood away from the periphery to core organs.

To understand how sympathetic stimulation results in vasoconstriction of the arterioles, we need to examine their structure, in particular the bands of tiny smooth muscle cells that lie in layers around the arterioles. Sympathetic stimulation causes these cells to contract in unison which, in turn, causes the arteriole to contract, reducing its diameter and increasing systemic vascular resistance. These muscle cells respond to the sympathetic neurotransmitter noradrenaline plus a variety of chemical messengers that circulate in the blood. Each of these chemical messengers has its own receptor on the smooth muscle cells that initiates contraction (Table 5.1 and Figure 5.5). We will meet some of these receptors again later in the chapter as they are the target for antihypertensive drugs.

## Cardiac output (heart rate × stroke volume)

Cardiac output, the amount of blood ejected from the left ventricle in one minute, is determined by two factors – heart rate and stroke volume. If either heart rate

**Table 5.1** The chemical messengers that cause contraction of smooth muscle cells on the peripheral arterioles

| Chemical messenger | Source of messenger | Target receptor on smooth muscle cell | Action on smooth muscle cell |
|---|---|---|---|
| Noradrenaline | Sympathetic neurons | $\alpha_1$ adrenergic receptor | Contraction |
| Adrenaline | Adrenal gland | $\alpha_1$ adrenergic receptor | Contraction |
| Angiotensin II | Circulating | Angiotensin-II receptor | Contraction |
| ADH-vasopressin | Posterior pituitary | ADH-vasopressin receptor | Contraction |

Figure 5.5 Control of arterioles by neurotransmitters and messengers such as noradrenaline, adrenaline, angiotensin-II and ADH-vasopressin, each binding to its own specific receptors resulting in vasoconstriction.

or stroke volume increase, then cardiac output will increase (and so BP increases). If either heart rate or stroke volume decrease, then cardiac output will decrease (and so BP decreases). Heart rate is the rate that the heart beats each minute, so the faster the heart beats, the more blood it will pump. Stroke volume is the amount of blood ejected from the left ventricle with each beat (around 70 ml at rest). A more forceful contraction, such as occurs during exercise, will eject even more blood − up to 100 ml or so in a normal individual. Sympathetic stimulation increases both heart rate and stroke volume − as does an increase in circulating adrenaline from the adrenal gland.

DID YOU KNOW ... that during a 26 mile marathon race, the average runner's heart will have beaten over 35 000 times? Typical heart rate will be around 150 beats per minute and the heart will pump 100 ml of blood with each beat. This means that if a runner takes four hours to finish, their heart will have pumped over 3600 litres of blood! At rest, 1200 litres of blood would be typical in four hours.

Another factor in the control of stroke volume is the amount of blood that is returning to the heart. This is known as the *preload*. For example, during exercise when the heart is working harder, more blood returns to the heart. This increase

THE PHYSIOLOGY OF BLOOD PRESSURE

in end-diastolic volume or preload causes the heart muscle to stretch more, resulting in a more forceful contraction and a larger stroke volume. This effect is called *Starling's law* after Ernest Starling, an English physiologist who worked at University College London in the early part of the last century.

## The baroreceptor reflex

Arterial blood pressure is monitored by pressure sensors in the circulatory system called *baroreceptors*, the most important of which are found on the aortic arch and the carotid sinus (a dilation of the internal carotid artery that supplies the brain). These stretch receptors monitor changes in blood pressure and send nervous signals to the cardiovascular control centre in the medulla, a region of the brain stem. The medulla regulates blood pressure by adjustments to the cardiac output of the heart and the peripheral resistance of the systemic arterioles. This process is called the *baroreceptor reflex* and we will now examine how it responds to decreases and increases in blood pressure.

> *Baroreceptors* are small regions on the aorta and carotid sinus that respond to changes in the stretch of the vessel walls as blood pressure fluctuates by sending signals to the cardiovascular control centre in the brain stem.

A decrease in blood pressure can have many causes such as haemorrhage, dehydration, heart attack and even just standing up too quickly. This drop in BP is detected by the baroreceptors which send signals to the cardiovascular control centre in the medulla via *afferent* neurons. The medulla then increases sympathetic activity in the circulatory system. This has the effect of increasing both the stroke volume and heart rate, which increases the cardiac output. Sympathetic activity also causes vasoconstriction in the peripheral arterioles in the skin which increases systemic vascular resistance (Figure 5.6). All of these contribute to an increase in blood pressure.

If you remember our formula for blood pressure, BP = CO × SVR, where cardiac output is defined by CO = HR × SV, you can see that the baroreceptor response increases all of the factors involved in blood pressure regulation. Heart rate, stroke volume and systemic vascular resistance all increase and, consequently, so does blood pressure.

> *Afferent* neurons are those that travel from the periphery into the central nervous system (CNS). Neurons that travel out of the CNS into the periphery are called *efferents*. A good way of memorising these two words is that **E**fferents **E**xit the CNS (so afferents must go in the other direction).

**Figure 5.6** Control of blood pressure via the baroreceptor reflex showing factors that respond to a fall in blood pressure.

## ANOTHER WAY TO PICTURE THIS

Remember we compared the arterial system to a long, thin balloon with a small hole in the end. If pressure in the balloon fell you would blow harder and more frequently (increase cardiac output) and pinch the other end to reduce the amount of air escaping (increase systemic vascular resistance).

So how does the body respond to an *increase* in blood pressure which is normally an indication of exercise? Obviously, a response that reduced cardiac output would be undesirable as it would limit our ability to exercise. However, complex mechanisms in the central nervous system suppress the baroreceptor response and selective vasodilation occurs that redistributes blood to the exercising muscles. This lowers systemic vascular resistance so that blood pressure only increases moderately, even though cardiac output may have doubled.

**CASE STUDY**

After major thoracic surgery, Graham appears to be recovering satisfactorily when you notice that his pulse rate has increased, he looks pale and feels cold to the touch. You check his blood pressure and this is normal. What might be causing the observed changes?

*Comment on case study* An unexplained increase in a patient's heart rate needs investigating. It may be that Graham is anxious but it could be that his blood pressure is falling and he is compensating by increasing his heart rate. If he looks pale and has cold skin, this could be a sign of vasoconstriction of the peripheral arterioles in the skin. The fact that his BP is normal may be because his compensatory mechanisms are currently sufficient to maintain his blood pressure. There could be several problems that are causing his blood pressure to fall, but after major surgery, internal bleeding is a possibility.

**A QUICK RECAP on the short-term regulation of blood pressure**

- The short-term regulation of blood pressure is largely determined by two factors – cardiac output (CO) and systemic vascular resistance (SVR).
- Cardiac output in turn is determined by heart rate and stroke volume.
- If blood pressure falls then the body responds by increasing both CO and SVR.
- The baroreceptor reflex responds to a fall in blood pressure by activating the sympathetic nervous system. This acts on the heart and peripheral arterioles, increasing both CO and SVR, and so blood pressure is increased.
- Various chemical messengers such as adrenaline, angiotensin-II and ADH-vasopressin can bind to receptors on the arterioles and cause vasoconstriction, so increasing SVR.

## The long-term regulation of blood pressure

The baroreceptor response's primary function is to respond to short-term changes in blood pressure. Long-term regulation involves adjusting sodium ($Na^+$) levels in the blood and this is done by the kidneys via the renin–angiotensin (RA) system.

The renin–angiotensin (RA) system operates in the background, maintaining blood volume and blood pressure. It also responds to falls in blood pressure via the kidneys, which detect a fall in blood pressure or a reduction in the flow of blood by increasing the release of the enzyme *renin* into the blood. This enzyme converts a circulating protein called *angiotensinogen* into *angiotensin-I*, which is further modified by *angiotensin-converting enzyme* (ACE) into *angiotensin-II* (Figure 5.7).

Angiotensin-II is the key protein in the long-term regulation of blood pressure. It circulates in the blood and has several actions, all of which act together to increase blood pressure.

**Figure 5.7** How angiotensin-II is produced in response to a fall in blood pressure.

1 Angiotensin-II causes the adrenal glands to release the hormone aldosterone. This hormone acts on the kidneys causing them to conserve sodium ($Na^+$) in the body by reducing the amount of $Na^+$ lost in the urine. The conservation of $Na^+$ by the kidneys increases levels of $Na^+$ in the blood and this increases the amount of water that the blood will hold. As the blood volume increases, the amount of blood returning to the left ventricle increases and so does the preload. With more blood in the left ventricle, the heart's muscle fibres become more stretched and under Starling's law, the force of contraction increases. The stroke volume increases and this in turn increases cardiac output and blood pressure. This might be more clearly explained in a flow chart (Figure 5.8).

Yes (before you ask), the renin–angiotensin system is complicated but ACE inhibitors, one of the most common group of drugs used in the treatment of high blood pressure and heart failure, act on the RA system. You need to understand this system in order to understand the action of ACE inhibitors.

2 Angiotensin-II is a potent vasoconstrictor that binds to angiotensin-II receptors on the smooth muscle cells of peripheral arterioles and causes them to constrict. Vasoconstriction increases systemic vascular resistance and as we know from our blood pressure formula, when SVR increases, so does blood pressure.

3 Angiotensin-II promotes the release of the hormone *ADH-vasopressin* from the anterior pituitary gland in the brain. ADH stands for 'antidiuretic hormone', and as the name implies, causes the kidneys to conserve water by reducing the amount of urine produced. Conserving water in the body helps to maintain blood volume and also blood pressure. The 'vasopressin' part of the name gives a clue to the hormone's other action; it acts on smooth muscle of the peripheral blood vessels as a vasoconstrictor and so increases systemic vascular resistance – and blood pressure.

Well, that's about all you need to know about blood pressure in order to understand how the various antihypertensive drugs work. However, before this we

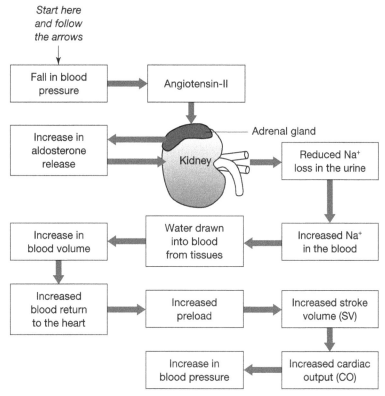

**Figure 5.8** How angiotensin-II (in response to a fall in blood pressure) acts on the kidneys to increase blood volume and blood pressure.

will need to understand something about the cause of hypertension and its consequences.

**A QUICK RECAP on the long-term regulation of blood pressure**

- The long-term regulation of blood pressure is primarily by the renin–angiotensin system.

- When blood pressure falls, renin production is increased by the kidneys and this converts angiotensinogen into angiotensin-I which is then converted into angiotensin-II by an angiotensin-converting enzyme.

- Angiotensin-II causes the hormone aldosterone to be released, and this makes the kidneys conserve sodium which increases blood volume, cardiac output and therefore blood pressure.

- Angiotensin-II causes vasoconstriction of the arterioles, resulting in an increase in systemic vascular resistance, and therefore blood pressure.

- Angiotensin-II promotes the release of the hormone ADH-vasopressin that causes the kidneys to reduce urine production and so conserve body fluids, helping to maintain blood pressure. ADH-vasopressin is also a vasoconstrictor.

## 5.2 The pathology of hypertension

This will be a rather short section because in over 90 per cent of cases of hypertension the cause is unknown. If you look in most books you will see most cases of hypertension described as *idiopathic*, which simply means that the cause is unknown. Idiopathic hypertension is also known as *primary* or *essential hypertension*. Hypertension is defined as having a systolic pressure of over 140 mmHg and a diastolic pressure over 90 mmHg. The problem gets more serious as pressures increase. Mild hypertension, between 140 and 159 mmHg, may initially be treated by changes in lifestyle, but more aggressive pharmacological treatment is needed as the problem gets worse.

**KEY FACT**

The cause of most hypertension is unknown. This means that generally we are treating the symptom rather than the cause.

Pathologies that cause an increase in cardiac output or an increase in systemic vascular resistance such as neurological or hormonal imbalances are the ones most likely to increase blood pressure – but in most cases the cause is unknown. Environment and lifestyle factors such as stress, smoking and obesity can exacerbate hypertension. Drugs such as alcohol, non-steroidal anti-inflammatory drugs (NSAIDS), steroids and even liquorice can also result in an increase in blood pressure. Particular ethnic groups may be more prone to hypertension, for example people of Afro-Caribbean origin are more likely to be hypertensive than other races. Age is an important risk factor as people are more likely to suffer from hypertension as they get older, especially after the age of 55 when around two-thirds of the population is hypertensive. *Secondary hypertension* is generally due to problems such as kidney disease, but again the cause is seldom identifiable.

**IN PRACTICE**

An interesting cause of hypertension in some individuals is a phenomenon known as *'white coat syndrome'* where their blood pressure increases rapidly when a nurse or doctor takes their blood pressure. As soon as the procedure stops, their blood pressure returns to normal!

People who are hypertensive may initially experience few symptoms, but over many years prolonged high blood pressure can damage organs, especially the brain, kidneys and cardiovascular system, and may result in *haemorrhagic stroke*, renal failure and myocardial infarction (heart attack). The development of atherosclerosis is accelerated in people with high blood pressure, especially if they are also diabetic. The heart itself can be affected over time as it is put under strain having to pump against high aortic pressure. The heart muscle gradually thickens and dilates, sometimes resulting in heart failure.

Because hypertension is generally symptomless, many people are not aware that they have high blood pressure until a routine check-up by their GP reveals the problem.

*Haemorrhagic stroke* is when the blood supply to the brain is interrupted by a bleed in the brain itself, often caused by the rupture of a blood vessel. Other types of stroke include ischaemic stroke, which is caused by the formation of a blood clot in the arteries of the brain.

**CASE STUDY**

Jane is 75 and has been diagnosed as hypertensive. When her GP checks Jane's blood pressure it is around 160/90 mmHg and he tells her that she may need to start taking drugs to reduce it. Strangely, when Betty, the community nurse, visits Jane at home and checks her BP, it is much lower – why might this be?

*Comment on case study* Jane's blood pressure may actually be within acceptable limits most of the time but the stress of visiting her GP's surgery may increase it to the point where she appears hypertensive – so-called 'white coat syndrome'. Betty, the community nurse, is visiting Jane in the relaxed surroundings of her own home and so is able to take her BP without stress temporarily increasing the reading. Current UK guidelines recognise this phenomenon and recommend ambulatory or home monitoring to provide a more accurate picture of the patient's typical resting BP.

## 5.3 Drugs used in the treatment of hypertension

The treatment of hypertension can be quite difficult because the choice of treatment for an individual patient is determined by so many factors, including the severity of the problem, the underlying pathology, other problems such as diabetes, the age and even the ethnic origins of the individual – not to mention their response to previous medication.

For mild hypertension where there are no complications, changes in lifestyle rather than drug therapy are to be preferred. Giving up smoking, losing weight, eating plenty of fruit and vegetables, taking exercise, and cutting down on both salt and excessive alcohol consumption can reduce blood pressure sufficiently to remove the necessity of long-term antihypertensive therapy. However, where blood pressure is significantly elevated or where there are complications such as diabetes, antihypertensive drugs may be the only solution.

Many drugs are used to treat hypertension and the choice of which is best for a particular patient is a clinical decision that must be made by the prescriber in accordance with local and national guidelines. In the UK, the National Institute for Health and Clinical Excellence (NICE) provides guidance on the treatment and care of people with hypertension and other diseases and conditions within the National Health Service. Currently, ACE inhibitors or angiotensin receptor blockers (ARBs), if ACE inhibitors are not tolerated, are the drugs of choice, followed by calcium channel blockers then thiazide-like diuretics. Patients over 55 years of age or of Afro-Caribbean descent (any age) are not recommended ACE inhibitors as initial treatment for reasons discussed shortly.

**CASE STUDY**

Mark is a reasonably fit and healthy, non-smoking 45 year old but at a recent visit to his GP, his blood pressure was found to be 150/90 mmHg. This was confirmed after home monitoring and Mark returned to his GP for a discussion as to the best course of treatment. What would you suggest?

*Comment on case study* If Mark is reasonably fit and healthy then he is probably asymptomatic with regard to his high blood pressure. It is good that he does not smoke as this would tend to increase his BP. Initially, lifestyle changes should be tried before resorting to drugs. Salt intake should be reduced, fresh fruit and vegetable intake increased and Mark should be encouraged to exercise more. Swimming, jogging or cycling are suitable but it should be an activity that Mark finds enjoyable otherwise he is unlikely to continue with it.

## Principles for the treatment of hypertension

If you remember back a few pages, you will recall that there was a simple formula that explained the factors regulating blood pressure:

$$BP = CO \times SVR$$
(Blood pressure = Cardiac output × Systemic vascular resistance)

where cardiac output is defined by

$$CO = HR \times SV$$
(Cardiac output = Heart rate × Stroke volume)

Remember that the body's response to a fall in blood pressure is to increase cardiac output and systemic vascular resistance, which returns the blood pressure to its normal level. We are now going to use this formula again to explain the action of antihypertensive drugs but instead of aiming to increase blood pressure we are going to reduce it.

**KEY FACT**

Antihypertensive drugs work by a variety of mechanisms but eventually all reduce either cardiac output or systemic vascular resistance – or both.

**Table 5.2** The effects of the main antihypertensive drugs on the factors that determine blood pressure

| Drug group | Action on SVR and CO | |
|---|---|---|
| | SVR | CO |
| ACE inhibitors and related drugs | Reduction | Reduction |
| Angiotensin-II receptor blockers (ARBs) | Reduction | Possible reduction |
| Thiazide-like diuretics | None | Reduction |
| Calcium channel blockers (CCBs) | Reduction* | Reduction* |
| Beta-blockers | Reduction | Reduction |
| Alpha-blockers | Reduction | None |

* Action varies with type of calcium channel blocker.

Table 5.2 shows the action of the main antihypertensive drugs on factors that determine blood pressure. Note that a reduction in either factor, systemic vascular resistance or cardiac output, will reduce blood pressure.

## Drug groups in the treatment of hypertension

### Antihypertensive group 1: angiotensin-converting enzyme (ACE) inhibitors (and related drugs)

These drugs are used to treat essential hypertension and some are also used for heart failure. This group of drugs includes **captopril, cilazapril, enalapril, fosinopril, imidapril, lisinopril, moexipril, perindopril, quinapril, ramipril** and **trandolapril. Aliskirin** is a related drug, introduced more recently, that has a slightly different action to the other ACE inhibitors.

ACE inhibitors interfere with the renin–angiotensin system that regulates long-term blood pressure. Remember that the body responds to a fall in blood pressure by converting angiotensin-I into angiotensin-II via angiotensin-converting enzyme (ACE). Angiotensin-II circulates in the blood where it has various actions that together increase blood pressure.

1 Aldosterone production is increased and this increases blood sodium, blood volume and so blood pressure.

2 Angiotensin-II also acts as a general vasoconstrictor and so increases systemic vascular resistance.

3 Angiotensin-II stimulates the release of ADH-vasopressin and, as well as acting as a vasoconstrictor, this hormone conserves water by reducing urine output.

ACE inhibitors are similar in molecular structure to angiotensin I and so bind to the active site of angiotensin converting enzyme and thus block its activity,

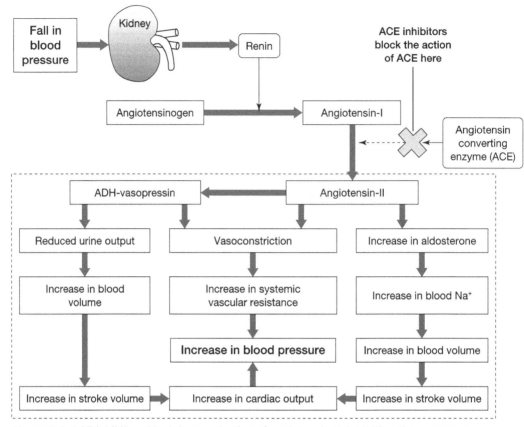

Figure 5.9 ACE inhibitors block the production of angiotensin-II, inhibiting the processes contained within the dotted line, and so reducing blood pressure.

preventing the conversion of angiotensin-I to angiotensin-II. Circulating levels of angiotensin-II fall and so does blood pressure (Figure 5.9).

**IN PRACTICE**

Remember that the NICE guidelines do not recommend the use of ACE inhibitors for patients over 55 years or of Afro-Caribbean descent of any age. The reason for this is that renin production by the kidney reduces with age and is naturally very low in Afro-Caribbean people so ACE inhibitors are less effective because the renin–angiotensin system will play a lesser part in overall blood pressure regulation.

*Side-effects* A persistent dry cough with ACE inhibitors is a common side-effect because these drugs not only inhibit angiotensin-converting enzyme but also enzymes in the lungs that metabolise bradykinin. This results in an accumulation of bradykinin in the bronchioles, which irritates the tissues, resulting in a dry cough. ACE inhibitors can also cause hypotension, especially in patients on diuretics.

## Antihypertensive group 2: renin inhibitors

**Aliskirin** is currently in a group on its own. A relatively recent drug, it interferes with the renin-angiotensin system but not by inhibiting the action of angiotensin converting enzyme. Instead it blocks the action of renin itself, so preventing it from converting angiotensinogen into angiotensin-I. The reduction in circulating levels of angiotensin-I results in a corresponding reduction in angiotensin-II and from here the effect is the same as that of an ACE inhibitor.

## Antihypertensive group 3: angiotensin-II receptor blockers (ARBs)

These drugs are used to treat essential hypertension and some are also used for heart failure. This group includes **candesartan, eprosartan, irbesartan, losartan, olmesartan, telmisartan** and **valsartan**. Patients who find the cough produced by many ACE inhibitors unacceptable may be better able to tolerate these drugs.

Angiotensin-II is a potent vasoconstrictor that causes an increase in systemic vascular resistance. Angiotensin-II targets angiotensin-II receptors on the smooth muscle cells that surround the arteries and arterioles. This causes the muscle cells to contract, resulting in vasoconstriction of the peripheral arterioles and an increase in SVR. Angiotensin-II receptor blockers (ARBs) bind to and block the angiotensin-II receptor and therefore reduce the vasoconstrictive effect of angiotensin-II (Figure 5.10). There is also some suggestion that ARBs acting on other angiotensin-II receptors reduce cardiac output.

**Figure 5.10** Angiotensin-II receptor blockers (ARBs) block angiotensin-II receptors from the vasoconstrictive action of angiotensin-II.

### Antihypertensive group 4: thiazide diuretics

There are several groups of drugs that produce diuresis, including loop diuretics, thiazides, thiazide-like diuretics and potassium sparing diuretics. Of these, the thiazide-like diuretics **chlortalidone** and **indapamide** are currently recommended by NICE as the diuretics of choice for essential hypertension. Other diuretics used for hypertension include the thiazides **bendroflumethiazide** and **cyclopenthiazide** and the thiazide-like diuretics **metolazone** and **xipamide**.

*Diuretics* stimulate the production of urine. In the kidneys, the blood is filtered in small filtration units called nephrons and, after processing, the filtered fluid becomes urine. This means that as urine production increases so more fluid is removed from the blood and therefore blood volume decreases. This in turn reduces preload in the left ventricle and a lower preload means a lower stroke volume and a lower cardiac output. Diuretics work by a common mechanism, altering the osmotic balance in the kidney and so increasing the amount of urine produced. The mechanism whereby the kidneys control the body's water balance is quite complex but you need to know the basic principles of diuresis in order to understand the pharmacological action of diuretics.

> **KEY FACT**
>
> *Diuretics* increase urine production and this reduces blood volume. As blood volume drops, so does stroke volume, cardiac output and blood pressure.

The kidneys are primarily a collection of millions of tiny tubes called nephrons. Within each nephron is a filtration unit called a *glomerulus*, a group of capillaries supplied with blood from a renal arteriole. The pressure in the glomerulus forces fluid from the blood through the glomerulus wall into the *Bowman's capsule* – Figure 5.11. This fluid is called *filtrate* and contains body waste such as urea and other small soluble molecules in the blood but not blood cells or plasma proteins. Around 140 litres of filtrate are produced each day by the millions of nephrons, but most of the water content of the filtrate is reabsorbed back into the blood. This leaves between 1 and 2 litres of urine to pass from the nephrons, down the ureters and into the urinary bladder from where it is voided from the body as urine.

The amount of filtrate produced each day is fairly constant but the amount of urine varies, depending on the hydration state of the individual. You have no doubt noticed that when you have been exercising on a hot day you do not produce much urine. On the other hand, if you have been out visiting friends and drinking tea or coffee socially, then you might be quite desperate to get home (and relieved when you do so). Urine production is controlled by the hormone ADH-vasopressin released by the posterior pituitary gland and its production increases as the body becomes more dehydrated. ADH-vasopressin is released into the bloodstream and acts on the tubules of the nephron, causing them to become more permeable to water, which leaves the nephron and is picked up by

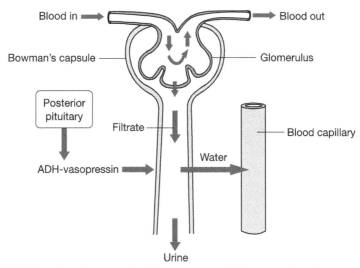

Figure 5.11 Schematic diagram of a kidney nephron. Water is reabsorbed from the filtrate under the influence of the pituitary hormone ADH-vasopressin.

adjacent capillaries. The more ADH is produced, the more water is reabsorbed from the filtrate and the less urine is produced (Figure 5.11).

> **DID YOU KNOW...** that the common dandelion *Taraxacum officinalis* has been used for centuries as a diuretic? The fresh leaves also taste nice in salads but there is a tradition that it causes nocturnal enuresis, hence the French name for dandelion, *pissenlit* or as we would say in English, 'wetting the bed'.

Diuretics inhibit water reabsorption from the filtrate, so more is lost as urine. They do this by blocking sodium and chloride ion pumps on the wall of the nephron. This has the effect of upsetting the osmotic balance in the tissue surrounding the nephron and this decreases the rate at which water is reabsorbed. As less water is reabsorbed from the filtrate, more water is lost as urine, and this causes a reduction in blood volume and blood pressure − as described above.

*Side-effects* As with most other antihypertensives, diuretics can tip the balance the other way, resulting in hypotension. Hypokalaemia (low potassium) and hyponatraemia (low sodium) can also be a problem as a consequence of interfering with the ionic balance of the kidney.

> **IN PRACTICE**
>
> Hypokalaemia and hyponatraemia can result from the use of diuretics or from severe sweating, vomiting or diarrhoea. Hypokalaemia can sometimes cause abnormal heart rhythms. Symptoms of hyponatraemia (low sodium) can include nausea, headaches and confusion.

> **CASE STUDY**
>
> Ben is 65 and was diagnosed with high blood pressure 5 years ago. He has gone to see his GP because of a persistent dry cough (despite having no chest infection) and is also concerned about his kidneys because he needs to go 'for a wee' two or three times during the night. His current medication is **ramipril** – 5 mg once daily and, more recently, **indapamide** – 2.5 mg once daily. Jim usually takes his medication around 9 o'clock at night with his evening cocoa.

*Comment on case study* It could be the ACE inhibitor that is causing the problem dry cough. Ben's GP could switch him to an angiotensin-II receptor blocker (ARB) such as **candesartan**. In fact, it was unusual for Ben to have been prescribed an ACE inhibitor as NICE guidelines consider patients over 55 are less likely to respond to this group of drugs. It is probably the diuretic **indapamide** that is causing Jim to visit the toilet during the night, which is why these diuretics are usually taken first thing in the morning to avoid this problem.

## Antihypertensive group 5: calcium channel blockers

Calcium channel blockers (CCBs) are a diverse group of drugs and exert their effects by different mechanisms. Drugs in this group that are licensed for the treatment of hypertension include **amlodipine, diltiazem, felodipine, isradipine, lacidipine, lercanidipine, nicardipine, nifedipine, nimodipine** and **verapamil**.

How come there are so many different types of drugs in this group?

If any group of drugs is successful this creates a market and manufacturers will develop their own drug to exploit that market. Also, as soon as a popular drug goes out of copyright then rival manufacturers will start to produce their own version. Currently, nine different drug manufacturers are producing **diltiazem**.

Calcium channel blockers act on calcium ion channels in various cells that have an important role in determining blood pressure. These cells include the myocytes (muscle cells of the heart), the heart's pacemaker cells and the smooth muscle cells of the peripheral arterioles. Calcium channels play an important role in the operation of these structures and blocking the channels with CCBs results in a fall in blood pressure – but by a variety of mechanisms. Ultimately, they reduce cardiac output or systemic vascular resistance and so reduce blood pressure.

*The heart's muscle cells* The entry of calcium ions into the myocytes of the heart initiates their contraction. CCBs block $Ca^{2+}$ channels in the myocytes' cell membrane and this reduces the cells' ability to contract. A reduction in the force of contraction reduces stroke volume, which reduces cardiac output.

*The heart's pacemaker cells* The entry of $Ca^{2+}$ ions into the heart's pacemaker cells is also an important determinant of heart rate, so blocking the $Ca^{2+}$ channels results in a slowing of the heart. A reduction in heart rate reduces cardiac output.

**Figure 5.12** The entry of calcium into the smooth muscle cells surrounding the arterioles induces contraction, so blocking Ca2⁺ channels with CCBs induces relaxation and vasodilation.

*The arterioles* The contraction of smooth muscle cells surrounding peripheral arterioles involves the entry of ions through $Ca^{2+}$ channels in the cell membrane. As CCBs block the $Ca^{2+}$ channels, contraction is inhibited and vasodilation promoted (Figure 5.12). Vasodilation reduces systemic vascular resistance.

Blocking calcium channels in the cardiovascular system therefore results in a reduction in systemic vascular resistance, heart rate and stroke volume and all of these factors combine to reduce blood pressure. Calcium channel blockers are divided into two groups defined by differences in the chemical structure. The *dihydropyridines* include all of the CCBs that end in 'ipine' such as **amlodipine**, **felodipine**, etc. This group act mainly on the smooth muscle of the arterioles, causing them to dilate and so reducing SVR. The remaining CCBs, **verapamil** and **diltiazem**, belong to the *non-dihydropyridine* group and are more cardio-selective, reducing cardiac output. **Diltiazem** is somewhat intermediate in its actions, causing a reduction in cardiac output and also peripheral vasodilation.

*Side-effects* Many, including GI disturbance, hypotension, palpitations, headache, dizziness, flushing, fatigue and so on. Constipation is commonly experienced with **verapamil**, most likely caused by the drug blocking $Ca^{2+}$ channels in the smooth muscle that encircles the gut. This reduces its contractility and therefore motility, leading to the sluggish passage of food through the gastro-intestinal system.

*Key interactions* Grapefruit juice inhibits gut enzymes that metabolise some CCBs, including **nifedipine**, **felodipine** and **verapamil**. This enhances the amount of drug absorbed and increases plasma concentration.

## Antihypertensive group 6: beta-blockers

Examples of this group include **acebutolol, atenolol, bisoprolol, carvedilol, celiprolol, labetalol, metoprolol, nadolol, nebivolol, oxprenolol, pindolol, propranolol** and **pindolol**. Selected members of this group of drugs are also used for angina and arrhythmias and as an adjunct in heart failure. For general antihypertensive therapy, current NICE guidelines relegate beta-blockers to the drug of fourth choice behind thiazide-like diuretics, calcium channel blockers and ACE inhibitors/ARBs.

We examined the anti-anginal action of beta-blockers in Chapter 4 and saw that they block $\beta_1$ receptors on the heart, thus reducing its responsiveness to activity by the sympathetic nervous system. As this keeps the heart rate low and reduces the workload of the heart, it is very useful in patients with angina and heart failure. However, the action of beta-blockers in hypertension is less well understood. Sympathetic activity is reduced during rest, so blocking the receptors to sympathetic activity has less effect on the resting heart, but beta-blockers certainly reduce cardiac output. There is evidence that some beta-blockers inhibit the release of renin from the kidneys, so reducing the hypertensive effects of angiotensin-II, and some also cause peripheral vasodilation. There is a suggestion that the baroreceptor response is less sensitive and beta-blockers may also have an effect on the central nervous system, reducing sympathetic activity.

*Side-effects* Many, including GI disturbance, postural hypotension, bradycardia, headache, fatigue and so on. Beta-blockers can also block the $\beta_2$ receptors in the lungs, causing brochoconstriction, explaining why they are contra-indicated in asthma.

## Antihypertensive group 7: alpha-adrenoceptor blockers

These drugs are generally used in combination with other hypertensives rather than on their own as mono-therapy. Selected members of the group are also indicated for benign prostatic hyperplasia (enlarged prostate gland) and congestive heart failure. The group includes **doxazosin**, **indoramin**, **prazosin** and **terazosin**.

The peripheral arterioles respond to a variety of vasoconstrictive chemical substances released in the body including, as we have seen, angiotensin-II, ADH-vasopressin and adrenaline. Both circulating adrenaline and noradrenaline, released as a neurotransmitter by the sympathetic nervous system, bind to alpha-1 ($\alpha_1$) receptors on the arterioles with the same effect. Blocking these receptors antagonistically means that neither adrenaline nor noradrenaline can bind and this results in relaxation of the smooth muscles of the arterioles and vasodilation (Figure 5.13).

**Figure 5.13** Alpha-adrenoceptor blockers such as **doxazosin** isolate smooth muscle cells of the arterioles from the vasoconstrictive action of adrenaline and noradrenaline.

These drugs also have a relaxing effect on the smooth muscle of the bladder and prostate gland, explaining their usefulness in the treatment of benign prostatic hyperplasia.

**A QUICK RECAP on drugs used in the treatment of hypertension**

- ACE inhibitors such as **captopril** block the action of angiotensin converting enzyme that converts angiotensin-I to angiotensin-II.

- Angiotensin-II causes vasoconstriction and an increase in cardiac output (by increasing blood volume). Blocking the production of angiotensin-II results in vasodilation and a fall in cardiac output which together cause a fall in BP.

- **Aliskirin**, a renin inhibitor, produces the same effect as ACE inhibitors by blocking the enzyme renin.

- Angiotensin-II binds to receptors on smooth muscle cells in the arterioles and causes vasoconstriction. Angiotensin-II receptor blockers such as **candesartan** prevent angiotensin-II binding to its receptors, resulting in vasodilation, a decrease in SVR and a fall in BP.

- Thiazide-like diuretics such as **indapamide** increase the production of urine and thus reduce the blood volume, which reduces cardiac output and thus BP.

- Calcium channel blockers have various actions. Some, such as **nifedipine**, cause peripheral vasodilation. Others, such as **verapamil**, result in reduced cardiac output.

- Beta-blockers such as **atenolol** have a not fully-understood action as antihypertensives, but probably inhibit the release of renin, reduce cardiac output and cause peripheral vasodilation.

- Alpha-adrenoceptor blockers such as **doxazosin** block $\alpha_1$-adrenergic receptors on the smooth muscle cells in the peripheral arterioles from the vasoconstrictive effect of adrenaline and noradrenaline, resulting in vasodilation.

## 5.4 Drugs used in the treatment of hypotension

High blood pressure is extremely common in our society and there are many drugs available for its treatment — as discussed above. At the opposite end of the blood pressure spectrum is hypotension — low blood pressure. This can result in fainting, palpitations and feelings of light-headedness, especially when standing from a sitting position. Unfortunately, there is little that can be done pharmacologically and currently there are no drugs licensed for moderate hypotension in the UK — although the alpha-1 antagonist **midodrine** is sometimes used off-licence for neuropathic postural hypotension. Treatment mostly involves lifestyle changes — wearing support stockings, increasing salt intake and ensuring adequate hydration.

Acute hypotension, a rapid fall in blood pressure, is a medical emergency and unless urgent action is taken, the patient can progress to irreversible shock and death. Treatment depends on the cause of the problem but if it is loss of body fluids (hypovolaemic shock) then volume replacement is of prime importance to maintain stroke volume and cardiac output. When fluids have been replaced then vasoconstrictor sympathomimetics such as **noradrenaline** can be administered. These act on alpha-1 adrenergic receptors, increasing peripheral vasoconstriction and so raising blood pressure.

## REFERENCES AND FURTHER RECOMMENDED READING

Books

Opie, L.H. and Gersh, B.J. (2008) *Drugs for the Heart* (7th edn). Saunders.

Websites

All recommended websites are open access (but free registration is sometimes required).

Bandolier: hypertension – http://www.medicine.ox.ac.uk/bandolier/

British Heart Foundation – http://www.bhf.org.uk/

Medscape: cardiology – http://emedicine.medscape.com/cardiology

National Centre for Health and Clinical Excellence (2011 Guidelines for the treatment of hypertension) – http://www.nice.org.uk/Guidance/CG127

Student, BMJ cardiology – http://student.bmj.com/student/student-bmj.html

# Test yourself

That was quite a testing chapter to work through, but hypertension is a very common problem and you will find patients on antihypertensive medication in many clinical scenarios. Not only is it important to understand the pharmacology of hypertension but the chapter will also have given you a good refresher in the physiology of blood pressure regulation. Try these questions to see how much you have remembered and understood of Chapter 5.

*The answers to these questions are at the end of the book (see p. 314).*

1 When you are checking someone's pulse in (say) the radial artery, is the pulse rate the same as heart rate?

2 Pressure in the arteries fluctuates between systole and diastole – which of these two is the higher pressure?

3 If cardiac output falls, what happens to blood pressure?

4 Name three substances carried in the blood that result in vasoconstriction.

5 What is the neurotransmitter released by sympathetic neurons that causes vasoconstriction?

6 If blood pressure falls because of haemorrhage, what would you expect to happen to heart rate?

7 If there is a general vasodilation of the systemic arterioles, what happens to blood pressure?

8 Name three effects of angiotensin-II.

9 ACE inhibitors inhibit the production of angiotensin-II and by so doing reduce aldosterone production – why might this reduce blood pressure?

10 Do diuretics increase or decrease the amount of water reabsorption in the tubules of the nephron?

11 Are diuretics most likely to lead to hypernatraemia or hyponatraemia?

12 What is the effect of blocking calcium channels in arteriole smooth muscle cells?

13 By what mechanism might CCBs cause constipation?

14 How do beta-blockers reduce blood pressure?

15 Why are beta-blockers contra-indicated in asthma?

Answers to the questions on p. 111.

1 Aorta
2 Right
3 Atria
4 Systole
5 Oxygenated
6 Vein

## Chapter 6

# Pain and its management

This chapter explains the anatomy and physiology of pain pathways, the inflammatory response and the pharmacological action of the major drug groups used for relief from inflammatory, trauma-induced, neuropathic and perioperative pain.

CONTENTS

The chapter contains some brief case studies and finishes off with some self-test questions in order that you can make sure that you have understood the physiology, pathology and pharmacology of pain and pain relief.

> **IN PRACTICE**
>
> You will encounter patients who are experiencing pain and being treated for it. In surgical wards, patients will have undergone operations that may be causing post-operative pain. In medical wards, patients may have infections and conditions such as cancer that cause pain. Midwives will be looking after women experiencing the pain of childbirth. In the community, elderly patients may be experiencing pain from chronic problems such as arthritis or sciatica. Pain is often the reason that patients seek medical help, so one of the first stages in the diagnosis of a problem is to ask the patient to describe the source and type of pain. This is why you need to understand the nature of pain and also the drugs that are used to help people who are experiencing pain.

## Introduction

Undoubtedly, everyone reading this chapter will have had some experience of pain. Hopefully it will have been fairly minor, arising from the bumps, grazes, toothache and nettle stings that most of us experience at one time or another. For others the pain may have been more severe, caused by accidents such as falling off a bicycle or perhaps the pain associated with childbirth. Most people would agree that pain is unpleasant and it is fortunate that medical science has developed techniques in pain management that reduce it to bearable levels. This has in itself led to major advances in surgical techniques that would be impossible without adequate pain control. Less than 200 years ago, operations were conducted without anaesthetic (or with copious amounts of alcohol), patients were forcefully restrained and surgeons had to operate very quickly indeed. Contrast that with the complex, life-saving procedures that modern surgeons perform, thanks to advanced anaesthesia.

Many philosophers have pondered on the subject of pain, asking why we should have to experience such a seemingly unnecessary and unpleasant phenomenon. Pain appears to serve no function except to aggravate an already unpleasant situation such as an injury or infection, so why should pain pathways have evolved in humans and probably all animals that possess a nervous system?

The answer becomes apparent when we consider the fate of those few individuals who are born without the ability to experience pain, a condition called *congenital analgesia*. You might think that it would be wonderful never to have toothache again or experience wasp or nettle stings but there is a downside. If you do not know that you are about to sustain an injury then you may not take the appropriate action to avoid that injury. Think what happens when you accidentally touch a hot domestic iron or a hotplate on a kitchen cooker. Almost before your skin touches the hot object you experience an unpleasant sensation and quickly withdraw your hand. Imagine what would happen if you did not experience that pain — there could have been quite a lot of tissue damage before you discovered that your hand was on fire! Similarly, if your finger touches a thorn on a rose bush, you feel the pain as the thorn pricks your finger and very quickly move your finger away. If you did not experience that sharp immediate pain then the thorn could easily pierce your flesh and the wound could become infected. Pain also teaches us to avoid potentially painful and thus dangerous situations such as fierce dogs, swarms of bees, etc.

Pain is also a useful mechanism for informing us that we have sustained an injury or developed an infection. We can then take the appropriate action to protect the injury from further damage, clean and dress the wound and possibly seek medical assistance.

In this chapter we will explore the way that the body detects pain and relays that information to the brain where the pain is conceptualised. Inflammation is associated with many clinical situations such as injury, infection and surgical procedures so we explore the nature of inflammation and how it may result in pain. Finally, we look at a very important but diverse group of drugs that relieve or prevent pain. These drugs range from over-the-counter analgesics for minor to moderate pain such as **paracetamol** to opioids such as **morphine** that are used to control severe pain. Because inflammation is a common source of pain we examine the mechanism of action of the non-steroidal anti-inflammatory drugs (NSAIDs) such as **ibuprofen** and also anti-inflammatory corticosteroids such as **prednisolone**. Finally, we examine the local anaesthetics such as **lidocaine**, widely used in dentistry and minor surgery, and take a brief look at the principles of general anaesthesia.

## WHERE ARE WE STARTING FROM?

In this chapter we will be discussing the nervous system and how it transmits pain signals to the brain. We will also be examining the action of drugs on pain pathways, so it is important that you understand the basic layout of the nervous system and how nervous impulses are transmitted along neurons (nerve cells). Let's start off with a short quiz to find out how much you know before we begin:

1   The nervous system can primarily be divided into two divisions, the central nervous system and the . . . ?

2 Do afferent neurons carry information into or out of the central nervous system?

_____

3 What is the difference between a neuron and a nerve?

_____

4 Name the two divisions of the autonomic nervous system.

_____

5 Motor neurons control which type of tissues?

_____

*Answers are at the end of the chapter on p. 166.*

How did you do? If you got most of the answers correct, you obviously have a basic knowledge of the nervous system. Otherwise, you might do well to open your favourite physiology book and brush up on the nervous system to make sure you understand the first section of this chapter. This is not the easiest of the body's systems to learn but you will need a good grasp of it to understand pain and how pain-relieving drugs work.

## 6.1    The physiology of pain and pain pathways

The experience of pain differs between individuals and will vary according to the nature of the noxious stimulus, previous exposure and the reaction to pain of that individual. The definition of pain accepted by most clinical practitioners goes something like:

> *'Pain is whatever the patient informs you that they are experiencing.'*

This is because no one can truly appreciate the pain that another person is experiencing. Some people are (or say they are) relatively impervious to pain while others seemingly over-react to the smallest painful stimulus. This means that whatever your belief about a patient's pain, he or she is the only one who really knows what it is like, so you have to respect the patient's description of their experience.

We generally divide pain into two types – **nociceptive** and **neuropathic** – and each type requires different clinical approaches and drugs.

**Nociceptive** pain usually has an identifiably physiological cause such as inflammation or injury. The pain from this source is transmitted along pain neurons into the spinal cord and up to the brain where the pain is conceptualised. Drugs that block the transmission of nervous impulses along the pain pathways will prevent pain messages from reaching the brain. This is perhaps the most common cause of pain and its treatment is perhaps the most straightforward.

**Neuropathic pain** is caused by neurological dysfunction that results in the perception of pain. Various conditions can affect nerves and these can cause neuropathic pain as a consequence of the problem. These conditions include trigeminal neuralgia, shingles, multiple sclerosis and diabetic neuropathy. Neuropathic pain can manifest itself in hyperalgesia (severe pain from a stimulus that would normally cause only slight discomfort), paresthesia (unpleasant or painful feelings such as pins and needles with no apparent stimulus) and allodynia (pain from a stimulus that should not normally cause pain). Symptoms such as depression and anxiety may also result from neuropathic pain. The physiology, pathology and treatment of neuropathic pain is often uncertain and problematical so Chapter 6 focuses primarily on nociceptive pain and gives a brief résumé of the drugs that are used to treat neuropathic pain towards the end of the chapter.

**KEY FACT**

Nociceptive pain generally has an identifiable cause such as injury and involves pain signals travelling to the brain along pain pathways. Neuropathic pain is caused by problems within the nervous system itself. It is generally more difficult to identify the cause of neuropathic pain – and to treat it.

## Acute and chronic pain

Another way that pain can be categorised is by separating it into acute or chronic. These divisions refer to the length of time that the pain is experienced by the individual and makes no reference to its intensity. Acute pain is short term and lasts a definite period of time before, for example, an injury is resolved and the pain subsides. Chronic pain is defined as pain that lasts more than six months. It may be neuropathic or nociceptive in origin, and caused perhaps by a long-term degenerative disease such as osteoarthritis.

**DID YOU KNOW ...** that the word 'chronic' is widely misused as meaning severe when it simply refers to the long duration of a problem or pain? The word comes from the Ancient Greek word *khronos* meaning time. This is the origin of words such as *chronometer* (accurate clock) and *chronological* (in date order).

## The neuroanatomy of pain

Nociceptive pain is transmitted along a relay of neurons, from the site of injury, into the spinal cord and up to the brain where the signals are conceptualised as pain. At the *distal* end of afferent nociceptive neurons (pain neurons) there are

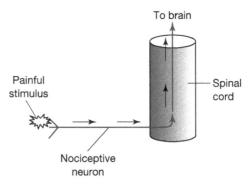

**Figure 6.1** A noxious stimulus is transmitted along an afferent nociceptive neuron into the spinal cord and from there to the brain.

nociceptors (pain receptors) that respond to painful stimuli such as heat, mechanical pressure and chemical stimulation. Once stimulated, these neurons send nervous impulses into the spinal cord and from there to the brain (Figure 6.1).

*Distal* refers to the point on an anatomical structure furthest away from the centre of the body. If you think of the human arm, the fingers are distal to the elbow. A point nearer to the centre is *proximal*, so the elbow is proximal to the fingers.

Nociceptors, found in most tissues, are nerve endings that respond to chemical, thermal and mechanical stimuli. There are various types of nociceptors and various types of nociceptive neurons, some of which transmit fast impulses representing sharp, well-localised pain while others, perhaps associated with inflammation, transmit slower impulses that signify a more diffuse, dull aching type of pain.

Let us now follow in some detail the neural pathways that take pain signals from the site of injury into the spinal cord and up to the brain. Firstly, we have the painful stimulation, perhaps a minor cut to a finger. The nociceptor is stimulated by the tissue damage and this initiates nervous impulses that are sent along the arm via the afferent nociceptive neuron and then into the spinal cord. Arriving via the dorsal root of the spinal cord, the nociceptive neuron sends signals across a *synapse* (nerve junction) to an ascending neuron that ascends to the *thalamus* in the brain where the signal crosses another synapse and finally reaches the *cerebral cortex* via a *thalamic–cortical* neuron (Figure 6.2). Some of the neurons that convey dull, aching pain ascend to the brain by a slightly different route but, essentially, all pain pathways lead eventually to the cerebral cortex where the information is processed into a form of conscious pain experience.

*Synapse* – where two neurons meet you will find a synapse. Nervous impulses jump from one neuron to another across these interesting structures by means of chemical messengers called neurotransmitters.

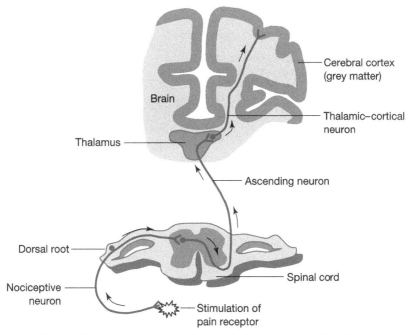

**Figure 6.2** Nociceptive pathways conveying pain signals from a site of injury to the cerebral cortex of the brain.

## The body's own analgesic system

Animals have evolved their own analgesic system that becomes activated when they are injured. This in-built analgesia provides short-term relief from pain that enables an animal to escape from predators or extract themselves from a dangerous situation without being crippled with pain. The mechanism is not fully understood but it is believed to originate deep within the brain from where efferent neurons descend down the brain stem and spinal cord where they meet with incoming afferent nociceptive neurons. Here the descending neurons release opioid-like peptides which block the transmission between the afferent nociceptive neurons and so inhibit the experience of pain (Figure 6.3). As we will see later in the chapter, this in-built analgesic system is utilised by opioid drugs such as **morphine** and **codeine** so it is important that we spend a few moments to explain how the opioid-like peptides work on the synapses in the spinal cord.

**DID YOU KNOW ...** that opioid-like substances are released during sustained strenuous exercise such as running or cycling? It is believed that these substances cause a sense of well-being or even euphoria that some endurance athletes experience, and may even lead to them becoming addicted to exercise.

Figure 6.3 Descending neurons inhibit pain transmission pathways in the body's own analgesic system.

## The synapse

We need to examine briefly how synapses operate because they are key targets for opioid drugs. When a nervous impulse arrives at the axon terminal of a neuron, it cannot simply jump to the next neuron because at the junction between the neurons there is a small gap that forms part of a structure called the synapse (Figure 6.4). The synapse comprises the axon terminal of the transmitting neuron and the cell membrane of the receiving neuron, separated from each other by a small gap called the synaptic cleft. Communication across the synaptic cleft is via neurotransmitters released by the transmitting neuron. As you can see from Figure 6.4, the neurotransmitters are pre-packed into small bubble-like structures called vesicles. When a nervous impulse arrives at the end of the transmitting neuron, this causes calcium ions to enter the terminal which stimulates the release of the neurotransmitters. These diffuse across the cleft and bind to receptors on the post-synaptic membrane of the cell receiving the message and this either stimulates or inhibits the receiving cell.

These synapses are complicated - are they targeted by other drugs beside opioids?

Synapses are indeed complex, perhaps one of the most complex structures in the body. They are targeted by many drugs, especially those used to treat mental health problems. Our four protein drug targets − receptors, ion channels, enzymes and carrier proteins − are all found in synapses and can be targeted by various drugs.

### A QUICK RECAP on the physiology of pain and pain pathways

- We can divide pain into various categories: nociceptive and neuropathic describe the origin of the pain; chronic and acute describe the duration of the pain.

- In nociceptive pain, signals are transmitted along a relay of nociceptive neurons from the origin of the injury or disease, up the spinal cord to the brain.

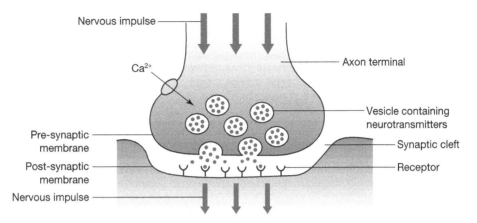

**Figure 6.4** Schematic diagram of a synapse. Nervous impulses are transmitted across the synapse via neurotransmitters (note that some types of neurotransmitter inhibit the forward transmission of nervous impulses).

- The body has its own analgesic system that reduces pain immediately after injury.
- The analgesic system inhibits pain transmission in the synapses of the spinal cord.

## 6.2 The pathology of inflammation and pain

When you hit your thumb with a hammer or cut yourself with a kitchen knife, you notice the area surrounding the injury becomes red, warm, swollen and painful – this is inflammation. You might think that what you are observing is the random consequence of tissue damage but this is not the case. Inflammation is a carefully programmed, non-specific immune response to injury, noxious chemical agents and microbial pathogens. The inflammatory response occurs immediately after trauma or infection and prevents the spread of pathogens, minimises further damage to cells and tissue and finally enhances repair and healing.

Inflammation manifests itself by the following symptoms:

- Redness
- Heat
- Swelling
- Pain
- Alteration of function.

The inflammatory response involves three key processes:

1 The vasodilation of small blood vessels in the area of damage, resulting in an increase in blood flow.

147

2  An increase in *vascular permeability* that causes *plasma* (the liquid, non-cellular part of the blood) to leak from small blood vessels into the area of damage.

3  The emigration of neutrophils (white blood cells) from the blood into the damaged area.

These processes can explain some of the symptoms of inflammation mentioned earlier. For example, vasodilation increases the blood flow to the damaged area and blood makes the area red and warm (Figure 6.5). Inflammation results in plasma leaking from the small blood vessels into the area of damage or infection and this causes oedema (swelling). This can also cause pressure on pain neurons and results in the dull, aching pain familiar in inflammation. Swelling can also impede muscle and joint movement and cause loss of function. Chemicals released in inflammation can add to the sensation of pain, and these will be discussed later.

> *Vascular permeability* – Vascular relates to the blood vessels and permeability is a measure of how easily fluid will pass through a membrane, etc. In this case an increase in vascular permeability means that the blood vessels become leaky.

The leaking of plasma from the small blood vessels brings plasma proteins into intimate contact with the damaged area. These proteins include the clotting proteins that help to stop bleeding and various immune proteins that help to destroy any microbes that may have been introduced into the area with the injury. Also introduced are proteins called kinins that promote vasodilation, increase the permeability of blood vessels and stimulate pain receptors. We will meet the kinins later when we examine how inflammation causes pain.

> **CASE STUDY**
>
> Geoff was playing football when he tripped and twisted his ankle. Still in his football strip, he presents in casualty with an ankle that is severely swollen, red and warm to the touch. It is also extremely painful and Geoff can't bear to put his foot on the ground. What are the processes triggered by the sprain that have caused Geoff's symptoms?

*Comment on case study* This is a classic presentation of inflammation. The tissue damage caused by the accident has triggered the inflammatory process resulting in oedema, loss of function and pain. Vasodilation has brought extra warm blood to the area giving it a flushed, red appearance. The extent of the damage needs proper clinical assessment but often sprains look and feel worse than they actually are. Hopefully, with rest, anti-inflammatories and TLC, Geoff will be back playing football in a few weeks' time.

## Mast cells

Mast cells are key components in the inflammatory response. They are found in connective tissue adjacent to blood vessels and injury or stimulation by the

**Figure 6.5** Small blood vessels in the inflamed area dilate and become leaky. This increases blood flow to the area, making it red and warm. Plasma leaking into tissues causes swelling.

immune system causes mast cells to release various mediators (locally acting chemicals) – Figure 6.6. Mast cells are part of the granulocyte family of white blood cells, so-called because they contain granules of pre-packed mediators that can be released very quickly once the mast cell is stimulated to do so, perhaps by injury.

Mast cells release various mediators by degranulation, including histamine. Histamine causes vasodilation and also increases the permeability of small blood vessels, making the area red, warm and swollen – as discussed above. Other mediators released by mast cells attract circulating *neutrophils* from the blood, which squeeze through the walls of the small blood vessels and migrate towards the area of inflammation. Here, the neutrophils mature and *phagocytose* micro-organisms that may have caused the infection or have been introduced into a wound during the initial injury (Figure 6.7).

*Phagocytose* – literally translated, means eating cells. Neutrophils and macrophages are large immune cells that engulf and destroy bacteria.

**Figure 6.6** Mast cells release mediators either by degranulation or more gradually by synthesis.

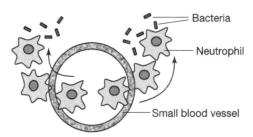

**Figure 6.7** Neutrophils are attracted by mediators released by mast cells and migrate from the blood to the area of inflammation where they phagocytose bacteria.

Other chemical mediators require synthesis and consequently are released some time after histamine, and these include *prostaglandins, thromboxanes* and *leukotrienes*. These mediators are very important pharmacologically because there are many groups of drugs that are targeted at either blocking their production or inhibiting their action.

## Prostaglandins

Prostaglandins are important mediators in the inflammatory process. They are members of a large family derived from arachidonic acid (a fatty acid) and are found in most tissues of the body. Prostaglandin biochemistry is complex, as are the actions of prostaglandins themselves. They belong to a family that includes prostaglandins, thromboxanes and leukotrienes which have important roles, unconnected with inflammation in maintaining cell and tissue homoeostasis.

Prostaglandin $E_2$ ($PGE_2$) is the main prostaglandin involved in inflammation. It is secreted by mast cells and other immune cells, and reinforces the action of histamine and bradykinin, resulting in vasodilation of small blood vessels, an increase in vascular permeability and the stimulation of nociceptive neurons.

$PGE_2$ also plays a less well-defined role in the transmission of pain signals in the spinal cord and in the *hypothalamus* of the brain. It can affect the body's thermostat, resulting in pyresis (fever). Prostaglandins also have many roles unconnected with inflammation, including the maintenance of the gastric mucosa (lining of the stomach), the inhibition of gastric acid secretion, smooth muscle contraction and dilation, coagulation, synaptic modulation and sleep regulation.

*Hypothalamus* Situated at the base of the brain, the hypothalamus has a key role in maintaining the internal environment of the body. The hypothalamus regulates the sympathetic and parasympathetic nervous system as well as the release of pituitary hormones.

Because anti-inflammatory drugs inhibit prostaglandin synthesis, it is necessary to examine briefly how they are produced by mast and other immune cells.

The raw material is the phospholipid membrane of the cell. This is converted into arachidonic acid, then into a *cyclic endoperoxide* and finally into a prostaglandin or thromboxane (Figure 6.8).

The key enzyme in this process is a cyclo-oxygenase (COX) that has arachidonic acid as its substrate. There are several forms of cyclo-oxygenase but the two that have known pharmacological significance are COX-1 and COX-2. Prostaglandins and thromboxanes are produced extensively in the body and have many roles unconnected with inflammation. These are produced by the enzyme COX-1, which can be thought of as a housekeeping enzyme, producing prostaglandins and thromboxanes that are involved in many important body functions such as gastric acid regulation, synaptic modulation, blood clotting etc. The production of COX-2 is increased during inflammation, resulting in large amounts of prostaglandin $PGE_2$ in the inflamed area.

> **KEY FACT**
>
> COX-1 is an enzyme that is produced in many tissues where it produces prostaglandins and thromboxanes involved in homeostasis. COX-2 is an enzyme found primarily in inflamed tissues where it produces prostaglandin $E_2$, which contributes to the symptoms of inflammation.

**Leukotrienes** are closely related to prostaglandins and thromboxanes and have been implicated in asthma. Their synthesis uses a similar pathway but does not involve the cyclo-oxygenase enzyme. Their role in inflammation is still being determined but they are known to activate and sensitise some white blood cells and cause bronchoconstriction.

Yes, prostaglandin chemistry is quite complex but it is the major target of non-steroidal anti-inflammatory drugs (NSAIDs) such as **diclofenac** and **ibuprofen**. Thromboxanes are targets of **aspirin** in the prevention of clotting and the action of leukotrienes is inhibited by anti-asthma drugs such as **montelukast** and **zafirlukast**.

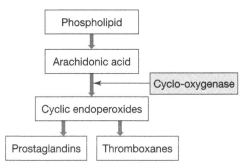

**Figure 6.8** Outline pathway for the synthesis of prostaglandins and thromboxanes.

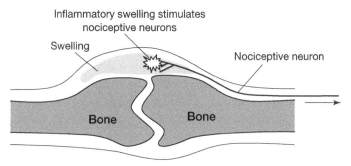

Figure 6.9 Pressure from inflammatory swelling stimulates nociceptive neurons.

Figure 6.10 PGE$_2$ sensitises nociceptors to the action of bradykinin.

## The role of prostaglandins in inflammatory pain

There are two key mechanisms whereby prostaglandin E$_2$ increases pain. Firstly, PGE$_2$, along with histamine and bradykinin, increases vascular permeability and the resulting swelling increases pressure in the inflamed area that stimulates nociceptive neurons (Figure 6.9).

Prostaglandin E$_2$ also increases pain by making nociceptive neurons more sensitive to the bradykinin produced in inflammation (Figure 6.10). Bradykinin is a potent stimulator of nociceptive neurons and its action is enhanced by the presence of PGE$_2$.

## Headaches and migraine

Headaches and migraine are two of the most common pain problems and probably the most frequent reasons for people taking pain-relieving drugs. These problems do not easily fit into either category of nociceptive or neuropathic pain as generally the pain does not arise from trauma, inflammation or neurological damage. Sometimes we can identify the cause of a headache, such as a stressful day at work or commuting in a hot and noisy bus, but the actual mechanism that causes the pain is poorly understood. Migraines are a particularly unpleasant form of headache as they are frequently accompanied by nausea and visual disturbance.

**A QUICK RECAP on the pathology of inflammation and pain**

- Inflammation is a programmed response to infection or injury.

- The key signs of inflammation are redness, heat, swelling, pain and alteration of function.

- Vasodilation brings more blood to the inflamed area, making it red and warm.

- Plasma leaks out of small blood vessels into tissues, making them swollen and painful, and reducing their ability to function.

- Mast cells and other immune cells produce histamine and prostaglandins that are key players contributing to vasodilation and causing small blood vessels to leak plasma.

- Prostaglandin $E_2$ is the main inflammatory prostaglandin, produced in a pathway where COX-2 is a key enzyme.

- The body produces many prostaglandins in other tissues that are unconnected with inflammation, produced in a pathway where COX-1 is the key enzyme.

- Headaches and migraine are two of the most common pain problems but the mechanisms that cause the pain and other symptoms are poorly understood.

## 6.3 Drugs used in the management of inflammation and pain

### Non-steroidal anti-inflammatory drugs (NSAIDs)

There are many non-steroidal anti-inflammatory drugs (NSAIDs) available, including ibuprofen, diclofenac, aceclofenac, acemetacin, dexibuprofen, dexketoprofen, etodolac, fenoprofen, flurbiprofen, indometacin, ketoprofen, mefenamic acid, meloxicam, nabumetone, naproxen, sulindac, tenoxicam and tiaprofenic acid. There are minor differences between these drugs with regard to indications but most can be used to reduce inflammation and relieve pain in rheumatic disease, musculoskeletal problems, osteoarthritis, etc. **Ibuprofen** and **diclofenac** are perhaps the most common NSAIDs for relief of general aches and pains, dental pain, dysmenorrhoea, etc. Pain relief starts within a few hours but their full anti-inflammatory action may take several days.

**Aspirin,** a NSAID in the pharmacopoeia for many years, has largely been superseded by more modern drugs. It has, however, had a revivial as an antiplatelet drug, used for the prevention of thrombosis in patients with cardiovascular disease.

All NSAIDs have a similar action, reducing inflammation, swelling and pain by inhibiting the production of prostaglandins, especially $PGE_2$. The key target for NSAIDs is the cyclo-oxygenase enzyme COX-2, the form that is produced during inflammation and contributes to the production of copious amounts of $PGE_2$ in the inflamed area. This prostaglandin contributes to the increase in vascular permeability that allows plasma to leak from the blood into the area of inflammation. The resulting swelling can increase pressure on nociceptive neurons, stimulating them and causing the familiar inflammatory aching pain. $PGE_2$ also sensitises nociceptors to the pain-producing mediator bradykinin, contributing to the pain experienced. For these reasons, it is obviously desirable to inhibit the action of COX-2 and so reduce the production of $PGE_2$ to help relieve inflammatory pain.

### KEY FACT

Non-steroidal anti-inflammatory drugs block the enzyme COX-2, found primarily in inflamed tissues where it is part of the pathway that produces prostaglandin $E_2$.

*Side-effects* The side-effects of NSAIDs are numerous and vary between patients in severity and frequency. The gastro-intestinal tract (GIT) appears to be particularly vulnerable, resulting in discomfort, diarrhoea, nausea and sometimes ulceration and bleeding. Some patients exhibit hypersensitivity to NSAIDs and can experience rashes and oedema. NSAIDs can worsen their symptoms for some asthmatics.

Prostaglandins have a role in regulating stomach acid and also in the maintenance of the gastric mucosa, so the inhibition of prostaglandins by NSAIDs explains their adverse gastro-intestinal effects. Figure 6.11 shows how closely related are the pathways that produce inflammatory and non-inflammatory prostaglandins. The two forms of cyclo-oxygenase, COX-1 and COX-2, are very similar in structure so it is little wonder that NSAIDs targeted at the inflammatory enzyme COX-2 may also block and inhibit the action of the non-inflammatory enzyme COX-1 that maintains tissue homoeostasis.

### IN PRACTICE

Although some NSAIDs are available OTC (over the counter) from chemists and even supermarkets, they are not as safe as many would believe. This is especially so in elderly patients who are more susceptible to bleeding as a side-effect of NSAIDs and for whom the consequences of bleeding are more likely to be serious. NSAIDs also increase risk in elderly patients suffering from cardiac or renal disease.

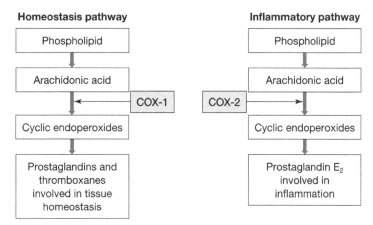

**Figure 6.11** Showing how closely related are the inflammatory and non-inflammatory pathways that produce prostaglandins. Drugs targeted at COX-2 may also bind to and inhibit the action of COX-1.

## Selective COX-2 inhibitors

This group of drugs includes **celecoxib** and **etoricoxib** and has the same basic mechanism of action as other NSAIDs such as **ibuprofen** and **diclofenac**. The key difference is that this group has a high specificity for COX-2 and so is useful in the treatment of chronic inflammatory diseases such as osteoarthritis and rheumatoid arthritis where the long-term use of conventional NSAIDs could prove problematical. Because these drugs are highly specific for COX-2, they do not inhibit COX-1 appreciably and therefore should not affect the production of those non-inflammatory prostaglandins involved in normal tissue homeostasis. In particular, they should not cause gastro-intestinal problems as can the long-term use of conventional NSAIDs.

Unfortunately these drugs have had a chequered history and over the past few years several have been withdrawn because of concerns over their safety due to evidence that they caused an increase in the rate of heart attacks and liver toxicity. At the time of writing (2012) only **celecoxib** and **etoricoxib** remain on licence as general analgesics and neither of these drugs is recommended for patients with coronary artery disease. **Parecoxib** is licensed only for short-term post-operative use.

## Paracetamol

**Paracetamol** is a non-anti-inflammatory, non-steroidal that has mainly antipyretic (fever reducing) and analgesic properties. Its mechanism of action is by no means well understood but current research suggests that as well as inhibiting COX-2, one of its metabolites may act as an agonist for cannabinoid receptors in the central nervous system. Because it has little effect on normal prostaglandin production, it is relatively free of those side-effects commonly caused by conventional NSAIDs, in particular gastro-intestinal irritation.

Although the short-term use of **paracetamol** at therapeutic doses produces relatively few side-effects, liver damage can unfortunately occur at only two to three times the therapeutic dose. This is due to the build-up in the liver of *N-acetyl-para-benzoquinoneimine*, a hepatotoxic metabolite of **paracetamol** that at normal doses is usually present only in small amounts. Permanent liver damage can result unless the patient is treated quickly with an antidote such as intravenous **acetylcysteine**. People who are malnourished or taking liver-enzyme inducing drugs (see Chapter 3) are particularly at risk of liver damage.

Prescribing **paracetamol** to very young children needs to be done with care, especially if they are being given over-the-counter medication by their parents who may not appreciate that common cough and antipyretic remedies can contain appreciable amounts of **paracetamol**.

Go on then, why are there no analgesics in Africa?

> Why are there no analgesics in Africa?

**Because the parrots eat 'em all**

I'll need an analgesic after that joke . . . !

---

**CASE STUDY**

Anne is 60, has been admitted to hospital for a hip replacement and complains of post-operative pain. You are aware that she suffers from angina and has had a stomach ulcer and are worried that conventional NSAIDs such as **diclofenac** are likely to cause gastric bleeding. Would a COX-2 inhibitor such as **etoricoxib** be suitable to help ease Anne's pain?

---

*Comment on case study* The use of conventional NSAIDs such as **diclofenac** where someone is at risk from gastro-intestinal bleeding is not advised and even selective COX-2 inhibitors should only be used with caution. However, Anne also has angina, which is indicative of coronary artery disease. This means that she is at risk of a heart attack so COX-2 inhibitors are definitely not suitable for her as they increase the risk of coronary problems. **Paracetamol**, which is not associated with gastric bleeding or a heart attack, might be a better choice. If the pain is severe then an opioid may be indicated, perhaps **co-codamol**, a compound of **codeine** and **paracetamol**. Oral solutions of **morphine** could be considered if **codeine** is not well tolerated.

## Anti-inflammatory steroids

Anti-inflammatory steroids mimic the action of natural glucocorticoids such as hydrocortisone and corticosterone – stress hormones secreted by the adrenal gland in response to injury, stress, severe infection and pain. They have a general immunosuppressive activity, as well as increasing the metabolism of carbohydrate and protein and reducing inflammation. Glucocorticoids increase the supply of glucose, triglycerides and amino acids to ensure the nutrient supply to key organs such as the brain and to provide materials for the repair of tissues. Although it may seem strange, glucocorticoids also limit the inflammatory response during injury, presumably to limit damage that may occur from excessive activity in the immune system.

Anti-inflammatory corticosteroids include **beclometasone**, **betamethasone**, **cortisone**, **hydrocortisone**, **prednisolone** and **dexamethasone** that have a variety of uses including the reduction of inflammatory pain in rheumatoid arthritis, the prevention of asthma attacks, the treatment of psoriasis and also immunosuppression after transplantation to prevent rejection.

Being derivatives of cholesterol, corticosteroids are lipid in nature and can therefore pass through the cell membrane without requiring a transporter protein. They act deep inside the cell, in the nucleus where they bind to receptors that control the production of proteins. Their anti-inflammatory action is thought to be due to the fact that they reduce the release of *cytokines* – chemical signals released by immune cells such as neutrophils, mast cells and macrophages. As we saw earlier in the chapter, inflammation results in pain, so any group of drugs that have an anti-inflammatory action will reduce nociceptive pain.

### IN PRACTICE

The long-term use of systemic glucocorticoid drugs can suppress the activity of the adrenal gland, resulting in reduced levels of natural glucocorticoids. If steroid drugs are withdrawn abruptly, this can leave the adrenal cortex insufficient time to recover, and circulating glucocorticoids, both synthetic and natural, can be so low as to cause severe hypotension and even death. Patients on long-term systemic steroids should carry a Steroid Treatment Card that explains this risk.

The long-term use of systemic glucocorticoids is problematical. Elevated blood glucose levels can result in Type 2 diabetes, and immunosuppression can result in infections. Bone metabolism can be adversely affected, resulting in *osteoporosis*, thinning of the bones, and growth can be retarded in children. Metered dose inhalers used in asthma deliver corticosteroids in a formulation that produces the maximum anti-inflammatory effect in the bronchioles with the minimum systemic effect, thus allowing their safe long-term use.

*Osteoporosis* is a condition where the bones become porous and weak. It is more common in women and often progresses more quickly after the menopause when female hormone levels begin to decline.

## Drugs for chronic inflammatory diseases

Rheumatoid arthritis is a complex and unpleasant disease whose pathophysiology is still not fully understood. It is essentially an auto-immune disease where the body's immune system malfunctions, producing inflammation, especially in the synovial joints of the hands and feet which become swollen, deformed and painful. The treatment of arthritis is a specialist area and the drugs involved are often complex in their action, expensive and their availability (or lack of it) via the NHS is sometimes a matter of controversy. Whilst non-steroidal anti-inflammatory drugs can help control the symptoms of rheumatoid arthritis, disease-modifying anti-rheumatic drugs (DMARDs) may actually slow the progression of the disease. Most of the drugs used have an immunosuppressive and anti-inflammatory action. The most commonly encountered are **methotrexate, sulfasalazine, penicillamine** and **sodium aurothiomalate**. Although these drugs have been used for many years, their mechanism of action is still not fully understood. Newer drugs have been developed more recently based on monoclonal antibodies, including **adalimumab, certolizumab pegol, golimumab** and **infliximab**, that target the inflammatory cytokine, *tumour necrosis factor-alpha* (TNFα). **Rituximab** targets a protein on B lymphocytes and **tocilizumab** targets *interleukin-6* (IL-6) receptors. **Abatacept, anakinra** and **etanercept** are all relatively new *fusion proteins* with immunological targets within the inflamed joint. Whilst the targets of these new, high-tech drugs have been characterised, their precise mechanism of action is still being investigated.

Should we be using drugs if we don't know how they work?

Ideally we should understand how drugs work but if we insisted on this for all our drugs, we would find some big gaps in the pharmacopoeia. Often drugs are in use for many years before scientists discover their mechanism of action. Most importantly, we need to be assured of their efficacy and safety.

## Opioid analgesics

**Morphine** and its relatives make up the opioid analgesics, perhaps the strongest and most effective painkillers in current use. It is closely related to the illegal narcotic heroin but as **morphine** is less lipid-soluble, it is slower to cross the blood–brain barrier and produce the euphoric effects of heroin. **Morphine** is obtained from opium, the sap of the poppy *Papaver somniferum* that is grown in a band of south Asian countries from Afghanistan to Thailand. Current opioids include **morphine, buprenorphine, codeine, diamorphine** (heroin), **dipipanone, fentanyl, hydromorphone, meptazinol, methadone, oxycodone, pethidine, tapentadol** and **tramadol**. Each opioid drug has its own benefit with regard to speed of onset, duration of effect and side-effects, but **morphine** itself is generally thought of as the most valuable analgesic for severe pain.

As we saw earlier in this chapter, the body possesses its own analgesic system which damps down incapacitating pain immediately after injury. This involves the release of opioid-like peptides that block the transmission of nervous impulses between the afferent nociceptive neurons, thus inhibiting the experience of pain. Efferent neurons from the brain descend the spinal cord to synapse with the afferent nociceptive neurons in the dorsal horn. Here they release the opioid-like peptides such *as β-endorphin, dynorphin and enkephalins* that block the synaptic transmission of the afferent neurons and thus reduce the experience of pain.

The opioid-like peptides inhibit synaptic transmission by binding to opioid receptors on the pre-synaptic membrane and the post-synaptic membrane of the synapse. On the pre-synaptic membrane they inhibit the opening of the calcium channels and so prevent the release of the neurotransmitter that sends the signal to the receiving neuron. On the post-synaptic membrane, the opioid-like peptides bind to opiate receptors and make the membrane less responsive to stimulation by neurotransmitters. As **morphine** and other opioid drugs are similar in molecular structure to the opioid-like peptides, they bind to the same opioid receptors and produce the same effect – inhibition of the pain transmission across the synapse (Figure 6.12).

*Side-effects* Any drug that has such a strong effect on the nervous system will almost inevitably be associated with unwanted effects. There are opioid receptors on various parts of the body and it is the action of opioid drugs on these receptors that is responsible for most of the side-effects. Nausea and vomiting, especially after initial administration, can be a problem, as can respiratory depression with some opioids, believed to be due to a reduction in the sensitivity of respiratory centres in the brain stem to carbon dioxide, the main driver of breathing. A decrease in gastro-intestinal motility is another problem with opioids, especially **codeine**.

**CASE STUDY**

Stan has terminal cancer and is receiving palliative care at home, which includes oral **morphine** to help with the pain. He is relatively pain free with the prescribed medication but complains of constant nausea and also constipation. What would you advise?

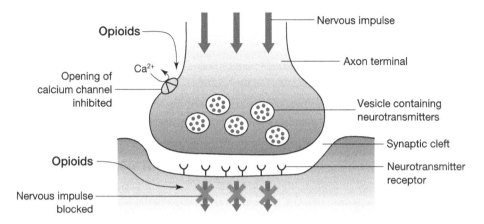

**Figure 6.12** Opioids bind to opioid receptors (not shown) and inhibit the transmission of nervous impulses across the synapses between pain neurons in the spinal cord.

*Comment on case study* Nausea and constipation are common side-effects of **morphine** but Stan's pain is under control, which is important for patients with terminal cancer. Pain control in palliative care is a specialist area and any changes to his medication should be done with caution. Exercise often helps with constipation but this is unlikely to be possible for Stan so dietary changes or a laxative might help. There are anti-nausea drugs such as **metoclopramide** and **haloperidol** that might help with the nausea.

## Drugs used for neuropathic pain

Neuropathic pain is pain caused by neurological dysfunction rather than the stimulation of nociceptive neurons by injury, inflammation, etc. This makes pain relief problematical because the pain is not following the normal neural pain pathways that can be targeted by conventional analgesics. Sometimes analgesics such as **paracetamol**, non-steroidal anti-inflammatory drugs (NSAIDs), **codeine**, etc., have an effect on neuropathic pain but the results are unpredictable. Anti-depressants such as the tricyclic **amitriptyline** can be effective but they work by a poorly understood mechanism, separate to their action on depression. Anti-epileptic drugs such as **gabapentin**, **pregabalin**, **carbamazepine** and **sodium valproate** inhibit excitable neurons in epilepsy and have a similar action in neuro-pathic pain. Generally the treatment of neuropathic pain can be difficult because the mechanism that causes the pain is poorly understood. It is, therefore, often a matter of carefully trying different drugs and monitoring their effects to see which works best.

## Drugs for headaches and migraine

Occasional, mild headaches generally respond to over-the-counter (OTC) analgesics, as single drugs or compound proprietary formulations. Sometimes, caffeine is included with **paracetamol** or **ibuprofen** but the evidence for its efficacy is weak. Regular or severe headaches need proper medical assessment to exclude a more serious underlying problem. Migraine headache may also respond to simple OTC analgesics such as **aspirin**, **paracetamol**, **ibuprofen** or perhaps **tolfenamic acid**, a non-steroidal licensed specifically for migraine. Where other symptoms are present anti-migraine drugs such as serotonin (5-HT) agonists can be used. These bind to specific receptors on cranial arteries, inducing vasoconstriction and so reducing blood flow to areas of the brain associated with migraine symptoms. These drugs include **almotriptan**, **eletriptan**, **frovatriptan**, **naratriptan**, **rizatriptan**, **sumatriptan** and **zolmitriptan**. Ergot-derived drugs such as **ergotamine tartrate** are now used less frequently due to their side-effects.

Various drugs can be used for the prophylaxis of migraine to help those who experience frequent attacks but only the antihistamine and 5-HT agonist **pizotifen** is currently licensed or recommended. In these patients, some thought should be given to identifying and avoiding the potential migraine trigger.

### CASE STUDY

Dave works as a journalist on a local newspaper; his hours are irregular and his job stressful. He spends a lot of time driving and meals during the day are mostly snacks – sandwiches or chips. Recently, the occasional headaches he suffered from have become more frequent and intense, some of them developing into migraines. He says he needs to take painkillers nearly every day but they no longer seem to help much. What would you suggest?

*Comment on case study* Dave's stressful lifestyle is probably a contributory cause of his headaches. Paradoxically, the regular use of analgesics can sometimes cause headaches. More drugs are not the answer to Dave's problem. He can't do much about his demanding job but he could try to make time for activities that help reduce stress. Swimming or jogging before or after work are both good for relieving stress – and a healthier diet should help. If the headaches persist then Dave should talk to his GP as further tests may be necessary.

## Local anaesthetics

All local anaesthetics in current use are derivatives or analogues of cocaine, a drug extracted from leaves of the coca plant, *Erythroxylum coca,* grown in South America. For thousands of years South American Indians have chewed the leaves of the coca plants to relieve fatigue in the harsh climate of the high Andes. Its numbing effect was later utilised in Europe to relieve pain in surgical procedures. Current local anaesthetics in common use include **lidocaine**, **bupivacaine**, **levobupivacaine**, **mepivacaine**, **prilocaine**, **ropivacaine** and **tetracaine**.

Local anaesthetics are relatively uncomplicated in their action, blocking nervous impulses in the nociceptive neurons. All nervous impulses depend on sodium channels opening in the neuron membrane. As the nervous impulse arrives at a section of the neuron membrane, sodium channels open and this allows the impulse to move to the next section of membrane where sodium channels open, allowing the nervous impulse to move to the next section of membrane ... and so on (Figure 6.13). Potassium channels are also involved in the nervous impulse, but we will concentrate on the sodium channels as they are the main targets for local anaesthetics.

Local anaesthetics block Na⁺ channels in the membranes of nociceptive neurons. This prevents the nervous impulse travelling along the nociceptive neuron and the subsequent neurons in the pain pathway on its way to the brain. If pain signals do not reach the brain, the individual will not experience any pain (Figure 6.14).

Local anaesthetics block conduction primarily in the small-diameter afferent nociceptive neurons rather than the larger motor neurons, and this means that motor control is less affected than pain perception. However, some loss of motor function occurs, depending on procedure and dose, as anyone who has tried to eat or talk after a local anaesthetic for dental work will testify.

*Epidurals* are useful for a variety of procedures where anaesthesia of a large region of the body is required or where general anaesthesia is contra-indicated or undesirable, for example in childbirth. Epidurals can be used in general surgical procedures in the pelvic region or legs, for example hip replacement. **Lidocaine** and **bupivacaine** are used at concentrations that produce dense sensory block and usually induce moderate to dense motor block. For analgesia during labour, **bupivacaine** is used at lower concentrations than for surgical procedures and is popular as it produces less interference with motor function.

**Figure 6.13** A nervous impulse travels along a neuron as Na⁺ channels open in the cell membrane.

**Figure 6.14** A local anaesthetic blocks Na⁺ channels and halts the nervous impulse.

**IN PRACTICE**

Epidurals are very effective for operations where a general anaesthetic is undesirable. The epidural is delivered by injection into the epidural space surrounding the spinal cord. Needless to say, this is a procedure requiring special training and is invariably performed by an anaesthetist.

*Side-effects* The most significant unwanted effects result from local anaesthetics entering the circulatory system, and to prevent this problem they are often combined with **adrenaline**, a vasoconstrictor which inhibits blood flow to the area being anaesthetised – thus limiting seepage of the drug into the general circulation.

## General anaesthetics

The development of safe and reliable general anaesthesia, together with antiseptic techniques, has revolutionised surgery. Early anaesthetics involved large amounts of alcohol, which, together with a surgeon whose reputation relied on his speed, resulted in a mortality rate that persuaded many patients that the disease was preferable to the cure. The outlook for the patient improved with the introduction of anaesthetics such as chloroform and the aseptic techniques pioneered by Joseph Lister in the nineteenth century. Modern anaesthesia under the control of skilled anaesthetists now allows surgeons to perform ever more complex operations that would previously have been thought impossible.

The use of general anaesthetics is mostly confined to the operating theatre, where the drugs are invariably administered by specialist anaesthetists or under their direct supervision. Being such a specialist area, this section will just cover the basic principles of anaesthetics and the interested reader who needs greater depth is recommended to seek out one of the more specialist publications on this subject. Some suggestions for further reading are provided at the end of this chapter.

The key aims of the effective general anaesthetic are first to achieve unconsciousness (hypnosis) so that patients are unaware of the procedure and second to ensure that the procedure is pain-free (analgesia). In addition, the anaesthetic should provide a degree of sedation, render the patient immobile and ensure they have no memory (amnesia) of what occurred between the induction of anaesthesia and waking in the recovery suite. Often, a combination of drugs is used to fully achieve these aims.

General anaesthetics can be divided broadly into two groups, the intravenous anaesthetics and the inhalational anaesthetics. The intravenous anaesthetics include **propofol, thiopental sodium, etomidate** and **ketamine**. These are often used to induce anaesthesia, which is then maintained for the duration of the procedure by inhaled anaesthetics. **Propofol** on its own is also sometimes used to maintain anaesthesia.

Inhalational anaesthetics, generally used to maintain anaesthesia, include **desflurane, halothane, isoflurane, sevoflurane** and **nitrous oxide**.

Human consciousness is not well understood and consequently the mechanism of action of general anaesthetics is not well understood. Apart from **ketamine** and **nitrous oxide**, the anaesthetics mentioned above are all believed to enhance the action of GABA (gamma-aminobutyric acid) synapses in the CNS by binding to GABA (subtype A) receptors – GABA$_A$. It has been found that sub-classes of the GABA$_A$ receptor are present in different parts of the brain, which may explain the different action of anaesthetics on the brain. For example, an anaesthetic binding to the GABA$_A$ receptors in the *hippocampus* and *amygdala* may cause amnesia while binding to the GABA$_A$ receptors on the thalamus and cortex may cause unconsciousness. **Ketamine** is a non-competitive inhibitor of NMDA (N-methyl-D-aspartate) receptors in the spinal cord which interferes with pain transmission. **Nitrous oxide** appears to have an effect that enhances the action of endogenous opioids in the spinal cord but its precise mechanism of action is not well understood.

**DID YOU KNOW . . .** that the propensity of nitrous oxide to cause euphoria and giggling gave nitrous oxide the popular name of 'laughing gas'? Developed as an anaesthetic in the early nineteenth century by the engineer James Watt, it was quickly adopted by the British upper classes and 'laughing gas parties' became very popular for a time.

Other associated drugs that may be found in the operating theatre include sedatives, generally benzodiazepines such as **diazepam, lorazepam, midazolam** and **temazepam** (see Chapter 11). These help relieve the anxiety and fear that patients naturally experience before undergoing an operation. Opioid analgesics such as **alfentanil, fentanyl** and **remifentanil** have a rapid onset of action and are used to ensure a pain-free procedure. Muscle relaxants such as **atracurium, rocuronium, vecuronium** and **suxamethonium** are used to prevent spasm during surgery and also to allow the insertion of a tracheal tube to assist breathing (intubation). As with the general anaesthetics themselves, the use of these adjunctive drugs is a specialist area.

**A QUICK RECAP on drugs used in the management of inflammation and pain**

- Non-steroidal anti-inflammatory drugs (NSAIDs) target the COX-2 enzyme responsible for producing the inflammatory prostaglandin PGE$_2$.

- NSAIDs can also inhibit COX-1 enzyme, which has a variety of non-inflammatory functions in the body. This may produce some of the side-effects associated with NSAIDs.

- Paracetamol is a widely used analgesic drug without an anti-inflammatory action.
- Anti-inflammatory steroids such as prednisolone act by suppressing activity in the immune cells involved in inflammation.
- NSAIDs can help relieve symptoms in chronic inflammatory diseases but specialist disease-modifying anti-rheumatic drugs (DMARDs) can slow the progression of the disease.
- Opioid drugs mimic natural opioid-like peptides that work in the synapses between nociceptive neurons to dampen pain after injury.
- Neuropathic pain is often idiopathic and difficult to treat.
- Headaches can be treated with analgesics and migraines may respond to serotonin (5HT) agonists.
- Local anaesthetics block sodium ion channels in nociceptive neurons, and this inhibits the transmission of pain signals to the brain.
- General anaesthetics have actions in the central nervous system that induces analgesia, hypnosis and amnesia.

## REFERENCES AND FURTHER RECOMMENDED READING

Books

Bennett, M. (2010) *Neuropathic Pain* (Oxford Pain Management Library). Oxford University Press.

Peck, T.E., Hill, S.A. & Williams, M. (2008) *Pharmacology for Anaesthesia and Intensive Care* (3rd edn). Cambridge University Press.

Smith S., Scarth, E. & Sasada, M. (2011) *Drugs in Anaesthesia and Intensive Care* (4th edn). Oxford University Press.

Websites

All recommended websites are open access – but free registration is sometimes required.

Medscape: rheumatology – http://emedicine.medscape.com

The Oxford Pain Internet Site – http://www.medicine.ox.ac.uk/bandolier/

The British Pain Society – http://www.britishpainsociety.org/

## Test yourself

Now you have finished reading this chapter it is worthwhile finding out how much you have learned and remembered. Pain control is an important part of clinical practice so it is important that you understand the action of the various anaesthetics and analgesics.

*The answers to these questions are at the end of the book (see p. 315).*

1 What is the usual clinical definition of pain?

2 We generally divide pain into two types: *nociceptive* and _____.

3 Another way that pain can be categorised is into *acute* and _____.

4 What kind of stimuli would activate nociceptive neurons?

5 Describe the route of signals to the brain of a painful stimulus to a finger.

6 What is the function of opioid-like peptides?

7 Name the five key symptoms of inflammation.

8 Outline the pathway that results in the synthesis of prostaglandins and thromboxanes.

9 The synthesis of prostaglandins and thromboxanes depends on a cyclo-oxygenase enzyme that exists in two forms. Which form is involved in inflammation?

10 What is the role of prostaglandin $E_2$ in inflammation?

11 Why might an NSAID cause the side-effect of gastro-intestinal bleeding?

12 Why is overdosing with **paracetamol** dangerous?

13 List five common side-effects of opioid drugs.

14 How do local anaesthetics such as **lidocaine** prevent pain during minor surgical procedures?

15 Name the two main classes of general anaesthetics.

Answers to the questions on p. 142.

1 Peripheral nervous system.

2 Afferents carry information into the CNS.

3 A neuron is a single nerve cell whereas a nerve is a collection of neurons protected by a sheath of connective tissue.

4 Sympathetic and parasympathetic.

5 Motor neurons control muscles.

# Chapter 7

# Disorders and drugs of the digestive system

This chapter explains the structure and function of the digestive system, the disorders and pathologies associated with the digestive system and the action of the major drug groups used in their treatment.

**CONTENTS**

The chapter contains some brief case studies and finishes off with self-test questions so you can make sure you have understood the physiology of the digestive system, associated disorders and the pharmacology of drugs used to treat those disorders.

**IN PRACTICE**

Whatever your branch of clinical practice, you will encounter patients with digestive problems. Sometimes digestive disorders will be the prime reason for them seeking treatment while other patients regard problems such as indigestion, heartburn or constipation as normal and would self-medicate with over-the-counter proprietary medicines. Frequently, digestive problems are *iatrogenic* – a direct consequence of treatment. Examples would be nausea caused by drugs or constipation caused by prolonged stays in hospital. Whatever their cause, digestive disorders are very common and this is why you need to understand the processes of digestion, the nature of common disorders and the drugs available to treat them.

*Iatrogenic* is when a patient suffers adverse consequences from treatment. This could be a hospital-acquired infection such as MRSA or adverse reactions from a clinical procedure or drug.

## Introduction

Have you ever regretted eating that second helping of pudding? Have you ever thought the hygiene of the fast-food restaurant may have left something to be desired? Perhaps a change in diet on holiday left you feeling bloated and less regular than normal? We have all experienced these problems occasionally and may well have used some over-the-counter (OTC) medications such as indigestion tablets or laxatives to help to ease the symptoms. While unpleasant, these problems of the gastro-intestinal tract are generally temporary and not serious. Within a few hours or days they resolve themselves and we are back to normal. For this reason in this chapter, some problems such as indigestion, constipation and diarrhoea are being referred to as disorders rather than pathologies. Some disorders, of course, can develop into something more serious, truly deserving of the term pathology. Diarrhoea, for example, can have many causes and mostly the problem is just mildly irritating but sometimes, especially in the very young or very elderly, it can be a life-threatening crisis requiring hospitalisation and IV fluid replacement. Heartburn can affect most people occasionally and most sufferers would regard it as a minor problem that can be alleviated with a proprietary antacid from the local pharmacy, but it can occasionally develop into the more serious condition, *ulcerative oesophagitis*. Those problems truly deserving of the pathology title such as *peptic ulcers, ulcerative colitis* and *Crohn's disease* generally require specialist treatment and although some of the drugs mentioned later in the chapter are part of the treatment regime, detailed discussion of their use is beyond the remit of this introductory book.

**WHERE ARE WE STARTING FROM?**

In this chapter we shall examine the digestive system in relation to the common disorders that can affect most of us – indigestion, constipation, etc. Most of us will be familiar with the basic structure and function of the digestive system but let's start off with the usual short quiz to find out how much you know before we begin.

1   What is the name of the muscular tube that transfers food from the mouth to the stomach?

_____

2   What organ secretes digestive enzymes into the duodenum?

_____

3   What is the large organ that produces bile?

_____

4   Proteins are important nutrients and the digestive system breaks them down into their component parts called . . .

_____

5   Would semi-digested food leaving the stomach first encounter the large or small intestine?

_____

*Answers are at the end of the chapter on p. 186.*

How did you do? If you got all five correct, then you will find this chapter relatively straightforward. If not, then we cover the basic physiology of the digestive system in the first part of this chapter.

## 7.1   The physiology of the digestive system

The principal task of the digestive system is to transfer the nutrients from the food we eat into our body, where those nutrients will be used for processes such

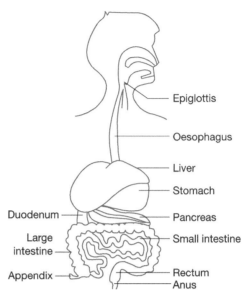

Figure 7.1 Layout of the digestive system.

as energy, protein production and general tissue maintenance. The digestive system is basically a tube that runs from the mouth to the anus (Figure 7.1). During the passage of food along this tube, various chemicals and enzymes are added to break down the food into its component parts. The muscular walls of the gut squash and squeeze the food along the system, which aids the process of breakdown.

There are various accessory organs associated with the digestive system such as the pancreas that secretes a variety of digestive enzymes into the duodenum to assist with the breakdown of food into its component parts. The liver also deserves a mention as it plays a key role in lipid metabolism; it is therefore targeted by drugs such as statins and, as we saw in Chapter 3, the liver plays a key role in drug metabolism. The gall bladder stores the bile produced by the liver and secretes it into the duodenum via the bile duct where it assists in the digestion of lipids.

In Chapter 1 we examined the three main groups of nutrients – carbohydrates, proteins and lipids. We discussed how they need to be in their smallest component parts in order to be suitable for use by our cells. Thus, polysaccharides such as starch need to be broken down into monosaccharides such as glucose, and the proteins need to be disassembled into their component amino acids. Lipid digestion is quite complex but most are broken down into fatty acid molecules that eventually find their way into the bloodstream via the lymphatic system. This is the prime role of the digestive system; to make unpromising chunks of organic matter such as pizza, sausages, salad and chips into molecules small enough to be absorbed from the gut into the body (Figure 7.2).

**Figure 7.2** Nutrients are broken down in the digestive system into their main component parts that can then be absorbed into the bloodstream and transported to the cells of the body.

> **KEY FACT**
>
> The digestive system contributes to homeostasis by maintaining the supply of essential nutrients to the body.

The first stage of the digestive process starts in the mouth. Teeth accomplish mechanical digestion by chewing and chemical digestion is achieved by saliva produced by salivary glands. As food is passed to the back of the mouth it triggers the *swallowing reflex*.

Saliva, produced by salivary glands in response to the taste and smell of food, has several functions. It begins the digestion of carbohydrates by the enzyme *amylase*, which breaks down polysaccharide starches into more simple sugars – disaccharides and monosaccharides. Saliva also moistens food, allowing it to be swallowed. Antibacterial enzymes in saliva keep the mouth clean and kill bacteria present on food. Saliva also rinses away food debris that may serve as a nutrient source for bacteria.

> **IN PRACTICE**
>
> Any diseases or drugs that inhibit the production of saliva can result in recurrent mouth infections. AIDS patients and those receiving chemotherapy for cancer are at particular risk.

After chewing, food is swallowed and passes down the oesophagus by a ripple of muscular activity called *peristalsis*. At the junction of the oesophagus and trachea, a small flap of cartilage called the epiglottis prevents food and drink entering the lungs.

> *Peristalsis* explains how you can swallow food even when hanging upside down. The muscles surrounding the digestive tract contract sequentially like a Mexican wave that pushes the food along (even defying gravity).

**Figure 7.3 Cross-sectional diagram of the stomach.**

The stomach is basically a large, muscular bag that stores food before releasing it gradually into the duodenum and small intestine at a rate appropriate for optimal digestion and absorption (Figure 7.3). Muscular contractions by the stomach help to break down food mechanically, while hydrochloric acid (HCl) and the enzyme *pepsin* start to break down proteins chemically. The lining of the stomach, the *gastric mucosa*, is protected from its own acid digestive juices by a layer of mucus that is produced by secretory cells. The *gastro-oesophageal sphincter* (also called the *cardiac sphincter*) at the entrance of the stomach prevents regurgitation into the oesophagus and the *pyloric sphincter* between the stomach and the duodenum controls the passage of food between the two regions. Sphincters are bands of muscle cells that contract to form a kind of one-way valve. The acidic pulp that empties from the stomach into the duodenum is called chyme.

### IN PRACTICE

The lumen of the stomach is generally free of bacteria because they are killed by its acidity of pH 2–3. However, one bacterium, *Helicobacter pylori*, seems to thrive at this high level of acidity. *H. pylori* were originally thought of as relatively harmless, but are now known to be one of the main causes of peptic ulcers.

In order to understand the mechanism of certain key drug groups discussed later in section 7.3, it is necessary to explain the mechanism whereby the gastric mucosa produces hydrochloric acid (HCl).

Hydrochloric acid is made up of hydrogen ions ($H^+$) and chloride ions ($Cl^-$). These are secreted separately by the parietal cells of the gastric mucosa and form HCl in the lumen of the stomach:

$$H^+ + Cl^- \rightarrow HCl$$

Note that as the positive charge on the hydrogen ion is cancelled out by the negative charge on the chloride ion, HCl is written without a charge symbol. The hydrogen ion is quite important because its concentration in a solution deter-mines the acidity of that solution. The hydrogen ion is in fact the 'H' in pH and the more hydrogen ions there are, the more acidic is the solution. A hydrogen ion is also effectively a proton. In Chapter 2 we discussed ions and found that they are (usually) atoms that have gained or lost a negatively charged electron. Figure 7.4 shows the structure of a hydrogen atom (one positively charged proton and one negatively charged electron) and the hydrogen ion, a single, naked proton.

The hydrogen ion is a hydrogen atom that has donated its electron so that there only remains a naked, positively charged proton, i.e. a hydrogen ion. The hydrogen ions are actively pumped by the *parietal* cells of the gastric mucosa into the lumen of the stomach via a proton pump driven by ATP. The movement of positively charged ions into the lumen pulls the negatively charged chloride ions in the same direction, into the lumen of the stomach where they combine to form hydrochloric acid. The parasympathetic nervous system stimulates digestion by increasing the release of HCl and pepsin, especially after the consumption of food. Receptors on the secretory cells of the mucosa are stimulated by acetylcho-line released by parasympathetic neurons, the hormone *gastrin* and histamine released by adjacent mast cells (Figure 7.5).

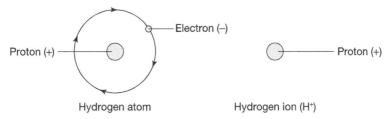

Figure 7.4 A hydrogen atom, showing the relationship of the proton and electron (not to scale) in comparison with a hydrogen ion.

Figure 7.5 The release of hydrochloric acid by the parietal cells is promoted by acetylcholine, histamine and gastrin.

**KEY FACT**

The secretion of pepsin and HCl is stimulated by histamine, the hormone gastrin and the parasympathetic nervous system releasing acetylcholine.

Moving on from the stomach we come to the duodenum and the pancreas – an important accessory digestive organ that secretes a variety of enzymes, including *amylase*, *proteases* and *lipase* into the duodenum. Amylase breaks down starch into simple sugars and proteases break down proteins into amino acids. Lipases break down fats with the aid of bile, secreted by the liver, stored in the gall bladder and then released into the duodenum. Alkaline bicarbonate is also secreted by the pancreas to neutralise the acid chyme and provide a pH more suitable for the pancreatic enzymes. The pancreas also has an endocrine function, secreting the hormones *insulin* and *glucagon* involved in the regulation of blood glucose.

**Insulin** and **glucagon** are released by the pancreas to regulate blood glucose. High blood glucose causes insulin to be released, whereas glucagon is released when blood glucose is low. Insulin lowers blood glucose by stimulating cells to take it in from the blood. Glucagon causes the liver to release stored glucose into the blood.

The small intestine consists of the *duodenum*, *jejunum* and *ileum*. It is the part of the digestive system where most food is broken down into its basic component parts then absorbed into the bloodstream for distribution to the tissues and cells of the body. The walls of the small intestine contain many folds and projections that increase its surface area in order to optimise the absorption of nutrients (the larger the surface area, the faster the rate of absorption). From the small intestine the remaining undigested material passes into the *caecum* and the colon or large intestine.

**DID YOU KNOW ...** that the folds and projections inside the small intestine increase its surface area over 500 times compared to a smooth-walled tube? The length of the small intestine is around 6 metres but without the folds and projections it would need to be around 3 kilometres in length (which would not do much for your waistline).

The main function of the large intestine is the processing and storage of faecal matter, prior to its ejection from the body. The essentially liquid material that enters the colon is transformed into more solid faeces via water reabsorption. Little nutrient absorption occurs in the large intestine except for some vitamins, including vitamin K produced by the gut bacteria and important in blood clotting. Faeces are predominantly water (75 per cent), the remainder being the indigestible components of food, bacteria and cells sloughed from the wall of the digestive tract.

The faeces are expelled by downward pressure on abdominal muscles, generally in response to the *defecation reflex*, triggered by faeces congregating at the end of the colon and stimulating stretch receptors.

**A QUICK RECAP on the physiology of the digestive system**

- The principal function of the digestive system is to break down food into its component parts that can be easily absorbed into the blood for distribution to the cells of the body.
- Starches are broken down into simple sugars, lipids into fatty acids and proteins into amino acids. The breakdown of food is done chemically and mechanically.
- Accessory organs such as the liver and pancreas secrete enzymes and other chemicals into the digestive tract to help to break down food.
- Most absorption takes place in the small intestine consisting of the duodenum, the jejunum and the ileum.
- Faecal matter in the large intestine is mainly undigested food, bacteria and cells from the lining of the digestive tract.
- Water is absorbed as the faeces move through the large intestine along with some vitamin K produced by resident bacteria.

## 7.2    Disorders of the digestive system

Diseases can affect any part of the digestive system from the mouth to the anus, and although some can be serious, many common problems such as indigestion, heartburn, diarrhoea and constipation are relatively minor but unpleasant enough to detract from our enjoyment of life.

### Disorders of the upper digestive system

Stomach problems are often of uncertain origin and symptoms can be rather vague in nature, including discomfort, bloating, pain and nausea. Common names for these problems include indigestion and heartburn, which are referred to clinically as *dyspepsia* and gastro-oesophageal reflux. Before resorting to drugs to manage stomach problems, it is generally recommended that lifestyle changes be tried such as reducing alcohol consumption, dietary modification to avoid aggravating foods, weight reduction and smoking cessation. Using pillows to elevate the upper torso in bed can reduce reflux and help patients sleep better.

Gastro-oesophageal reflux disease (GORD) affects nearly everyone at some time and is caused by stomach acid leaking back through the gastro-oesophageal sphincter into the oesophagus and causing inflammation and pain. Remember that the stomach has a structure that enables it to withstand acid but the oesophagus does not have this protection, so if acid is regurgitated then this can cause damage, inflammation and pain. Symptoms may be worsened by coughing, lifting or by certain foods. Generally, dyspepsia and GORD are temporary problems but, as they can become chronic and perhaps indicate a more serious underlying pathology, persistent symptoms may need further clinical investigation.

**Peptic ulcers** can occur in both the stomach and the duodenum. They are caused by erosion of the gastric mucosa that exposes the underlying tissue to the corrosive influence of stomach acid. Many years ago, stress and spicy foods were considered the main causes of peptic ulcers, but we now know that the bacterium *Helicobacter pylori* is responsible for over 70 per cent of cases. Non-steroidal anti-inflammatory drugs (NSAIDs) discussed in Chapter 6 also contribute to the problem. Symptoms include pain, vomiting, a reduction in appetite and weight loss.

### CASE STUDY

Wendy is complaining of abdominal pains and nausea that have been getting worse over the past few weeks. She already suffers from rheumatoid arthritis and regularly takes OTC *ibuprofen* in addition to the anti-rheumatoid medicines prescribed by her GP. She buys her analgesics from the supermarket as they are cheaper than the high-street chemist. What would you advise?

*Comment on case study* There is a possibility that **ibuprofen** may be causing the beginning of a peptic ulcer, if Wendy has been taking it regularly for a long time. Self-medication with over-the-counter (OTC) drugs is not always advisable – especially with a long-term problem. If Wendy bought her analgesics from the high-street chemist that dispenses her GP-prescribed medicine, the pharmacist would check for side-effects or interactions. Wendy should consult her GP for a check-up and a review of her medication. There are analgesics such as **paracetamol** and **etoricoxib** that may help with the pain without causing stomach problems.

## Disorders of the lower digestive system

We now move to the other end of the digestive system and discuss two problems that will have affected nearly everyone at some time in their lives – diarrhoea and constipation.

**Diarrhoea** is the frequent passage of liquid faeces and can range from minor discomfort to an emergency requiring fluid and electrolyte replacement. Acute diarrhoea can have several causes, including food poisoning resulting in *gastro-enteritis*, inflammation caused by infection of the gastro-intestinal tract. This infection can be caused by bacterial pathogens such as *Campylobacter*, *Salmonella* and *Escherichia* and viral pathogens including *norovirus, astrovirus, adenovirus*

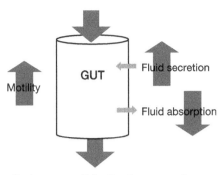

**Figure 7.6** Mechanisms that can result in diarrhoea – an increase in motility or fluid secretion or a reduction in fluid absorption.

and *rotavirus*. Chronic diarrhoea has many causes including *irritable bowel syndrome* (IBS), *Crohn's disease, diverticular disease, diverticulitis* and intolerance to foods such as milk (lactose intolerance) and wheat (*coeliac disease*).

In the large intestine there is much reabsorption of water along its length, so that by the time they are ready to be excreted, faeces should be reasonably (but not too) firm. Diarrhoea interferes with the normal processing of faecal matter by either increasing motility, resulting in insufficient time for absorption, increasing fluid secretion into the gut, or reducing fluid absorption from the gut (Figure 7.6).

**Constipation** is difficult or infrequent defecation that can have many causes, generally a reduction in motility or excessively hard faeces that may be caused by dehydration. Retention can be a problem where, for some reason, people are reluctant to defecate, perhaps finding it painful with haemorrhoids or after abdominal surgery. Dietary causes of constipation are common, especially due to lack of fibre, the indigestible cellulose part of plants. Lack of exercise and various drugs such as opiates, antispasmodics (see below) and some antidepressants can inhibit gut motility, which reduces the frequency of defecation.

**IN PRACTICE**

Constipation is very common in hospitals because the patient's mobility is restricted, their diet may be different from normal and pre-operative fluid restriction can add to the problem. Many drugs can cause constipation as a side-effect. Opioids, calcium channel blockers and many anticholinergic drugs all interfere with gut motility.

**Haemorrhoids** (piles) are enlarged and engorged blood vessels in or around the anus. They are a common and painful problem that affects most of us at some time in our lives. Generally they arise as a result of constipation, pregnancy or inactivity. Symptoms include pain on defecation, bright blood-streaked stools and itching. Piles are unpleasant but in themselves not serious and generally they clear up within a week or so, especially if constipation, a common cause, can be resolved.

> **CASE STUDY**
>
> Andy visits Jenny the practice nurse at her weekly surgery. He has been suffering from depression on and off for several years, accompanied by chronic constipation. Andy's diet appears to be acceptable but you notice that his antidepressant drug, *amitriptyline*, has anticholinergic effects. Could this be contributing to the problem of constipation?

*Comment on case study* As the name suggests, drugs with anticholinergic activity inhibit the action of acetylcholine, either blocking acetylcholine receptors or reducing general parasympathetic activity. As digestive motility and secretion are stimulated by parasympathetic activity, anticholinergic drugs such as **amitriptyline** are quite likely to reduce gut motility. If lifestyle changes do not help, a review of Andy's medication may be needed. **Amitriptyline** is no longer recommended for depression so changing to a more recent antidepressant such as **citalopram** or **fluoxetine** could help as these are less likely to cause constipation.

**Irritable bowel syndrome** (IBS) is a relatively mild problem characterised by abdominal pain and discomfort, accompanied by constipation or diarrhoea, but no observable abnormalities show up in investigative tests such as *colonoscopy*. The problem remains enigmatic in its origins which may not have a single cause. Food intolerance, stress and immune dysfunction have all been implicated. This problem should not be confused with *inflammatory bowel disease*, which includes Crohn's disease and ulcerative colitis. This is a serious problem that causes ulceration and inflammation in the lower digestive tract and, in extreme cases, perforation of the bowel wall resulting in a clinical emergency. *Antibiotic-associated colitis* is caused by the bacterium *Clostridium difficile* that flourishes after antibacterial drugs have killed off its more susceptible competitors.

**Diverticular disease** is quite common, especially in the elderly. Small pouches called *diverticula* develop in the walls of the large intestine, resulting in periodic pain in the lower abdomen. A change in eating habits to include more fibre in the diet often helps, ensuring regular bowel movements and reducing pressure on the colon wall. Less common, but more serious, is *diverticulitis*, caused by inflammation of the diverticula which can sometimes result in perforation of the large bowel.

> *Colonoscopy* is a procedure to examine the large intestine for signs of disease. After an enema to clear the bowel, a catheter with a spotlight and small video camera linked to a display screen is introduced into the colon.

**A QUICK RECAP on disorders of the digestive system**

- Dyspepsia and gastro-oesophageal reflux (indigestion and heartburn) are very common problems affecting the upper digestive tract.
- Diarrhoea is another common problem that can be acute, often caused by food poisoning, or chronic, from problems such as food intolerance or irritable bowel syndrome.

- Constipation can be caused by diet, dehydration, inactivity or drugs such as opiates.
- Haemorrhoids generally have constipation as their cause.
- Irritable bowel syndrome is a relatively common problem whose cause is poorly understood.
- Inflammatory bowel disease can be a serious problem resulting in inflammation and ulceration of the colon.
- Diverticular disease is common, especially in the elderly, and can lead to the more serious problem of diverticulitis.

## 7.3 Drugs used in the management of digestive system disorders

Mild or occasional heartburn or dyspepsia will have been experienced by most people at some time. Generally, these problems do not require a GP prescription and the local chemist will have a wide range of OTC remedies available, most of them alkaline salts, aimed at reducing the acidity of the stomach.

> **KEY FACT**
>
> Most drugs that treat gastro-oesophageal reflux disease and dyspepsia aim to reduce the acidity of the stomach contents.

### Antacids

Antacids usually contain aluminium or magnesium compounds, which, being alkaline, increase the pH of stomach chyme, making it less acid and reducing its irritating effect on the oesophagus. Common preparations include **aluminium hydroxide**, **magnesium carbonate** and **magnesium trisilicate**. Alginates extracted from seaweed are quite commonly combined with the antacids. They are believed to form a raft that floats on top of the stomach contents, reducing reflux and protecting the oesophagus from stomach acid. Most of these preparations can be obtained without prescription and their proprietary names (such as Acidex® and Gaviscon®) may already be familiar to you.

### H$_2$ receptor antagonists

This group of drugs is used to treat GORD, peptic and duodenal ulcers. Examples include **cimetidine**, **famotidine**, **nizatidine** and **ranitidine**.

As the name implies, these drugs work by blocking H$_2$ receptors in the gastric mucosa. As we saw earlier in the chapter, gastric secretions are stimulated by

**Figure 7.7** Showing how $H_2$ receptor antagonists and proton-pump inhibitors reduce the secretion of hydrochloric acid from the parietal cells of the mucosa into the lumen of the stomach.

various chemical messengers – including histamine. Histamine binds to the $H_2$ sub-class of histamine receptors on the parietal cells of the gastric mucosa and stimulates the release of hydrochloric acid. $H_2$ receptor antagonists work by blocking the $H_2$ receptors from the stimulatory effect of histamine and thus reduce the secretion of hydrochloric acid (Figure 7.7). The stomach contents become less acidic which relieves the symptoms of discomfort.

**IN PRACTICE**

**Cimetidine** especially can interact with other drugs by inhibiting P450 cytochrome enzymes in the liver (see Chapter 3). These enzymes metabolise various drugs and blocking their action can increase the serum levels of drugs such as **warfarin, phenytoin** and **aminophylline.**

## Proton-pump inhibitors

This group of drugs is used for the treatment of peptic ulcers, dyspepsia and GORD. They are also indicated for use with antibacterial drugs in the eradication of *Helicobacter pylori*. Examples of the group include **esomeprazole, lansoprazole, omeprazole, pantoprazole** and **rabeprazole.**

These drugs work by irreversibly inhibiting the proton pump in the parietal cells of the mucosa, thus preventing hydrogen ions being pumped into the lumen of the stomach, and slowing the formation of hydrochloric acid (Figure 7.7). Proton-pump inhibitors selectively accumulate in the parietal cells of the mucosa, and despite having a relatively short half-life can exert their effect for several days. The most common side-effect of these drugs is gastric discomfort, nausea, etc.

## Drugs used in the treatment of peptic ulcers

Peptic ulceration, either NSAID-induced or as a result of *Helicobacter pylori* infection, requires specialist attention so we will outline the drugs used in their treatment without going into too much detail on their mechanism of action. As discussed in Chapter 6, a side-effect of NSAIDs is gastric irritation caused by inhibiting the production of prostaglandins that maintain the gastric mucosa. **Misoprostal** is a prostaglandin analogue that helps prevent NSAID-induced ulceration, especially in those elderly patients who rely on NSAIDs for pain relief. **Tripotassium dicitratobismuthate** helps heal peptic ulcers, possibly inhibiting the formation of the gastric enzyme pepsin. **Sucralfate** reacts with hydrochloric acid to form a protective barrier around the ulcer. For peptic ulcers resulting from *Helicobacter pylori* infection, a treatment regime that eradicates the infection is recommended, combining two antibacterial drugs such as **amoxicillin**, **clarithromycin** or **metronidazole** with a proton-pump inhibitor such as **lansoprazole**.

## Drugs used in the treatment of diarrhoea

In developed countries, acute diarrhoea is unpleasant but not generally life-threatening, although neonates and the elderly may be at particular risk. In severe cases, rehydration can be required but generally the problem resolves itself in a few days. Except in cases of serious bacterial infection, it is not generally recommended that antibacterial drugs are prescribed for diarrhoea. This is because it can be difficult to determine if the problem is indeed bacterial in origin, and most cases are self-limiting. If the cause of diarrhoea is viral, no suitable antiviral drugs are available. Antimotility drugs can be used in cases of uncomplicated acute diarrhoea but are not recommended for young children.

Antimotility drugs are mainly based on drugs that have constipation as a side-effect and include **codeine phosphate, co-phenotrope, loperamide hydrochloride** and **morphine**. Opiates are well known for causing constipation by reducing gut motility and so this allows more time for the gut to reabsorb water, making the faeces less liquid and reducing the frequency of evacuation.

Some of the preparations mentioned above are combination drugs. **Co-phenotrope** is a combination of the opiate **diphenoxylate** and the anticholinergic drug **atropine**. **Morphine** is generally combined with **kaolin**, a type of clay that holds moisture and increases the viscosity of the gut contents.

## Drugs and preparations used in the treatment of constipation

Constipation is often associated with lifestyle or pathologies not directly related to the gastro-intestinal system. Treatment therefore is usually first directed at lifestyle changes where possible. Exercise, adequate fluid intake and a diet containing plenty of fresh fruit, vegetables and fibre-containing cereals are a formula for keeping the bowels regular and avoiding constipation. Many drugs such as opioids and antidepressants are well-known causes of constipation but it may not be practical or safe to change medication in the short term. Haemorrhoids make defecation painful, encouraging retention of faeces, so treating the haemorrhoids may relieve the constipation. Where pharmacological treatment is the only option to relieve constipation, there are four classes of laxatives:

- **Bulk-forming laxatives** – these are preparations high in insoluble plant cellulose. They increase the faecal mass and stimulate peristalsis. Examples include **ispaghula husk**, **methylcellulose** and **sterculia**.

- **Osmotic laxatives** – these modify the osmotic environment and pull water into the colon, which softens stools and increases faecal mass. Examples include **lactulose** and **macrogols** (polyethylene glycols).

- **Stimulant laxatives** – these increase fluid secretion into the gut, softening the stools and also stimulating peristalsis. Examples include **bisacodyl**, **dantron**, **docusate**, **sodium picosulfate** and **senna**. **Glycerol** administered via a suppository also acts as stimulant laxative.

- **5-HT$_4$ receptor agonists** – **prucalopride** stimulates peristalsis in the large intestine.

**Prucalopride** is the only drug in its class of 5-HT$_4$ receptor agonists. A relatively recent introduction to the pharmacopoeia, it is used for chronic constipation in women. This drug mimics 5-hydroxytryptamine (5-HT)/serotonin, binding to the 5-HT$_4$ sub-class of receptor on parasympathetic neurons in the gut. This promotes the release of acetylcholine which in turn stimulates peristalsis. Its women-only licence does not reflect any pathophysiological differences between the sexes, simply that the clinical trials on which the licence was based recruited mainly women.

## Drugs and preparations used in the treatment of haemorrhoids (piles)

As constipation is a common cause of haemorrhoids, the first line of treatment may be to treat the constipation, either with lifestyle changes or the drugs and preparations mentioned above. Preparations for haemorrhoids are generally designed to reduce inflammation, pain and itching. They are sold in combination preparations that may contain anti-inflammatory steroids such as **hydrocortisone**, local anaesthetics such as **lidocaine** and mild astringents such as **zinc oxide**. All may be combined into ointment or suppositories.

## Drugs used in the treatment of irritable bowel syndrome

Irritable bowel syndrome is usually managed by a variety of lifestyle modifications before resorting to drugs. Changes in diet often help with the problem but, failing that, antispasmodic drugs such as **atropine, dicycloverine, hyoscine** and **propantheline** are available. Motility is promoted by the parasympathetic stimulation of muscarinic acetylcholine receptors so inhibiting these receptors reduces gut motility. For obvious reasons, constipation is a common side-effect of these drugs.

**Alverine, mebeverine** and **peppermint oil** are also used to relieve abdominal colic and distension in IBS and diverticular disease. They relax abdominal smooth muscle but their precise mechanism of action is uncertain.

**A QUICK RECAP on drugs used in the management of digestive system disorders**

- Dyspepsia and gastro-oesophageal reflux are generally treated with drugs that reduce stomach acid, either by neutralising it with alkaline preparations or inhibiting its secretion.
- Drugs that inhibit the secretion of stomach acid include $H_2$ receptor antagonists such as **cimetidine** and proton-pump inhibitors such as **omeprazole.**
- Peptic ulceration as a result of *Helicobacter pylori* infection is usually treated by a combination of antibacterial drugs.
- Drugs used to treat diarrhoea are generally based on opioids that cause constipation as, in this case, a useful side-effect.
- Constipation is primarily treated with adjustments to lifestyle but bulk-forming, osmotic and stimulant laxatives may be useful.
- Haemorrhoids are treated with combination compounds of anti-inflammatory steroids, local anaesthetics and mild astringents.
- Treatment of IBS usually involves antimuscarinic drugs such as **dicycloverine,** and **hyoscine** that reduces gut motility and therefore spasm-induced pain.

### FURTHER RECOMMENDED READING

All recommended websites are open access (but free registration is sometimes required).

Bandolier: gastroenterology − http://www.medicine.ox.ac.uk/bandolier

Medscape: gastroenterology − http://emedicine.medscape.com/gastroenterology

NHS website − http://www.nhs.uk/Conditions/

## Test yourself

Now you have finished reading through this chapter, try answering these questions to see how much you have learned.

*The answers to these question are at the end of the book (see p. 316).*

1 Name the three sections of the small intestine.

2 Proteins are broken down into their component parts called ... ?

3 What is the enzyme in saliva that breaks down starches?

4 Name the two sphincters in the stomach.

5 Name the digestive enzyme secreted into the stomach that denatures proteins.

6 Name three chemical messengers that stimulate the release of hydrochloric acid.

7 Which organ secretes digestive enzymes into the duodenum?

8 Heartburn is the commonly used name for what disorder?

9 Which bacterium is responsible for most cases of peptic ulcer?

10 Would a reduction in motility in the large intestine be most likely to cause constipation or diarrhoea?

11 How do alginates help to reduce the symptoms of gastro-oesophageal reflux?

12 What type of receptor is targeted by **cimetidine**?

13 How do proton-pump inhibitors reduce stomach acid?

14 A side-effect of which group of drugs is useful in the treatment of diarrhoea?

15 How do osmotic laxatives work?

Answers to the questions on p. 169.

1 The oesophagus.
2 The pancreas.
3 The liver.
4 Amino acids.
5 The small intestine.

# Chapter 8

## Infection and antimicrobial drugs (bugs and drugs)

This chapter starts off with some basic microbiology, examining the nature of microbes and how they are classified into different groups, especially the pathogens. We then consider the consequences of infection, the diseases caused by microbes and finally the pharmacological action of the drugs used to treat microbial infection.

## CONTENTS

The chapter contains some brief case studies and finishes off with self-test questions to enable you to make sure that you have understood the nature of microbes, associated disorders and the pharmacology of antimicrobial drugs.

### IN PRACTICE

Drugs that treat microbial infections are extensively used in most areas of clinical practice, both in primary care and the hospital setting. In primary care, infections are very common and you will encounter patients with coughs, colds, sore throats, flu, cystitis and numerous other unpleasant but rarely fatal diseases – except perhaps in vulnerable patients such as the elderly. In hospitals, staff not only treat patients with infectious diseases but also put considerable effort into preventing uninfected patients from contracting diseases. This means that you may well find yourself in an area of clinical practice where your patients have contracted an infection or are vulnerable to contracting infections. It is important, therefore, that you have a good understanding of the nature of the various pathogenic microorganisms, the diseases they cause and how the drugs work that we use to treat microbial infections.

## Introduction

Everyone reading this will undoubtedly have suffered from a bacterial, viral or fungal infection at some time in their lives. In our environment, we are surrounded by innumerable small organisms, collectively called microbes. Although most of them are perfectly harmless, some cause disease and in our crowded world it is very easy to pick up infections. Different microbes cause different diseases, so if you have had a cold then it was caused by a virus, probably rhinovirus, which affects the upper respiratory tract (not the large African animal with a horn on its head). If you have had a sore throat, then that may have been a bacterial infection caused by *Streptococcus*. Candidiasis, commonly called thrush, will have been caused by a fungus called *Candida albicans*. All of these organisms can cause disease in humans but they are very different from each other. A bacterium is as different from a fungus or virus as we are from a dandelion. This means that the methods whereby they cause disease are different and, very importantly, the drugs that we use to combat them are very different. So, to understand antimicrobial pharmacology you really need to know something about the microbes themselves. You need to understand their structure, how they reproduce, how they are spread and how they cause infection.

Another important feature that will be covered in this chapter is how microbes, especially bacteria, can develop resistance to antimicrobial drugs. Hospital infections are constantly in the news, especially those caused by organisms such as meticillin resistant *Staphylococcus aureus* (MRSA) and *Clostridium difficile*. These organisms are causing significant problems because they quickly develop resistance to new antibacterial drugs and the use of these drugs is now much more carefully controlled in an attempt to prevent resistant strains from developing and spreading.

*Antimicrobial* drugs are widely used in hospitals and primary care, so it is important that you understand how they work and why they must be used with caution.

> *Antimicrobial (drug)* refers to any drug that is targeted at a microbe. Drugs targeted at specific groups of microbes now have specific names, thus we have antibacterial drugs, antiviral drugs, antifungal drugs, etc. The term 'antibiotic' is used less often these days.

We are going to subdivide the microbes into their various groups, but first let us define our terms. Microbes, or microorganisms, are very small organisms that can only be seen using a microscope. There are many types of microbes but most of them that cause disease belong to the following groups:

- Bacteria
- Fungi
- Viruses
- Protozoa.

There are also other small, parasitic organisms such as *helminths* (worms) that cause disease, but whether these truly fit into the category of microbes is open to debate. From a pharmacological view, these organisms cause infections, and as they are usually grouped in the pharmacopoeia with bacteria, fungi and viruses, we will include them in this chapter.

## WHERE ARE WE STARTING FROM?

In this chapter we will be exploring the wonderful world of germs, how they cause disease and, finally, how we thwart their plans with antimicrobial drugs. Even if you have a reasonable knowledge of human physiology, it may be that you have not studied microbial physiology, so you might like to try our usual short quiz to see what you know.

1   Is *Candida albicans* (the organism that causes thrush) a bacterium, a fungus or a virus?

2   What does MRSA stand for?

_____

3   Which organism is bigger: a bacterium or a virus?

_____

4   What type of organism causes the common cold?

_____

5   Is penicillin the drug of choice for a cold?

_____

*Answers are at the end of the chapter on p. 210.*

How did you do? Don't worry if you couldn't answer all of these questions – microbiology is not an everyday subject. However, you need to know the basics in order to understand microbial disease and treatment, and the following few pages will provide a good starting point for your studies.

## 8.1   How do microorganisms fit into the scheme of life?

There are many chemicals such as disinfectants and bleaches that are very effective at killing microbial cells and these are used widely to ensure that our environment, especially our hospitals, is relatively free from germs. Unfortunately, microbial cells that cause disease also live in our bodies, alongside human cells, so disinfectants and bleaches would not make very good drugs – they might kill the microbes but they would also kill us . . . ! The principle here is that antimicrobial drugs must differentiate between microbial cells and human cells – otherwise the human cells will be damaged by the drugs. Fortunately, there are some structures and proteins found within microbial cells that make them sufficiently different from human cells to allow us to target them with antimicrobial drugs. Because different groups of microbes have different structures or targets, it is first necessary to establish how the various groups fit into the scheme of life. When we have done this, we can then decide how to deal with them.

All life on the planet appears to reside within one of the five kingdoms of organisms, as shown in Figure 8.1. Bacteria form the oldest kingdom and were one of the first organisms to evolve on Earth, some three billion years ago. It is believed that all other organisms on the planet evolved from bacterial ancestors. Plants, animals, fungi and a kingdom of (mostly) single-celled organisms called *protoctista* evolved more recently, and are much more closely related to each other than they are to bacteria.

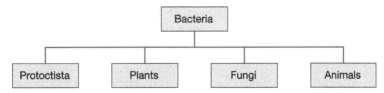

Figure 8.1 All life on Earth can be allocated to one of the five kingdoms.

That's five kingdoms − what about the viruses?

Good question. Viruses are a problem because there is some dis-agreement as to whether or not they can be classified as being alive, let alone them having a kingdom of their own. There is also uncertainty about how they are related to the other five kingdoms.

As well as dividing life into the five kingdoms, there is a more fundamental division between bacteria and other cellular organisms. Bacteria are all single-celled organisms and their cell structure is relatively simple. They do not have a nucleus and are called *prokaryotes*. All other cellular organisms such as plants, animals, fungi and protoctista have more complex cells with nuclei and are called *eukaryotes*. As viruses are not cellular they do not really fit into either category. Let us now examine our five groups of organisms that are responsible for most infectious diseases in humans, starting with bacteria.

*Prokaryote* means 'pre-nucleus' (*karyon* being Greek for nucleus). *Eukaryote* means 'true nucleus'. Bacteria are prokaryotes; all other cellular organisms (including humans) are eukaryotes.

## 8.2 Bacteria

Bacteria are undoubtedly the most successful group of organisms ever to have evolved on planet Earth. The mighty dinosaurs ruled supreme for tens of millions of years but their reign was short compared to the bacteria that emerged from unknown origins over three thousand million years ago and are still with us today. Bacteria make up the greatest biomass on the planet, bigger than all of the rainforests put together. They have adapted to live almost everywhere on the planet, from hot springs to frozen tundra, from the deepest seas to the highest mountains − so it is hardly surprising that our bodies make very pleasant, comfortable homes for bacteria.

Bacteria are small, generally between 1.0 and 2.0 μm (1 μm = 1/1000 mm), which means that they are invisible to the naked eye. They grow rapidly by cell division: one bacterium splits into two, then each of those split into two, and so on − less than 20 minutes for each cell cycle in ideal conditions. Believe it or not, in 12 hours one bacterium could theoretically divide 36 times and produce around

35 billion new cells. This is why it is dangerous to leave cooked food unrefrigerated overnight because a few hundred bacteria that settled on the food the day before have become trillions of bacteria by the next day. Our digestive enzymes and stomach acid that were quite sufficient to deal with a few hundred bacteria may be overwhelmed by the sheer numbers produced by uncontrolled overnight proliferation. The bacteria pass through the stomach into the small intestine and can cause infection along with the symptoms of food poisoning. Of course, the constant doubling rate described above is seldom encountered outside the laboratory, but even so, given the right conditions, a small colony of bacteria can quickly become a big colony.

So refrigeration doesn't kill bacteria then?

No, low temperatures slow down bacterial metabolism and so reduce the rate at which they multiply. The body's defences can cope with the small numbers of bacteria that we inevitably consume with our food every day.

## The structure of bacteria

Bacteria are diverse and come in many different shapes but they all have some common characteristics. Bacteria are single-celled organisms and although some bacteria do form aggregations, each cell is essentially self-sufficient. Also, unlike eukaryotic cells, bacteria do not have membrane-bound organelles such as mitochondria, endoplasmic reticulum, Golgi apparatus or a nucleus. Bacteria do have DNA that codes for their proteins but it is not grouped into a nucleus enclosed by a nuclear membrane. The cell wall is another unique feature of bacteria, and this is described shortly in more detail as it is an important target for some drugs.

Some bacteria are motile (able to move) and, while they are not likely to chase you down the street, they can move a few micrometres towards a more promising source of nutrients. This limited locomotion is achieved by means of *flagella*, fine whip-like structures that propel the bacteria along. The *fimbriae*, fine hair-like structures that can be seen on some bacteria, are not used for movement but are believed to be involved with attachment to the host's tissue. Figure 8.2 shows the structure of a typical bacterium.

Some bacteria such as *Clostridium* can undergo a form of hibernation by forming tough outer coats called *endospores*. These dormant structures can survive

**Figure 8.2** Structure of a typical bacterium.

long periods without water and are highly resistant to our attempts to eradicate them with detergents and disinfectants. This means that rooms and equipment that appear clean can harbour bacterial endospores that can eventually re-emerge into fully functional pathogens that can cause disease.

Most bacteria do not invade human cells but are found on the skin or epithelial tissue that lines mucus membranes. A few bacteria such as *Chlamydia* are *obligate* intracellular parasites that can only reproduce within their host's cells.

*Obligate* is a word frequently encountered in microbiology that refers to microbes with very specific nutritional or environmental requirements. Consequently, obligate intracellular parasites cannot reproduce outside of their host's cells.

## The classification of bacteria

Of all organisms, bacteria are perhaps among the most diverse and difficult to classify. Despite them all being relatively simple, single-celled organisms, they exhibit much variety in their structure and metabolism. If you look at the currently available antibacterial drugs as listed in the BNF you will see that these drugs tend to target specific groups of bacteria. These groups are described in specific terms such as *streptococcal*, *Gram positive* or *aerobic* so it is important that you spend a little time understanding basic bacterial classification.

There is a multitude of different bacteria in the environment and while most of them are relatively harmless to humans, there are quite a few that are pathogenic, i.e. they have the ability to cause disease. Common pathogenic bacteria and the infections they cause include:

- *Escherichia coli* – diarrhoea, vomiting and cystitis
- *Enterococci species* – bacteraemia (bacteria in the blood), bacterial endocarditis (infection in the heart)
- *Staphylococcus aureus* – wound infection and septicaemia
- *Salmonella species* – diarrhoea and vomiting
- *Streptococci species* – sore throat, scarlet fever, rheumatic fever, meningitis
- *Helicobacter pylori* – stomach ulcers
- *Pseudomonas aeruginosa* – pneumonia and septicaemia
- *Clostridium difficile* – colitis
- *Campylobacter species* – diarrhoea
- *Chlamydia trachomatis* – sexually transmitted infection
- *Haemophilus influenzae* – pneumonia and bacterial meningitis.

Some of these bacteria are called *opportunistic pathogens* because they only cause disease when the opportunity arises, perhaps because someone's immune system has been suppressed, either by illness or immunosuppressive drugs.

Otherwise, these bacteria live in and on us as *commensals*, generally without causing any problems. From a clinical view, it is important to know something about the different groups because to some extent, the group that a bacterium belongs to will determine the antibacterial drug chosen to target it. We could spend the whole of this book examining the classification of bacteria but we will limit ourselves to groupings that have relevance to the type of antibacterial drugs used, starting with the bacterial cell wall.

> *Commensals* are bacteria that live in and on us, benefiting from our body in terms of nutrients but not doing us any harm. They sometimes inadvertently benefit us by out-competing pathogenic bacteria and in the gut may produce useful substances such as vitamin K.

## Classification by cell wall

The structure of the bacterial cell wall can influence the type of antibacterial drug used and you will find two broad categories mentioned in the BNF – *Gram positive* and *Gram negative*. Christian Gram was a Danish microbiologist (1853–1938) who developed a technique of staining bacteria so that they could be viewed under the optical microscope. Normally, bacteria are colourless and you have to stain them with a chemical pigment such as crystal violet in order to see them. Gram found that all the bacteria he tested seemed to fall into two groups; those that were stained by his staining technique and those that were not. This proved such a useful tool in classifying bacteria that the two groups were named Gram positive and Gram negative in his honour. It was later found that the reason for each group's different reaction to Gram's stain was that their cell wall was significantly different in structure.

The bacterial cell wall contains a substance unique to bacteria called *peptidoglycan*. This is a complex molecule containing proteins, sugars and acids. Its purpose is to provide integrity and strength to the cell wall of the bacterium. Gram-positive bacteria have a cell wall comprising mainly of peptidoglycan whereas Gram-negative bacteria have a thin layer of peptidoglycan sandwiched between two membranes. Figure 8.3 shows a much simplified depiction of the Gram-positive and Gram-negative bacterial cell wall.

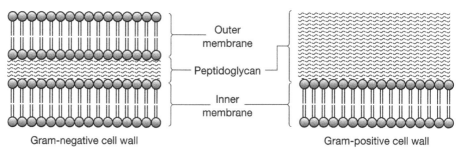

Gram-negative cell wall

Outer membrane

Peptidoglycan

Inner membrane

Gram-positive cell wall

**Figure 8.3** Simplified structure of the Gram-positive and Gram-negative cell wall.

We also need to be aware of the bacterial enzyme *transpeptidase*. This has a central role in the production of peptidoglycan and it is this enzyme that is targeted by antibacterials such as penicillins and cephalosporins. The pharmacological relevance of the cell wall structure is that, generally, Gram-negative organisms are innately more resistant to antimicrobial drugs because their cell wall is more complex and this makes drug penetration more difficult.

Gram-positive species include:

- *Enterococci species*
- *Staphylococcus aureus*
- *Streptococci species*
- *Clostridium difficile.*

Gram-negative species include:

- *Escherichia coli*
- *Salmonella species*
- *Helicobacter pylori*
- *Pseudomonas aeruginosa*
- *Campylobacter species*
- *Chlamydia trachomatis*
- *Haemophilus influenzae.*

## Classification by oxygen requirement

Some antibacterial drugs are listed as being particularly suitable for anaerobic infections so we need a brief mention of this method of grouping bacteria. Bacteria such as *Pseudomonas* require oxygen and are called *aerobes* while others such as *Clostridium* and *Chlamydia* require an oxygen-free environment and are called *anaerobes*. Whether bacteria are aerobes or anaerobes can determine the choice of antibacterial drug.

As is usual with bacteria, they refuse to divide themselves into neat categories and you will come across some that are partially aerobic and partially anaerobic. These are the *facultative anaerobes* such as *Pseudomonas*, *Staphylococci* and *Escherichia* that can switch their metabolism depending on whether oxygen is present or not.

## Classification by shape

Bacteria come in various shapes and these are used in classification (Figure 8.4). The two largest groups are *bacilli*, which are rod shaped, and *cocci*, which are spherical. The cocci can group themselves further by the way that they form aggregations. *Diplococci* join together in pairs, *streptococci* form chains and *staphylococci* aggregate into groups that look rather like bunches of grapes.

Bacilli          Diplococci          Streptococci          Staphylococci

Figure 8.4 **Some common shapes and groupings of bacteria.**

## How bacteria cause disease

We know that many bacteria are opportunistic pathogens that can multiply when conditions are amenable, but how do they actually cause disease? How is it that organisms as small as bacteria can produce such unpleasant diseases in organisms millions of times their size? Some bacteria such as *Staphylococci*, *Streptococci* and *Clostridium* release toxins, which are chemicals that damage the host cells and their membranes. Other bacteria have components of their cell wall that appear to make the bacterial cell itself intrinsically toxic. These include many Gram-negative genuses such as *Escherichia*, *Pseudomonas* and *Salmonella*. For many bacteria, the precise mechanism whereby they cause disease is not fully understood.

**DID YOU KNOW . . .** that *staphyle* is Greek for bunch of grapes? *Staphylococci* are so named because they are cocci that aggregate into groups that look rather like bunches of grapes when viewed under the electron microscope.

**A QUICK RECAP on bacteria**

- Bacteria are single-celled organisms that can reproduce very quickly by cell division.
- Bacteria are prokaryotic organisms, meaning that they do not have a true nucleus.
- Bacteria can be classified by their cell wall into Gram-positive and Gram-negative species.
- Bacteria can also be classified by their shape, their motility and their ability to tolerate oxygen.
- Many bacteria live in and on us as commensals but can cause disease when the opportunity arises. These are called opportunistic pathogens.

## Antibacterial drugs

In 1928 the Scottish microbiologist Alexander Fleming was working at St Mary's hospital in London when he accidentally discovered penicillin, the first effective antibacterial drug. Fleming found that some of his cultures of *Staphylococcus aureus* had been contaminated by the mould *Penicillium notatum* and this had killed the bacteria. Unable to manufacture the antibacterial substance produced by the mould in any quantity, Fleming went on to other work but later his discovery was taken up by two other researchers, Howard Florey and Ernst Chain. They successfully produced the antibacterial substance, now named penicillin, in sufficient quantities to save many Allied soldiers' lives in the second part of World War II. In 1945, Fleming, Florey and Chain jointly received the Nobel Prize for Medicine for their discovery of penicillin.

## Principles of antibacterial action

Antibacterial drugs target bacterial cells that are living and reproducing within the human body so if these drugs are going to kill bacterial cells and leave human cells unharmed then they will have to target structures that are found in bacterial cells but not in human cells. This is called the principle of *selective toxicity* – where a drug kills the harmful bacteria without damaging the host's cells. Fortunately, humans are eukaryotic and bacteria are prokaryotic so there are quite a few differences that we can identify as targets.

> **KEY FACT**
>
> Antibacterial drugs must target bacterial cell structures that are different from those found in eukaryotic human cells.

Some drugs, the broad spectrum antibacterials, are effective against a wide range of bacteria, both Gram-positive and Gram-negative. Other antibacterials, termed narrow spectrum, are used against specific families or groups of bacteria.

> **IN PRACTICE**
>
> Broad spectrum antibacterials can be quite useful if a bacterial infection is diagnosed but the type of bacteria that is causing the infection has not been identified. This type of prescribing is sometimes called *blind therapy*.

## Bactericidal and bacteriostatic action

Bacteria can either be killed with a drug that has a bactericidal action or their growth inhibited with a drug that has bacteriostatic activity. The benefit of killing a bacterial colony is self evident but that of inhibiting its growth less so. In the latter scenario, the body's immune system is better able to recognise and destroy a static rather than expanding colony of invading bacteria. Drugs that attack the cell wall have a bactericidal action – and by definition a bacteriostatic action. Drugs that inhibit protein synthesis tend to be more bacteriostatic, although they may also be bactericidal at higher doses.

## Antibacterials 1: drugs targeting the cell wall

This group of drugs, sometimes called the beta-lactams (β-lactams), comprises the penicillins, cephalosporins and carbapenems which are widely used and contains some of the most commonly prescribed broad spectrum antibacterials. Penicillins include **amoxicillin**, **ampicillin**, **benzylpenicillin**, **phenoxymethylpenicillin**, **flucloxacillin** and **temocillin**. Cephalosporins include **cefaclor**, **cefadroxil**, **cefalexin**, **cefixime**, **cefotaxime**, **cefpodoxime**, **cefradine**, **ceftazidime**, **ceftriaxone** and **cefuroxime**. Both groups are effective when used for various common bacterial infections such as throat infections, tonsillitis, ear infections and urinary tract infections (UTI) as well as more serious problems such as septicaemia (systemic infections), endocarditis (heart infections) and meningitis (inflammation of the lining of the brain). **Aztreonam**, also a β-lactam, is the sole representative of its group and is effective against Gram-negative aerobes. The carbapenems have a wider spectrum of activity and include **doripenem**, **ertapenem**, **imipenem** and **meropenem**.

> ### CASE STUDY
>
> Devinder arrives at your practice with her son Manjit, aged 5, who is very ill with the classic symptoms of meningitis – stiff neck, fever, vomiting, headache, etc. His mother says he is allergic to penicillin – what would you do?

*Comment on case study* Urgent referral to the nearest hospital is required because meningitis can be life-threatening. Manjit needs immediate antibacterials so a broad spectrum cephalosporin such as **cefotaxime** could overcome the problem of his allergy to penicillins. This should be administered intravenously to hasten its effects. As the child is vomiting, oral antibacterials would not be appropriate.

The penicillins, cephalosporins and carbapenems belong to a group of drugs called *β-lactam* antibacterials, so called because their molecular structure contains a functional group called a *β-lactam ring*. We try to avoid molecular structures in *Introducing Pharmacology* but the term *β-lactam* is regularly used when discussing antibacterial drugs so we need to know what it means. Figure 8.5 shows the basic structure of penicillin and cephalosporin and you will see that

**Figure 8.5** Molecular skeletons of penicillin and cephalosporin showing β-lactam ring defined by a hatched line.

they are relatively simple molecules that both contain a β-lactam ring. This ring is of pharmacological importance because, apart from it being essential to penicillin's antibacterial action, bacteria have devised cunning mechanisms to deactivate it.

A key difference between bacterial and human cells is the bacterial cell wall containing the structural molecule peptidoglycan as one of its key components. Peptidoglycan is unique to bacteria so it makes a good target for antimicrobials as human cells will be unaffected. Bacteria make peptidoglycan with the help of the bacterial enzyme transpeptidase, again unique to bacteria, and it is this enzyme that is targeted by the β-lactam antibacterials. With the inhibition of transpeptidase, bacteria cannot make their cell wall properly so it becomes unstable, causing the bacteria to lyse (burst) and die.

**DID YOU KNOW ...** that penicillin is excreted unchanged in the urine? In its early days, penicillin was so difficult to produce that doctors would collect the patient's urine, extract the penicillin and re-inject it back into the patient.

## Bacterial resistance to the β-lactam antibacterials

Before we discuss the β-lactam antibacterials further, we need to have a brief diversion into bacterial resistance. The reason for this is that the choice of antibacterial drug can be determined by whether the target organism is one that has developed resistance – or not.

We tend to think of bacterial resistance as a relatively recent phenomenon. In fact, as early as the 1940s, isolated cases of resistance to the early antibacterial drugs had been observed. Strains of *Staphylococcus aureus* were among the first organisms to exhibit resistance, but by the 1980s resistance among pathogenic bacteria was becoming widespread and creating serious problems, especially in hospitals.

Bacteria are prone to genetic mutation and in any population of a particular strain, there are likely to be a few individual bacteria that exhibit resistance to a particular antibacterial drug. Normally, a few resistant bacteria in a population of trillions should not cause problems because their numbers are relatively insignificant. However, what happens when we treat a patient with an antibacterial drug and kill all of the susceptible bacteria, leaving behind only those that are resistant to that drug? When this happens the resistant bacteria can proliferate without the constraint of competition and, because of the speed at which they can multiply, very soon they become the predominant strain (Figure 8.6). Antibacterial drugs are unable to kill them and so the resistant strains can continue to cause disease and spread to other patients, especially those who are already sick and susceptible to infection – as you might find in a hospital.

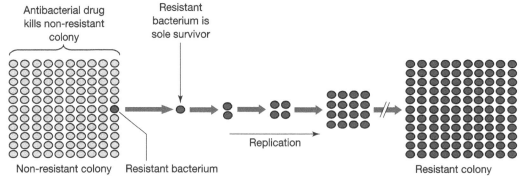

Figure 8.6 How bacterial resistance develops. An isolated resistant individual bacterium can quickly become the dominant strain when an antibacterial drug kills off the remaining bacteria in a non-resistant colony.

### IN PRACTICE

Few people like taking medicines and there is always the temptation for patients to discontinue a course of antibacterials when the symptoms start to subside. This can result in problems. Firstly, if not all of the pathogens are killed off then there is a good chance that they will re-grow and the infection will return. Secondly, the remaining bacteria may be those most resistant to the drug so the returning infection is caused by a resistant strain and more difficult to treat.

There are many ways that bacteria can develop resistance but one of the most common mechanisms is for them to produce enzymes that inactivate the antibacterial drugs. Such enzymes are the *β-lactamases*, produced by many resistant bacteria that inactivate β-lactam drugs such as penicillin and cephalosporin. The name of the enzyme group gives us a clue to the action of β-lactamases, which target and break the β-lactam ring, rendering the drugs ineffective (Figure 8.7).

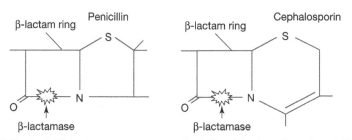

Figure 8.7 Bacterial β-lactamase enzymes attack the β-lactam ring of penicillins and cephalosporins, rendering them ineffective.

β-lactamases that have affinity for penicillins and cephalosporins are called *penicillinases* and *cephalosporinases* respectively.

> Penicillinases and cephalosporinases are enzymes of the β-lactamase family that target and denature some penicillins and cephalosporins, so rendering them harmless to bacteria.

### β-lactam antibacterials effective against resistant bacteria

Few β-lactam antibacterials are wholly immune from attack by β-lactamase-producing resistant bacteria. **Flucloxacillin** and **temocillin** are not inactivated by most β-lactamases and are thus generally effective against resistant *Staphylococcus* species. Because of the danger of resistance developing to these drugs, their use is reserved for infections caused by existing β-lactamase-resistant strains.

**IN PRACTICE**

**Meticillin**-resistant *Staphylococcus aureus*, or MRSA as it is popularly called, is a major problem in many hospitals, where it can cause post-surgical and other wound infections. **Meticillin** is now discontinued but MRSA continues its march of resistance through the pharmacopoeia and relatively few antibacterial drugs remain effective against it.

**Co-amoxiclav** is a clever combination of drugs that attempt to overcome bacterial resistance from β-lactamase-producing bacteria. The drug consists of a mixture of **amoxicillin**, an effective (but susceptible to penicillinase) broad spectrum antibacterial and **clavulanic acid**. The latter drug has no antibacterial action but is an effective inhibitor of bacterial β-lactamase. In other words, it binds to and blocks the action of β-lactamase, thus allowing **amoxicillin** to get on with its task of destroying bacteria. If you look at the molecular structure of **clavulanic acid** in Figure 8.8, you will note how close it is to the β-lactam skeleton of **penicillin** and related drugs. It is because of the structural similarity between **penicillin** and **clavulanic acid** that they are both targets for β-lactamase.

### Side-effects of β-lactam antibacterials

Probably the most serious side-effect of the penicillins is allergic hypersensitivity. Up to 10 per cent of the population is susceptible to adverse reactions from **penicillin** and its derivatives and can suffer from rashes and fever. In a few individuals, the reaction can be more severe, resulting in *anaphylaxis*, but this is fortunately quite rare. Individuals who already suffer from allergies, hay fever and asthma are at greater risk from hypersensitivity reactions.

Clavulanic acid

**Figure 8.8** Skeleton structure of clavulanic acid.

*Anaphylaxis* is a condition where a normally innocuous substance causes a severe immune response, resulting in general vasodilation and oedema in the lungs. This results in a fall in blood pressure and difficulty with breathing.

### IN PRACTICE

Sometimes antibacterial drugs can be the causative agent of bacterial diseases. *Clostridium difficile* in the gut is relatively unaffected by many of the broad-spectrum antibacterials that may kill other commensals, thus allowing *C. difficile* to flourish, free from competition. The proliferation of *C. difficile* can cause inflammation of the gut and even septicaemia.

## Antibacterials 2: drugs targeting ribosomes

There are many well-known antibacterial drugs in this category, such as tetracyclines, aminoglycosides, **chloramphenicol** and **erythromycin**. All of these drugs target bacterial ribosomes and prevent the bacterium from producing proteins.

The process of protein synthesis was discussed briefly in Chapter 1. A section of DNA, called a gene, codes for a protein and when the cell wants to make a particular protein, the gene is copied from DNA into mRNA. This is transported from the nucleus into the cytoplasm of the cell where the ribosomes translate the mRNA into a protein. The code contained in the mRNA tells the ribosome the order of the amino acids that make up the protein. Figure 8.9 is a greatly simplified portrayal of the process. It shows the ribosome tracking along a length of mRNA and reading the code. Each small section of mRNA contains the code for one of the 20 amino acids. The ribosome reads the code and then selects a corresponding free amino acid from the cytoplasm and adds it to the growing chain of amino acids.

The process of protein synthesis is of vital importance to any organism and any drug that interferes with the process will cause major problems for that

**Figure 8.9** A ribosome translates the code contained in a section of mRNA and assembles a chain of amino acids that form a protein.

organism. Growth in particular will be inhibited because cells need to make new proteins in order for them to undergo cell division. This is why drugs that target ribosomes inhibit bacterial growth – in other words, they are bacteriostatic.

Drugs such as the tetracyclines, aminoglycosides, etc. are able to target bacterial ribosomes because they are slightly different from the ribosomes found in eukaryotic human cells. This difference in structure, although relatively small, is just enough difference to make a target for antibacterial drugs.

**KEY FACT**
Bacterial ribosomes are slightly different from human ribosomes and therefore make a target for antibacterial drugs.

## Tetracyclines

This group includes **tetracycline** itself, **demeclocycline**, **doxycycline**, **lymecycline minocycline**, **oxytetracycline** and **tigecycline**. These are broad-spectrum antibacterials that are useful against a variety of organisms that can cause various diseases such as urinary tract, respiratory and oral infections. They are also widely used for *Chlamydia* infections and against *Neisseria meningitidis*, the causative agent of bacterial meningitis.

Resistance to tetracyclines is becoming increasingly problematical as bacteria find new ways of overcoming the drug. Many bacteria are able to pump the drug out of their cells and some produce a protein that appears to shield the ribosome from the effects of tetracycline. Others produce an enzyme that modifies tetracyclines, rendering them ineffective.

**IN PRACTICE**
Tetracyclines act as *chelating* agents for calcium in the body. In other words, they bind to $Ca^{2+}$ and prevent its use in physiological processes. They are contra-indicated in children under 12 and women who are pregnant or breast-feeding who need plenty of calcium, especially for bone growth in their unborn or newly born child.

## Aminoglycosides

This group includes **gentamicin**, **amikacin**, **neomycin** and **tobramycin**. None of this group is absorbed well orally and they are generally delivered IV or by intramuscular (IM) injection. They are effective against Gram-positive and Gram-negative aerobic bacteria and used for serious systemic infections, including bacterial meningitis. All aminoglycosides can cause damage to the inner ear and also damage to the nephrons of the kidney, so care is cautioned in those with renal problems. **Streptomycin**, a related drug, is reserved for tuberculosis.

**CASE STUDY**

Recently discharged from hospital where she underwent a hip replacement, Pam complains of a fever and severe discomfort when urinating. You suspect a urinary tract infection (UTI), possibly involving *E. coli*, one of the most common causative agents. What might be a suitable treatment?

*Comment on case study* There is just a possibility that the UTI was acquired in hospital and therefore might be a resistant strain. However, antibacterials effective against resistant bacteria should be reserved for infections where resistance is established. **Co-amoxiclav** might be a suitable choice where resistance is only a possibility. Because **clavulanic acid** has no antibacterial action, bacteria cannot develop resistance against it.

### Macrolides, lincosamides and chloramphenicol

These include **azithromycin**, **clarithromycin** and **erythromycin**, the latter being perhaps the most widely used of the macrolides as it has a similar spectrum of activity to **penicillin**. It is a useful alternative for patients allergic to **penicillin**.

**Clindamycin** is the sole representative of the lincosamides. Effective against Gram-positive cocci, it is recommended for staphylococcal joint and bone infections and peritonitis. **Chloramphenicol** is a potent broad spectrum drug that is reserved for serious systemic infections because it can severely suppress bone marrow activity in some individuals, resulting in anaemia. **Chloramphenicol** preparations are also available for topical application as eye and ear drops.

## Antibacterials 3: fluoroquinolones

Sometimes abbreviated to 'quinolones', this broad spectrum group includes **ciprofloxacin**, **levofloxacin**, **moxifloxacin**, **nalidixic acid**, **norfloxacin** and **ofloxacin**. They work by inhibiting topoisomerase II, an enzyme involved in uncoiling the DNA helix during DNA *replication* and mRNA *transcription*. The fluoroquinolones therefore prevent both cell division and protein synthesis. The group is particularly active against Gram-negative organisms in the treatment of infections of the respiratory and urinary tracts. **Ciprofloxacin** is used in the treatment of some sexually transmitted infections such as gonorrhoea and chlamydia.

*Replication* of DNA is the production of new DNA during cell (in this case, bacterial) division. *Transcription* is the copying of a section of DNA into mRNA during protein synthesis.

## Antibacterials 4: other antibacterial drugs

There are many different types of antibacterial drugs listed in the BNF, some of which are used regularly for common problems while others are for rarer diseases or have highly specific indications. It would be quite easy to devote a whole book to antimicrobial drugs, but as we have only one chapter, we will have to be selective and conclude this section on antibacterials with a brief summary of those drugs that are most regularly encountered in clinical practice.

**Vancomycin** and **teicoplanin** are used in the treatment of endocarditis and other serious infections from Gram-positive bacteria. These drugs inhibit peptidoglycan synthesis, causing rupture of the bacterial cell wall, but by a different mechanism from the β-lactam antibacterials.

**Trimethoprim** is used for urinary tract and lung infections. It works by inhibiting an enzyme responsible for synthesising DNA which prevents bacterial replication.

**Rifampicin** is useful for endocarditis and other serious infections, including tuberculosis and legionnaire's disease. It inhibits an enzyme that transcribes DNA into mRNA and so halts protein synthesis. **Rifampicin** is a potent inducer of hepatic enzymes that metabolise other drugs, including oral contraceptives, lowering their serum concentration.

**Metronidazole** is a widely used antimicrobial drug, effective against anaerobic bacterial infections including *Helicobacter*, *Clostridium*, bacterial vaginosis, leg ulcers, pelvic inflammatory disease etc. It is also used in dentistry to treat abscesses and ulcerative gingivitis. Unusually for an antibacterial drug, it is also effective against infections caused by protozoa. Metronidazole is activated specifically within anaerobic cells where it disrupts DNA and inhibits DNA replication.

**Nitrofurantoin** treats urinary tract infections. Its mechanism of action is not fully understood.

### A QUICK RECAP on antibacterial drugs

- Antibacterial drugs target structures that are different from human cells in bacteria.

- Some antibacterials are broad spectrum and target a wide range of bacteria. Some are narrow spectrum, targeting specific groups.

- Beta-lactam antibacterials include the penicillins, cephalosporins and carbapenems.

- Beta-lactam drugs block an enzyme involved in the production of peptidoglycan, an essential component of the bacterial cell wall. This bactericidal action causes the cell wall to rupture.

- Bacterial resistance is often due to bacteria-producing enzymes such as β-lactamases that denature the β-lactam ring of β-lactam drugs.

- Tetracyclines, aminoglycosides and related drugs target bacterial ribosomes and inhibit protein synthesis. This bacteriostatic action prevents replication.

- Fluoroquinolones prevent both cell division and protein synthesis.

- Many other antibacterial drugs are available, each having its own mechanism of action against the bacteria it targets.

## 8.3 Fungi

Fungi are a diverse group of organisms and the vast majority are non-pathogenic – some, such as chanterelles, are quite tasty and nice to eat. Other fungi, such as the yeast *Saccharomyces cerevisiae*, are used in brewing wines and beers and baking bread. Those that are pathogenic tend to be at the small end of the fungal size spectrum, often single-celled yeasts such as *Candida albicans*. Common pathogenic fungi include:

- *Candida albicans* – thrush (vaginal and oral)
- *Trichophyton* – athlete's foot
- *Aspergillus* – aspergillosis
- *Tinea capitis* – ringworm of the scalp and hair (a fungus, not a worm)
- *Tinea corporis, T. cruris* and *T. pedis* – skin and nail infections
- *Cryptococcus neoformans* – cryptococcosis.

Fungal infections in healthy individuals generally tend to be topical in nature and not life-threatening. Ringworm, thrush and athlete's foot are common and relatively easily treated, responding to antifungal drugs discussed below. Those in most danger from fungal infections are patients who are already severely ill or immunocompromised. Here fungi act as opportunistic pathogens and can cause serious and life-threatening conditions. *Candida albicans* is an example of an organism that rarely causes severe problems in healthy individuals beyond vulvovaginal candidiasis (thrush) in females and oral candidiasis in neonates and the elderly. However, *invasive systemic candidiasis* can develop in those whose immune system has been suppressed, such as human immunodeficiency virus (HIV) infected patients with acquired immunodeficiency syndrome (AIDS) or cancer patients receiving immunosuppressant drugs. This is a very serious disease with a high mortality rate that can result in organs of the body becoming infected. Systemic candidiasis is generally not encountered outside the intensive care unit.

Fungi are eukaryotic organisms, which means that their cell structure is similar to our own, and this makes them more difficult to target with drugs. Certainly, anti-bacterial drugs have no effect on them because bacterial targets are not found in fungi. However, as with bacteria, an antifungal drug has to target fungal structures that are unique to fungi and different from those found in human cells. A summary of the targets for antifungal drugs is shown in Figure 8.10.

**DID YOU KNOW . . .** that ringworm is caused by a fungus and has nothing to do with worms? The disease, more properly termed dermatophytosis, is most commonly the result of a *Trichophyton* infection of the skin, producing a ring-like lesion.

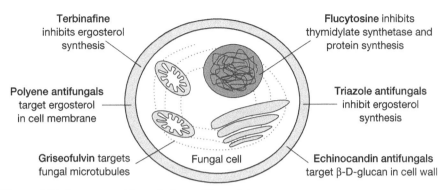

Figure 8.10 Summary of targets for antifungal drugs.

## Antifungal drugs

**Polyene antifungals (amphotericin)** target fungal cell membranes which contain *ergosterol* rather than the cholesterol found in human membranes. Like cholesterol, ergosterol is essential for the stability of the cell membrane. **Amphotericin** has an affinity for ergosterol and in binding to it disrupts the integrity of the membrane, causing the cell to lyse and die. **Amphotericin** is used for severe systemic fungal infections such as systemic candidiasis and *cryptococcosis*. It is acknowledged to be quite toxic and must be used with care.

**Triazole antifungals** include **fluconazole**, **itraconazole**, **posaconazole** and **voriconazole** that target fungal enzymes responsible for the synthesis of ergosterol. Membranes lose their integrity and this inhibits replication. Triazole antifungals are used for a wide range of fungal infections, topical and systemic, including oral and vaginal candidiasis plus invasive candidiasis and aspergillosis.

**Echinocandin antifungals** are relatively recent drugs and include **anidulafungin**, **caspofungin** and **micafungin**. They are used in the treatment of serious fungal infections such as systemic candidiasis and aspergillosis. These drugs inhibit the synthesis of a fungal polysaccharide *β-D-glucan*, an essential component of the fungal cell wall. The Echinocandins are large, complex molecules and have to be administered by IV infusion.

**Flucytosine** is an antifungal drug used for serious systemic infections. It inhibits the fungal enzyme *thymidylate synthetase*, an enzyme involved in protein synthesis. **Griseofulvin**, used for skin, scalp and nail infections, acts against fungal microtubules and prevents cell division. **Terbinafine**, an ergosterol synthesis inhibitor, is used for ringworm and nail infections.

## Topical antifungal drugs

There are many topical antifungals used to treat topical fungal infections such as ringworm, athlete's foot and candidiasis, including **nystatin**, **clotrimazole**, **econazole**, and **ketoconazole** and **miconazole**.

Unwanted effects of antifungals are usually mild and can include the ubiquitous nausea, vomiting, diarrhoea and rashes. Some of the azoles are cautioned in patients with hepatic impairment and congestive heart failure. Parenteral **amphotericin** also has many cautions, including anaphylaxis.

**CASE STUDY**

Darren is an IV drug user who has recently been diagnosed with HIV infection. He presents at surgery with white plaques on his tongue and gums. You suspect oral candidiasis. What would you prescribe?

*Comment on case study* **Fluconazole** is the drug of choice here and should resolve the problem. If Darren is susceptible to fungal infections, vigilance will be necessary as the HIV infection progresses because candidiasis and cryptococcosis can become invasive, causing serious problems in immunocompromised patients.

## 8.4 Viruses

Viruses are very, very small – around 10–100 nm (1000 nm = 1 μm) – so they can only be viewed with an electron microscope. They are obligate cellular parasites, meaning that they can only reproduce after invading a host cell and they are invariably pathogenic to their hosts. Most organisms are susceptible to attack by viruses; animals, plants, fungi and even bacteria are all viral targets. Viruses tend to be very specific to their hosts so, for example, humans cannot contract cat flu from their pets or hydrangea mosaic virus from their pot plants.

Common pathogenic viruses include:

- **Rhinovirus** – common cold
- **Orthomyxovirus** – influenza
- **Paramyxovirus** – measles
- **Varicella-zoster** – chickenpox and shingles (neural varicella-zoster)
- **Norovirus** – gastro-enteritis
- **Rotavirus** – diarrhoea (especially in children)
- **Astrovirus** – gastro-enteritis
- **Papillomavirus** – genital warts
- **Coronavirus** – Severe Acute Respiratory Syndrome (SARS)
- **Human immunodeficiency virus** – HIV – AIDS.

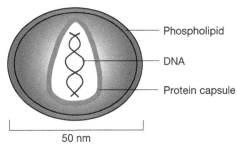

Figure 8.11 Typical structure of an encapsulated virus.

**DID YOU KNOW . . .** that viruses are so remote from other kingdoms and their relationships so problematical that they do not take normal nomencla-ture as devised by Carl Linnaeus (1707–1778)? These binomial (double) names identify organisms by their genus and species name respectively, as in *Homo sapiens* and *Escherichia coli*.

Viruses are very simple in their structure – often just a strand of DNA or RNA in a protein capsule or lipid envelope. Figure 8.11 shows a typical structure of an encapsulated virus but note that they exhibit great structural diversity.

Because viruses reproduce inside host cells, they are difficult to attack with drugs. A few drugs have been developed which target some of the proteins unique to viruses but our main defence is *vaccination*, which pre-programmes the body's immune system to defend it against a particular virus. A few drugs are available for the treatment of influenza and *respiratory syncytial virus* infections, generally for use only in high-risk patients.

## Human immunodeficiency virus (HIV)

Infection with human immunodeficiency virus (HIV) produces a complex, incur-able disease that results in a weakening of the body's immune response, with the eventual onset of a suite of diseases common in immunocompromised patients known as acquired immunodeficiency syndrome, or AIDS. This disease has spread inexorably across the world, infecting millions of people, especially in developing countries where sexual education is inadequate or ineffective. The development of drugs to combat HIV has been steady and while none of them produces a cure, it is now possible to slow the progression of HIV infection and give infected individuals a reasonable quality of life. It is an indication of the effort put into developing a cure for HIV that there are more drugs available to treat HIV than there are for all other viral infections combined. Generally anti-HIV drugs target viral enzymes or processes associated with viral replication in the cell. The drugs are always given in combinations termed HAART (highly active antiretroviral treatment). As HIV is a highly specialised area, you are recommended to access a specialist publication to investigate the pharmacology of the drugs used in the treatment of patients with this complex disease.

Why don't we just vaccinate against HIV?

For a vaccine to be effective, the virus it targets must have stable antigen markers that will be recognised by the immune system. HIV is a *retrovirus* and one characteristic of this group is their rapid mutation. This means that the protection conferred by a vaccination would be lost almost immediately because of the speed of mutation of the HIV antigen markers.

## Herpes virus infections

These infections are caused by viruses of the herpes group. Herpes simplex causes cold sores, conjunctivitis, mouth ulcers and genital infections. Varicella-zoster virus causes shingles and chicken pox. Drugs used to treat herpes infections are of the **aciclovir** (acyclovir) family that inhibit viral RNA polymerase, an enzyme that produces viral proteins. Protein synthesis is halted and so is viral replication.

### CASE STUDY

Charlie arrives in surgery with a streaming head cold. He says he feels 'rough' and wants some antibiotics to make him feel better and get him back to work. What would you do?

*Comment on case study* Charlie's problem is caused by a virus and is not bacterial in origin. The word *antibiotic* is popularly used to refer to antibacterial drugs and these will have no effect on Charlie's viral infection – in fact, there are currently no drugs available to treat the common cold. Having satisfied yourself that the problem is indeed a cold and that Charlie is not vulnerable to complications, he should be advised to stay at home, keep warm and not return to work until the symptoms have gone.

## 8.5    Protozoa

This group of single-celled organisms cause some unpleasant diseases that include malaria, amoebiasis and leishmaniasis. Fortunately, most of these diseases are usually found in the tropics so are less likely to be encountered outside a clinical setting specialising in tropical diseases. There are two common protozoal infections you are likely to encounter in the UK...

- Trichomoniasis is a fairly common sexually transmitted disease caused by the organism *Trichomonas vaginalis*. Treatment is by **metronidazole** or **tinidazole**.

- Toxoplasmosis is a disease caused by the protozoan *Toxoplasma gondii*. It is generally a self-limiting disease that can be caught from domestic pets. Pregnant women and immunocompromised patients are at more risk and require specialist clinical expertise.

## 8.6    Helminths (worms)

The threadworm (*Enterobius vermicularis*) is probably the most common cause of helmintic disease in the UK. The worms go through a cycle that requires the re-ingestion of worm eggs that are laid around the area of the anus. Pruritus (itching) results in scratching and the eggs can be transferred under the fingernails to the mouth – thus repeating the cycle. The obvious treatment involves education in basic hygiene followed by a dose of **mebendazole** or **piperazine**.

**Mebendazole** inhibits glucose uptake in the worms and **piperazine** paralyses muscles in the worms, allowing them to be expelled alive.

**A QUICK RECAP on drugs for fungal, viral, protozoan and helmintic infections**

- Antifungal drugs mainly target the fungal cell membrane that contains ergosterol rather than the cholesterol found in human cells.
- Viruses are obligate cellular parasites and therefore difficult to target with drugs. Vaccination is the most effective way to prevent viral infection.
- There are relatively few antiviral drugs for common viral infections such as colds and flu. Many drugs have been developed to combat HIV.
- Trichomoniasis, a sexually transmitted disease, is the most common protozoan infection in the UK, along with toxoplasmosis, a disease transmitted from domestic animals such as cats.
- Threadworms are relatively common in the UK, especially in children. They can be eliminated with good hygiene and drugs such as **mebendazole** or **piperazine**.

### FURTHER RECOMMENDED READING

All recommended websites are open access (but free registration is sometimes required).

NICE guidelines on infection control – http://guidance.nice.org.uk/CG139

National Electronic Library of Infection – http://www.neli.org.uk/

NHS Website (search for specific infection) – http://www.nhs.uk/Conditions/

Medscape – infectious diseases – http://emedicine.medscape.com/infectious_diseases

## Test yourself

Now you have finished reading through this chapter try answering these questions to see how much you have learned.

*The answers to these questions are at the end of the book (see p. 316).*

1 Name the four groups of microbes that can cause microbial infection.

2 Which was the first group of microbes to evolve on Earth?

3 What do you understand by the terms 'prokaryote' and 'eukaryote'?

4 Name three factors by which we can classify bacteria.

5 What is the name of the structural glycoprotein found in bacterial cell walls?

6 How do penicillins and cephalosporins kill bacteria?

7 What is the chief way that bacteria become resistant to penicillins and cephalosporins?

8 How does clavulanic acid help to evade bacterial resistance?

9 What is the difference between a bactericidal and a bacteriostatic drug?

10 What bacterial structure do tetracyclines and aminoglycosides target?

11 Why are tetracyclines contra-indicated in pregnant women?

12 What is the main target for antifungal drugs?

13 Why are viruses so difficult to target with drugs?

14 What is the most effective way to prevent viral infection?

15 What drug can treat both protozoan and bacterial infection?

Answers to the questions on p. 188.

1 A fungus (single-celled yeast).
2 Meticillin resistant *Staphylococcus aureus*.
3 A bacterium.
4 A virus.
5 No – a cold is caused by a virus and penicillin is only effective against bacteria.

# Chapter 9

# Disorders and drugs of the respiratory system

This chapter starts by examining the physiology of the respiratory system, its structure and function. We then look at the disorders and pathologies associated with the respiratory system and finally explore the pharmacology – the action of the major drug groups used in the treatment of respiratory disorders and pathologies.

## CONTENTS

The chapter contains some brief case studies and finishes off with self-test questions to ensure that you have understood the physiology of the respiratory system, associated disorders and the pharmacology of drugs used to treat those disorders.

**IN PRACTICE**

Whatever your branch of clinical practice, you will encounter patients with respiratory problems. Hay fever affects millions of individuals and can range from a minor irritation to a debilitating problem. Asthma is a common disease that generally originates in childhood and often persists into later life. Cystic fibrosis is an incurable genetic disease that can affect the lungs. It is less common than asthma but is also one that can continue from childhood into adulthood. Bronchitis and emphysema are relatively common chronic respiratory diseases that predominantly affect older people. All of the diseases just mentioned tend to be chronic problems that can persist for years but there are also many respiratory problems of a shorter duration. Some, such as pneumonia, can be very serious, especially in the elderly. Other diseases are unpleasant but usually less serious, and most people at some time will have succumbed to a cough or chest infection. Because the lungs are so important to the normal physiological functioning of the individual, any disease that interferes with gas exchange in the lungs can have a profound effect on the rest of the body. It is important, therefore, that you understand the basic physiology of the lungs, how associated pathologies can cause problems, and how the drugs at our disposal can help patients with respiratory problems.

## Introduction

Breathing is essential to life, every minute from the moment we are born until the final moment of our lives – often referred to as 'our last breath'. We breathe in and out around 13 times each minute, each breath delivering fresh, oxygen-containing air into the lungs and removing carbon dioxide. If we stop breathing for any reason the consequences are very serious indeed because after a few minutes we die – and things do not get more serious than that! Healthy lungs are essential for the well-being of the individual and any disease that compromises their efficient functioning is going to cause problems. The pattern of lung diseases in the UK has changed over the past decades, reflecting changes in wealth, health and lifestyle. Chronic obstructive pulmonary diseases (COPD) such as bronchitis and emphysema were originally industrial in origin, caused by poor working conditions in polluted factories. These days there are fewer heavy, polluting industries in the UK and health and safety regulations are much more tightly enforced. Even so, we have over half a million people in the UK with chronic bronchitis and emphysema but cigarette smoking is now the prime culprit. Hopefully, with fewer people smoking we may see a decline in these diseases. With a cleaner, less polluted environment most people might think that lung disease generally would be steadily declining but paradoxically one disease, asthma, has been steadily increasing in incidence. Sixty years ago, asthma was a relatively uncommon disease but today statistics released by the NHS indicate around five million people in the UK are being treated for this condition.

In this chapter we will first look at the anatomy and physiology of the respiratory system and then examine some common diseases such as asthma, bronchitis and cough. Finally, we look at the drugs available to help restore normal function when problems occur. There are also some diseases of the respiratory system that are caused by bacterial infections, such as pneumonia as well as viral infections, including severe acute respiratory syndrome (SARS) and influenza. These require specialist treatment beyond the scope of this introductory book but some of the antimicrobial drugs used to treat these infections were covered in Chapter 8. Lung cancer is another all too common disease, generally caused by cigarette smoking. As with lung infections, treatment requires the use of specialist drugs which are discussed in Chapter 12.

## WHERE ARE WE STARTING FROM?

In this chapter we will examine the respiratory system and the drugs that treat common disorders such as asthma, bronchitis and emphysema. You should already understand the basic anatomy and physiology of the respiratory system but let's start off with the usual short quiz to find out how much you do know before we begin:

1   What is the name of the main airway that connects the mouth to the lungs?

_____

2   Do we extract oxygen or carbon dioxide from the air we breathe in?

_____

3   When the ribs rise and the diaphragm falls, does air enter or leave the lungs?

_____

4   What is the name of the small air sacs at the end of the bronchioles where gas exchange takes place?

_____

5   What is the name of the membranes that surround the lungs?

_____

*Answers are at the end of the chapter on p. 231.*

How did you do? We cover the basics of the respiratory system at the beginning of this chapter but if you think you need to brush up on this topic then it might be an idea to visit your physiology book.

## 9.1 The anatomy and physiology of the respiratory system

The function of the respiratory system is primarily to facilitate the transfer of gas between the body and the atmosphere. Oxygen is a gas that is required by every cell of the body to make energy in the form of ATP. Without oxygen, cells are unable to make ATP in sufficient quantities and if the supply of oxygen is cut off for long enough then cells will die. This is what happens in heart attacks when a blood clot in the coronary arteries deprives heart muscle of oxygen-carrying blood and, unless the paramedics arrive quickly with thrombolytic drugs, cells and tissues start dying. The removal of carbon dioxide is an equally important task of the lungs. Carbon dioxide produced during cellular respiration is carried by the blood from the tissues to the lungs, where it is disposed of into the atmosphere. It will thus be obvious that any problem with the lungs will quickly affect gas exchange and, consequently, gas levels in the body. A fall in oxygen or a rise in carbon dioxide levels are both potentially serious and compensatory mechanisms exist in the body to restore normal gas levels. However, these mechanisms are dependent on lungs that are functioning normally.

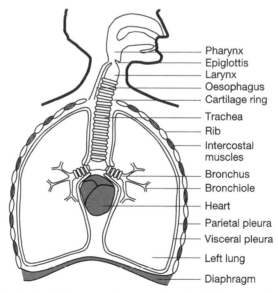

Figure 9.1 The structure of the respiratory system. Note that many branches of the bronchioles have been omitted for clarity, as have some of the ribs.

**Figure 9.2** Alveoli and associated capillaries form the respiratory membrane.

The structure of the respiratory system facilitates the movement of air between the outside of the body and the alveoli of the lungs where gas exchange takes place (Figure 9.1).

After entering the mouth or nose, air moves down the trachea to a point just underneath the midpoint of the sternum, where the trachea branches into the left and right bronchi. Each bronchus then divides and subdivides into bronchioles and these continue to divide, around 20 or so times, getting smaller with each division. At the end of the smallest bronchioles are the alveoli, small air sacs where gas exchange takes place. There are millions of alveoli in each lung, each surrounded by a network of small blood vessels called capillaries (Figure 9.2). The walls of the alveoli are only one cell thick, as are the adjacent capillaries, which means that air and blood are brought into very close proximity, separated by less than 1.0 μm. This area is called the *respiratory membrane*.

**DID YOU KNOW ...** that the adult human lungs contain almost 500 million alveoli, giving an average area of around 80 m² – about half the size of a tennis court? This large area provides spare capacity when there needs to be a dramatic increase in gas exchange – for example, during vigorous exercise.

## Gas exchange in the alveoli

Gas exchange takes place across the very thin respiratory membrane formed by the cells of the alveoli and capillaries. In the alveoli, the concentration of oxygen is high because breathing has brought in fresh air from the atmosphere. In the pulmonary capillaries, the concentration of oxygen in the blood is low because the tissue cells have extracted much of the oxygen to make energy in the form of ATP. This means that there is a *diffusion gradient* between the alveoli and the blood in the capillaries. Oxygen will therefore diffuse down this gradient from the alveoli to the blood (Figure 9.3).

The blood in the pulmonary capillaries has a high concentration of carbon dioxide because the cells of the tissues have produced carbon dioxide to make

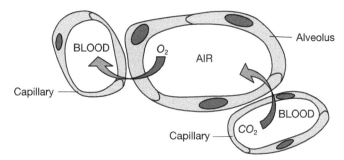

**Figure 9.3** The diffusion of oxygen and carbon dioxide across the respiratory membrane.

energy. In the alveoli, the concentration is low because breathing has brought in fresh air from the atmosphere and this contains very little carbon dioxide. This means that there is a diffusion gradient between the alveoli and the blood in the capillaries. Carbon dioxide will therefore diffuse down this gradient from the blood to the alveoli (Figure 9.3).

> The *diffusion gradient* is the difference in concentration of a substance such as a gas or an ion, separated by a permeable membrane. The substance tends to diffuse across the membrane from the area of high concentration to the area of low concentration. Breathing maintains the gradient and so ensures continuous diffusion of oxygen and carbon dioxide across the respiratory membrane.

## Ventilation and compliance

*Ventilation* is the physical movement of air into and out of the lungs. *Inspiration* is the movement of air into the lungs and requires the contraction of the external intercostal muscles that cause the ribs to rise and the flattening of the diaphragm. These two actions increase the volume of the lungs while, at the same time, decreasing the pressure. Air flows into the lungs down a pressure gradient from the higher atmospheric pressure outside to the lower pressure in the lungs.

*Expiration* is the movement of air out of the lungs and this also involves changes in volumes and pressures. However, in breathing when the body is at rest, no muscular effort or energy is required to contract the lungs because, being elastic in nature, they recoil automatically from their expanded state.

**ANOTHER WAY TO PICTURE THIS**

Think of a bath sponge, which is actually quite similar in structure to the lungs. If you stretch the sponge, as in inspiration, it will recoil of its own accord when released. The 'stretchability' of the lungs is called *compliance*.

The internal intercostal muscles, while not being used in quiet breathing, are necessary for forced expiration such as when coughing or during heavy exercise.

Healthy lungs with good compliance recoil automatically and easily, but certain disease conditions such as emphysema, bronchitis, tuberculosis and cystic fibrosis can compromise this process. *Mucus* that is produced in diseases such as bronchitis and asthma can partially block airways and result in ventilation problems.

*Mucus* is a viscous, slippery liquid that lines the mucous membranes of the body such as those of the respiratory, digestive and reproductive systems. Note the difference in spelling between the substance 'mucus' and the 'mucous' membranes that secrete it.

## Respiratory defences and maintenance

In the airways of the lungs, a mechanism exists for removing the bacteria, dust and detritus that we inevitably breathe in each day. *Goblet cells* in the walls of the bronchioles produce the thin layer of mucus that lines the trachea, bronchi and bronchioles. This mucus is constantly moved along by tiny cilia, hair-like projections on the epithelial cells lining the respiratory tract. This mucus traps any foreign matter that has entered the lungs and transports it to the top of the trachea where it is usually swallowed (Figure 9.4).

In the alveoli, white blood cells called *alveolar macrophages* patrol the alveoli and destroy any bacteria that they find.

## The control of breathing and compensatory mechanisms

When we are going about our daily tasks we are rarely conscious of the fact we are breathing in and out around 15 times each minute. Sometimes, when we are at the gym or running for a bus, we might notice that we are 'out of breath' and breathing more heavily and more rapidly than normal. These are examples of the control and compensatory mechanisms that maintain breathing and ensure adequate and efficient gas exchange in the alveoli of the lungs.

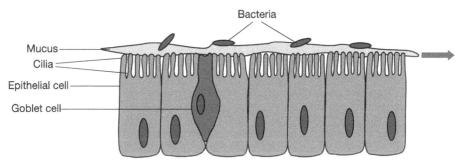

**Figure 9.4** Cilia on epithelial cells remove bacteria trapped in mucus from the respiratory tract.

The maintenance of normal, regular breathing is via the respiratory centres of the brain stem. These set a steady rhythm that maintains the rhythmical breathing in the lungs via efferent nerves that control the intercostal muscles and diaphragm. As these muscles steadily contract and relax, air is moved in and out of the lungs, bringing in oxygen and removing carbon dioxide. When we exercise, however, we need more oxygen for the muscles to make their ATP and in the process we produce more carbon dioxide that must be disposed of into the atmosphere. The rate and depth of breathing is increased to facilitate this need for increased gas exchange. The trigger for this change in rate is, perhaps surprisingly, primarily the increase in blood carbon dioxide levels rather than a fall in oxygen. This increase is detected by *chemoreceptors* in the medulla of the brain stem, which stimulates the rate and depth of breathing to pull more oxygen into the body and get rid of more carbon dioxide. When we stop exercising, levels of carbon dioxide fall and the rate and depth of breathing returns to normal.

### KEY FACT

The carbon dioxide level in the blood is the main driver of breathing. Exercise causes $CO_2$ levels to rise and this causes an increase in the rate and depth of breathing.

In chronic obstructive pulmonary disease (COPD), such as bronchitis and emphysema, a condition can develop where the patient's breathing is being maintained by what is called *hypoxic drive*. COPD is a long-term condition where gas exchange is continuously compromised, resulting sometimes in chronically high levels of carbon dioxide in the blood. Eventually the respiratory centres may start to disregard $CO_2$ as a stimulus for breathing and instead rely on low levels of oxygen as the prime driver of respiration.

### IN PRACTICE

When on hypoxic drive, the breathing of a COPD patient is being maintained by low levels of oxygen. This means it can be dangerous to suddenly give supplementary oxygen because the sudden rise in blood oxygen levels can remove the stimulus to breathe, resulting in respiratory failure.

*Chemoreceptors* are special receptor organs at the terminals of afferent neurons that detect changes in the chemical composition of the surrounding environment.

**A QUICK RECAP on the anatomy and physiology of the respiratory system**

- The prime function of the lungs is gas exchange between the body and atmospheric air. Oxygen is extracted from the air and carbon dioxide is disposed of into the air.

- Oxygen is transported in the blood from the lungs to the cells of the body where it is used in the production of energy in the form of ATP.

- Carbon dioxide is produced by cells when they make ATP and is transported in the blood to the lungs where it is disposed of into the atmosphere.

- At the end of the terminal bronchioles are small air sacs called alveoli, which form the respiratory membrane. This is where gas exchange between the air and the blood takes place.

- Breathing in and out is by movement of the ribs and diaphragm which, together, create pressure gradients that facilitate the movement of air.

- The lungs are kept clean by the production of mucus that traps bacteria and detritus from the air. The mucus is steadily moved out of the lungs by the ciliated epithelial cells that line the respiratory tract.

- The prime driver of breathing is the level of $CO_2$ in the blood. As levels rise so the rate and depth of breathing increases to remove $CO_2$ from the body – and bring in more $O_2$.

## 9.2 Disorders of the respiratory system

### Seasonal allergic rhinitis (hay fever)

Hay fever is very common and brings seasonal misery to millions of individuals in the UK. Caused by sensitivity to pollen, it triggers an inflammatory reaction, resulting in a runny nose, itching eyes and sneezing. Hay fever (as the name implies) is primarily associated with grass pollen. Rather than relying on bees and other insects for pollination, grasses reproduce by releasing vast amounts of pollen into the breeze. Only a tiny fraction of the pollen released succeeds in pollinating another grass so there is plenty left to pollinate your nose and start it running. Fortunately, plants only release pollen for a few weeks each year so the disorder is thankfully time-limited – at least until the following year's pollen fest.

### Asthma

**Asthma** is an inflammatory disease characterised by hypersensitivity of the airways resulting in periodic bronchospasm (narrowing of the airways). It is one of the most common respiratory diseases in the UK, where it affects around five million people, many of them children. The incidence of asthma has increased steadily over the past decades, which may be surprising considering that the atmosphere in the UK is now less polluted and health care has improved. The reason for this increase is not fully understood but is believed to be linked to the fact that our immune system is now challenged less often in infancy by disease-causing pathogens. Vaccination has all but eliminated many diseases such as diphtheria, measles and polio that were once common and our homes are generally clean and centrally heated. Consequently, children now are just not exposed to the immunological challenges of previous generations and somehow this may result in the immune system becoming more sensitive to challenges from substances such as dust mites and animal fur that present no real threat to their health. Whatever the reason, asthma is a very common disease and many drugs have been developed to make the lives of those who suffer from the problem more bearable.

In asthma, the bronchi and bronchioles become inflamed and sensitive to *allergens* such as dust mites, animal fur, pollen and a variety of otherwise innocuous substances. In addition to allergens, environmental factors such as cold air, stress and exercise can also exacerbate the problems of the asthma sufferer. When the asthmatic is exposed to particular allergens, this can cause an asthma attack. The allergen is carried into the airways, where it is recognised by mast cells of the immune system in the lining of the bronchioles. There then follows a sequence of events, typical of the inflammatory response that we examined in Chapter 6. Mast cells release chemical mediators such as histamine, prostaglandins and leukotrienes (Figure 9.5). This results in bronchoconstriction caused by contraction of the smooth muscle that surrounds the bronchioles. Plasma leaks out of the small blood vessels causing oedema and goblet cells in the bronchiole epithelium to release copious amounts of mucus. All of this has the effect of narrowing the airways and stimulating nerve endings, resulting in the feeling of irritation. In addition to bronchoconstriction and oedema, leukotrienes have a role in the attraction of

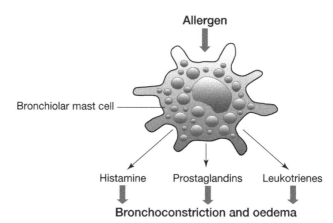

**Figure 9.5** Stimulation of a mast cell in the bronchioles by an allergen causes the release of histamine, prostaglandins and leukotrienes, resulting in bronchoconstriction and oedema.

*eosinophils*, white blood cells that amplify the inflammatory response and may eventually cause damage to the epithelial lining of the bronchioles.

*Allergens* are substances that trigger allergic reactions. The immune system recognises and responds to allergens by releasing chemical mediators such as histamine that are responsible for the symptoms of an allergic response such as swelling, sneezing and itching.

The onset of an asthma attack brings on dyspnoea (shortness of breath), tightness in the chest, coughing and wheezing – although symptoms will vary between individuals. Bronchoconstriction, swelling and excess mucus in the bronchioles impede the flow of air in and out of the lungs and this interferes with normal gas exchange in the alveoli. The uptake of oxygen into the blood is adversely affected, as is the removal of carbon dioxide, levels of which are elevated, resulting in an urgency to increase the rate of ventilation. Unfortunately, this is hampered by the narrow airways, resulting in the shortness of breath and distress experienced during an asthma attack. The initial attack is often followed by a *late-phase response* several hours later. This also involves bronchoconstriction and an increase in airway sensitivity but the mechanism behind it is less well understood.

**IN PRACTICE**

Narrowed airways cause breathing difficulties and perhaps the easiest way to monitor the efficiency of a patient's lungs is with a peak flow meter, a small hand-held device into which the patient blows hard. A scale gives the rate at which air is being exhaled in litres per minute. The reading can be checked against standardised figures for the patient's sex, age and height.

## Chronic obstructive pulmonary disease

Chronic obstructive pulmonary disease (COPD) includes bronchitis and emphysema and is characterised by a restriction of airflow both into and out of the lungs, which develops over a period of time, perhaps months or years. COPD differs primarily from asthma in that the restriction is permanent rather than episodic and reversible as in asthma. Although the pathologies of bronchitis and emphysema are somewhat different, they have a common set of breathing-related symptoms, including . . .

- Chronic cough
- Expectoration (coughing up) of mucus
- Breathlessness upon exertion
- Progressive reduction in the ability to exhale
- Increase in susceptibility to chest infections.

**Figure 9.6** Mucus, oedema and hypertrophy of smooth muscle can combine to reduce the size of the bronchiolar lumen.

The main cause of both bronchitis and emphysema is many years of smoking and it is the toxic chemicals in the smoke that cause permanent damage to the lungs. In bronchitis, smoking triggers chronic inflammation, which results in damage to the airways. The cilia, hair-like projections that move bacteria and foreign particles out of the lungs are damaged so that the lungs retain mucus. The mucous glands themselves become enlarged, resulting in an overproduction of mucus. Bacteria such as *Streptococcus pneumoniae*, *Haemophilus influenzae* and *Moraxella catarrhalis* become trapped in the excess mucus that accumulates in the lungs and this can result in chest infections. To add to the problem, *hypertrophy*, an overgrowth of the smooth muscle cells that surround the airways, will further restrict airflow. Figure 9.6 shows how oedema, mucus and hypertrophy can reduce the size of the bronchiolar *lumen* (air space).

In emphysema, the walls of the alveoli break down and this reduces the surface area of the respiratory membrane. Gas exchange is compromised, resulting in a lower intake of oxygen and a reduced removal of carbon dioxide. Bronchitis is a common complication of emphysema.

*Lumen* is a term used to refer to the space enclosed by any of the hollow organs of the body such as the bronchioles, small intestine or blood vessels.

**CASE STUDY**

Jim is 55 and presents at the clinic with a cough that has been troubling him for weeks and he says that he is producing a lot of phlegm. His breathing is noisy and he complains that it gets worse when he climbs the stairs. He says he has given up smoking but the smell of tobacco smoke on his clothes tells another story. What would you advise?

*Comment on case study* Jim's symptoms are indicative of early COPD. A peak flow test will give some indication of the state of his lungs. Jim needs to be honest about his smoking and perhaps be referred to a smoking-cessation clinic. If he can stop smoking now, there is a chance that the disease can be halted and he may be able to resume participation in normal physical activities.

## Cough

The cough is a defensive mechanism that can expel foreign bodies and mucus from the airways. It can also be triggered by irritation of the airways due to inflammation and infection. Irritation usually results in a dry cough where no mucus is expelled whereas in infection, the cough more often produces mucus. Some drugs such as ACE inhibitors (discussed in Chapter 5) can irritate the bronchioles, resulting in a dry cough. The cough mechanism itself is not well understood but is thought to operate via a poorly defined 'cough centre' in the brainstem. When this is activated, efferent nerves to the intercostal muscles of the ribs cause the rapid, forced expulsion of air, resulting in the familiar coughing sound.

**A QUICK RECAP on disorders of the respiratory system**

- Asthma is an inflammatory disease with hypersensitivity of the airways resulting in periodic bronchospasm.
- Symptoms of asthma are dyspnoea, coughing and wheezing and the production of excess mucus.
- The pathology of asthma involves the production of histamine, prostaglandins and leukotrienes, which cause bronchoconstriction and oedema.
- Chronic obstructive pulmonary disease (COPD) includes bronchitis and emphysema, chronic diseases that affect the movement of air in and out of the lungs.
- In bronchitis, excess mucus and trapped bacteria lead to recurrent infections.
- In emphysema there is an irreversible breakdown of the respiratory membrane in the alveoli, resulting in impaired gas exchange. Oxygen levels in the blood fall and carbon dioxide levels rise.
- Cough is a natural defence mechanism that expels foreign bodies from the airways but is also triggered by infection and inflammation.

## 9.3   Drugs used in the management of respiratory system disorders

There are various types of drugs used in the treatment of respiratory disorders. Drugs for hay fever are mainly antihistamines, damping down the inflammatory response in the nasal passages. For obstructive disorders, improving the movement of air through the bronchioles can be achieved by bronchodilators that relax the smooth muscle surrounding the bronchioles, and both long- and short-acting bronchodilators are available. Another approach is to reduce inflammation in the bronchioles, which can help make the airways less sensitive as well as reducing oedema and mucus production. For those with chronic asthma, the BNF provides a recommended protocol that outlines the best choice and combination of drugs to ensure effective management of the disease. Acute, severe asthma attacks can be life-threatening if the patient is unable to breathe properly and supplemental oxygen often needs to be administered as well as the specific bronchodilators discussed below.

## Drug group 1: antihistamines

As we saw in Chapter 6, inflammation starts with the stimulation of mast cells, causing them to release histamine and other inflammatory mediators. In the case of hay fever, it is pollen grains that stimulate the mast cells. The histamine released binds to $H_1$ receptors on the epithelium of the nasal passages resulting in rhinorrhoea (runny nose), itching and sneezing. The eyes are also frequently affected, causing itching and watering.

The oral antihistamines are divided into two groups; the sedating and non-sedating antihistamines. Both groups are antagonists, blocking $H_1$ receptors and reducing the inflammatory effects of histamine on nasal epithelium.

The more recent, non-sedating antihistamines indicated for allergic rhinitis include **acrivastine**, **cetirizine**, **desloratadine**, **fexofenadine**, **loratadine**, **mizolastine** and **rupatadine**. They only minimally cross the blood-brain barrier so are less likely to cause drowsiness. The older, more sedating antihistamines include **chlorphenamine**, **clemastine**, **cyproheptadine**, **ketotifen** and **promethazine**. These drugs also have an antimuscarinic activity which may help reduce mucus secretion. No prizes for guessing that the main side-effect of sedating antihistamines is drowsiness.

Other preparations used to treat hay fever include corticosteroid nasal sprays such as **beclometasone**, **budesonide**, **flunisolide**, **fluticasone**, **mometasone** and **triamcinolone**. These have an immunosuppressive effect on mast cells in the nasal passages, reducing their sensitivity to pollen allergens. This inhibits the production of histamine and other inflammatory mediators such as prostaglandins and leukotrienes. **Azelastine** is an $H_1$ antihistamine available as a nasal spray.

## Drug group 2: bronchodilators (indicated for asthma and COPD)

### Bronchodilators 1: selective beta$_2$ agonists

These include **salbutamol, terbutaline, bambuterol, formoterol, indacaterol** and **salmeterol**. They are sometimes termed sympathomimetics in that they mimic the action of the sympathetic nervous system. These drugs are indicated for asthma and chronic obstructive airway disease. **Salbutamol** and **terbutaline** are short-acting bronchodilators, reversing the symptoms of asthma. Others such as **formoterol** and **salmeterol** are longer-acting drugs used to control chronic asthma. **Indacaterol** is a bronchodilator used only for COPD. **Bambuterol** is a long-acting, orally delivered pro-drug of **terbutaline**, used where inhalation medication is difficult.

The autonomic nervous system controls the muscle tone in the bronchioles, allowing them to constrict and dilate. Parasympathetic nerves innervate the bronchial smooth muscle which causes bronchoconstriction. Sympathetic nerves are few in the lungs but activation of the sympathetic system causes the adrenals to release the circulatory hormone adrenaline. This binds to $\beta_2$ adrenergic (adrenaline) receptors on the smooth muscle cells of the bronchiole walls, causing the muscle cells to relax and the bronchioles to dilate (Figure 9.7). This is part of the suite of responses initiated by sympathetic activity and allows more air (and oxygen) to be drawn into the lungs during 'fight or flight' situations.

Selective beta$_2$ agonists such as **salbutamol** and **terbutaline** mimic the action of adrenaline but are selective for the beta$_2$ adrenaline receptors that occur mainly on the smooth muscle of the bronchioles. The effect of adrenaline or an agonist of adrenaline binding to these receptors causes the smooth muscle to relax and the bronchioles to dilate. Air can more easily move in and out of the lungs and so the feeling of breathlessness is relieved (Figure 9.8).

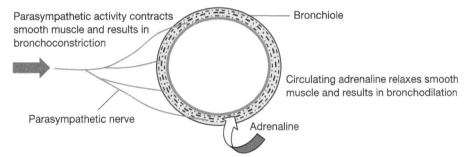

**Figure 9.7** The action of parasympathetic nerves and adrenaline on the bronchioles.

**Figure 9.8** Beta$_2$ agonists such as *salbutamol* mimic adrenaline and cause relaxation of bronchiolar smooth muscle, resulting in bronchodilation.

Most of the selective beta$_2$ agonists can be delivered by a self-administered, *metered dose inhaler* that delivers a predetermined quantity of the drug directly into the lungs. **Salbutamol** and **terbutaline** can also be delivered by a *nebuliser*, a face-mask adapted for drug delivery that converts a solution of the drug into an aerosol mist. Nebulisers can deliver higher doses of these drugs than can inhalers and are recommended for patients with an acute exacerbation of asthma. In specific cases, administration may be by tablet, syrup or injection.

*Side-effects* The side-effects of selective beta$_2$ agonists are mainly due to them interacting with other adrenergic receptors. Beta$_1$ receptors on the heart can be inadvertently targeted and result in tachycardia or palpitations. Binding to beta$_2$ receptors on the skeletal muscle cells can result in fine tremor.

### IN PRACTICE

Inhaled bronchodilators are generally less likely to cause side-effects than will oral or parenteral delivery. Smaller doses can be administered because the drugs are delivered directly to their target in the lungs.

## Bronchodilators 2: antimuscarinic bronchodilators

There are two drugs in this group – **ipratropium** and **tiotropium**. These drugs are antagonists that block muscarinic acetylcholine receptors on the smooth muscle cells of the bronchioles. Parasympathetic activity increases muscle tone in the bronchioles and so effectively acts as a bronchoconstrictor. Using an antagonist drug to block the muscarinic receptors from the effects of acetylcholine results in bronchodilation (Figure 9.9).

One of the most common side-effects of the antimuscarinic bronchodilators is dry mouth. Parasympathetic activity stimulates digestive processes including

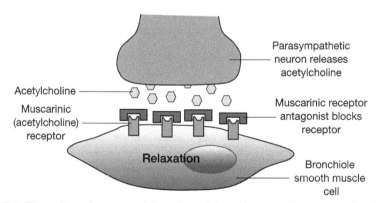

**Figure 9.9** The action of a muscarinic antagonist on the smooth muscle cells of the bronchioles.

salivation, so one effect of inhibiting the parasympathetic system is to reduce the production of saliva. Constipation may also be a problem.

> **CASE STUDY**
>
> Heidi, an asthmatic five-year-old, is brought to A&E in obvious respiratory distress. She is having difficulty breathing and her mother says that she has never had such a severe asthma attack. What should be done?

*Comment on case study* This is an emergency and needs immediate attention. There is no point trying to assess Heidi's lung function with a peak-flow meter because, if she is unable to breathe properly, she will not be able to blow into the device. Heidi should be given supplementary oxygen and **salbutamol** or **terbutaline**, possibly delivered by a **nebuliser**, until she stabilises and is able to breathe by herself.

## Bronchodilators 3: Theophylline and aminophylline

**Theophylline** is related to caffeine and acts as a bronchodilator but its mechanism of action is not fully understood, although it probably involves the relaxation of smooth muscle in the bronchioles as well as some anti-inflammatory action. It can inhibit both early and late phase response and can also be used as an adjunct to $\beta_2$ agonists. **Aminophylline** is a combination of **theophylline** and **ethylenediamine**, the latter increasing the solubility of the preparation and allowing it to be injected in cases of severe acute asthma.

    **Theophylline** has a very small window between the therapeutic dose and toxicity and both hepatic impairment and smoking can affect plasma concentration markedly. It interacts with other drugs such as antibacterials, calcium channel blockers, diuretics and many others.

> **DID YOU KNOW ...** that before modern bronchodilators were developed, doctors relied on atropine and adrenaline to treat asthmatics? A novel mode of atropine administration was to prescribe asthmatics 'stramonium cigarettes' made from the leaves of *Datura stramonium*, a plant containing various alkaloids including atropine. Amongst South American ethnic communities the plant was used in religious rituals and the 1960s saw its revival as an hallucinogenic drug during the 'psychedelic culture'. Unfortunately, the tropane alkaloids in Datura are toxic and deaths have resulted from its recreational use.

## Drug group 3: corticosteroids

Inhaled anti-inflammatory corticosteroids are primarily used to reduce bronchial inflammation in the management of asthma. Corticosteroids include **beclometasone**,

**budesonide, ciclesonide, fluticasone** and **mometasone. Prednisolone** may be given orally in certain cases.

Anti-inflammatory corticosteroids are related to natural glucocorticoids, stress hormones secreted by the adrenal gland that include hydrocortisone and corticosterone. When released during stress they increase the levels of glucose and lipids in the blood, as well as promoting the breakdown of protein. They also reduce inflammation and act as immunosuppressants and it is these characteristics that make them desirable for therapeutic purposes. Glucocorticoids are steroids, derivatives of cholesterol and therefore lipid in nature. As such, they are able to traverse the cell membrane and exert their effect by binding to intracellular receptors, deep within the cell itself. Not all of their actions are fully understood but it is believed that their anti-inflammatory and immunosuppressive action is due mainly to the inhibition of the release of cytokines (cell-signalling molecules) such as *interleukins* and *tumour necrosis factor alpha* (TNF-$\alpha$). We know that mast cells and eosinophils play a part in the inflammation and sensitisation of asthmatic airways and it is believed that corticosteroids inhibit the activity of these cells. This reduces inflammation and also represses eosinophil activity, giving the body's repair mechanisms the opportunity to restore the integrity of the endothelial lining of the airways.

Anti-inflammatory corticosteroids usually include the other actions of glucocorticoids as side-effects such as an increase in blood glucose, a decrease in protein metabolism and immunosuppression. The prolonged use of orally administered corticosteroids is associated with problems such as osteoporosis, an increased risk of diabetes and the suppression of growth – which could be a real problem for children with chronic inflammatory diseases. Fortunately, inhaled corticosteroids produce far fewer side-effects than with oral administration, especially if the asthma can be controlled with only moderate dosages. Oral candidiasis can be a problem with inhaled glucocorticoids because they produce localised immunosuppression, promoting infection from opportunistic pathogens such as the yeast, *Candida albicans*.

## Asthma preventers: miscellaneous

**Sodium cromoglicate** and **nedocromil sodium** are useful prophylactics against exercise-induced asthma. Their mechanism of action is uncertain.

**Leukotriene receptor antagonists** such as **zafirlukast** and **montelukast** block *cysteinyl leukotriene receptors* in the bronchioles. Leukotrienes are produced in inflammation and blocking their receptors has been shown to induce bronchodilation. They are not used as short-term bronchodilators and are somewhat less effective than other drugs such as **salbutamol** and the corticosteroids. However, as they have an additive effect they can be useful when used in combination with other drugs.

**Omalizumab** is a monoclonal antibody for use in patients suffering from severe persistent allergic asthma uncontrolled by steroids and beta agonists. It acts by blocking the interaction of IgE antibodies and mast cells, which in turn prevents the release of inflammatory mediators such as histamine. **Omalizumab**, like all drugs produced by *recombinant technology*, is relatively expensive so its use is restricted within NICE guidelines.

## COPD drugs: miscellaneous

**Roflumilast** is a relatively recent **phosphodiesterase type-4 inhibitor**, licensed in the UK for use in COPD associated with chronic bronchitis. By a complex mechanism **roflumilast** inhibits the release of inflammatory mediators in the bronchioles.

**Mucolytics** reduce mucus viscosity in COPD patients which enhances expectoration and include **carbocisteine**, **erdosteine** and **mecysteine**. The mechanism by which these drugs work is not fully understood.

## Cough relievers

Coughs may result from temporary upper respiratory infections or they may be a symptom of a more serious underlying disorder. In the latter case it is recommended that the main pathology is addressed before suppressing the cough. In COPD such as chronic bronchitis, cough suppressants may provide relief from cough but sputum retention can be a problem and increase the risk of infection. Smokers' cough is best treated by giving up smoking.

Two drugs are recommended for a dry or painful cough – **codeine phosphate** and **pholcodine**. Both are opiates and work by a poorly defined suppressive action on the 'cough centre' in the brainstem. When taken in larger doses, side-effects include constipation and respiratory depression.

**Expectorants** are medicines that promote the expulsion of bronchial secretions. There are many proprietary expectorant preparations and cough remedies available OTC, containing a range of drugs in various combinations, but evidence for their efficacy is poor.

**A QUICK RECAP on drugs used in the treatment of respiratory disorders**

- There are two principal approaches to treating asthma and COPD. Bronchodilators open the airways, making breathing easier. Asthma-preventing drugs such as corticosteroids reduce inflammation, mucus production and oedema.

- Selective beta$_2$ agonists such as **salbutamol** and **terbutaline** mimic adrenaline and cause smooth muscle in the bronchioles to relax – and the bronchioles to dilate.

- Antimuscarinic bronchodilators such as **ipratropium** block acetylcholine receptors and cause smooth muscle in the bronchioles to relax – and the bronchioles to dilate.

- Corticosteroids such as **beclometasone** act as immunosuppressants and reduce the activity of mast cells and eosinophils which cause inflammation and long-term damage to the lining of the airways.
- Severe dry cough can be treated using **codeine**-based drugs, but suppressing a cough is not always desirable in COPD due to sputum retention.

## FURTHER RECOMMENDED READING

All recommended websites are open access (but some may require free registration).

Asthma UK – http://www.asthma.org.uk/

British Lung Foundation – http://www.lunguk.org/

Medscape – pulmonary diseases – http://emedicine.medscape.com/pulmonology

NICE Guidelines on COPD – http://www.nice.org.uk/guidance/CG12

NHS website (asthma) – http://www.nhs.uk/conditions/asthma/

NICE Guidelines on Omalizumab for severe persistent allergic asthma – http://www.nice.org.uk/guidance/TA133

## Test yourself

Now you have finished reading through this chapter try answering these questions to see how much you have learned.

*The answers to these questions are at the end of the book (see p. 316).*

1 List the airways through which air flows from the mouth to the alveoli.

2 What is the average area of the alveoli? (Square metres or tennis courts will do.)

3 What happens to the rate and depth of breathing as carbon dioxide levels rise?

4 Where are the central chemoreceptors located?

5 Explain the term *hypoxic drive*.

6 What is the normal function of mucus in the airways?

7 Name five possible triggers of an asthma attack.

8 What is dyspnoea?

9 Explain the key difference between emphysema and bronchitis.

10 What is the main causative agent of emphysema and bronchitis?

11 Which cells are targeted by both **salbutamol** and **ipratropium**?

12 What receptor is the main target for **ipratropium**?

13 How are corticosteroids useful in asthma?

14 Why would long-term systemic use of corticosteroids be problematical in children?

15 What common side-effect might be caused by a cough reliever such as **codeine**?

Answers to questions on p. 213.

1 The trachea.
2 Oxygen.
3 Air enters the lungs.
4 The alveoli.
5 The pleural membranes.

# Chapter 10

# Disorders and drugs of the endocrine system

This chapter starts by examining the physiological functions of the endocrine system, especially the regulation of blood glucose, the function of the thyroid gland and the hormonal regulation of the female reproductive cycle. We then consider disorders and pathologies associated with the endocrine system including diabetes, osteoporosis, post-menopausal symptoms and thyroid disorders. Finally we investigate the pharmacology, the action of the major drug groups used in the treatment of key endocrine disorders, for contraceptive purposes and reproductive dysfunction.

## CONTENTS

This chapter is organised slightly differently from previous chapters. Normally we would discuss the physiology of a system, followed by associated disorders and finally the drugs used to treat those disorders. The endocrine system, however, is not a tightly integrated system like the nervous system. The various hormones discussed in this chapter, although contributing to general homeostasis, are not closely related and control different physiological processes. As a consequence, their associated pathologies affecting blood glucose, bone, reproduction and thyroid function are also not interrelated (other than being associated with the endocrine system). Therefore, to make this chapter more coherent, we will group the pathologies and drugs into separate, discrete topics.

As usual, the chapter contains some brief case studies and finishes off with self-test questions to enable you to ensure that you have understood the physiology of the endocrine system, associated disorders and the pharmacology of drugs used to treat those disorders. The chapter also discusses one of the most commonly prescribed groups of drugs in the UK – hormonal contraceptives. Whilst on the subject of reproduction, we will also visit drugs used to treat sexual dysfunction in men.

### IN PRACTICE

Whatever your branch of clinical practice, you will undoubtedly encounter patients who have been prescribed drugs that act on the endocrine system. Some of these patients will suffer from diabetes, a disease that affects at least 2.5 million people in the UK. You may come into contact with these patients for reasons other than their diabetes, but it is still important to understand both the disease and the associated drugs to avoid potential problems such as drug interactions. Hormonal contraceptives are another common group of drugs that could be prescribed to any woman of child-bearing age. Closely related are drugs used as hormone replacement therapy (HRT) for older women for the treatment of post-menopausal symptoms. Again it is important to understand their action as there is the possibility that their effectiveness may be compromised by other drugs – with obvious and unfortunate consequences where they are prescribed for contraceptive purposes! As hormonal contraceptives can also have an effect on blood clotting, you need to appreciate the consequences for a patient undergoing surgical procedures.

# Introduction

The endocrine system and the nervous system together coordinate and control most physiological processes in the body. In Chapter 11 we will examine drugs prescribed for disorders of the nervous system, specifically for patients with mental health problems. In this chapter we will discuss drugs that help patients with endocrine disorders.

There are a variety of problems that can affect the glands of the endocrine system. Most of these disorders result in either the over-production or under-production of the hormone normally secreted by that gland, and this can have serious consequences for homeostasis. For example, diseases of the thyroid gland can result in hyperthyroidism, where circulating levels of thyroid hormone are abnormally high, or hypothyroidism, where circulating levels of thyroid hormone are abnormally low. The pancreas is another gland that can be affected by disease. This often results in a reduction in the release of insulin − a causative factor in diabetes. The ovaries secrete the steroid hormones oestrogen and progesterone, which fluctuate in a monthly cycle until menopause around the age of 45, when levels start to decline. This can result in unpleasant symptoms such as hot flushes − unpredictable episodes of sweating, accompanied by a feeling of intense warmth.

In this chapter we will be examining the many drugs prescribed for problems affecting the endocrine system. We will also be discussing hormonal contraceptives, which are not used to treat or prevent a disease, but are widely used by women as a safe and effective method of controlling their fertility and preventing unwanted pregnancies.

## WHERE ARE WE STARTING FROM?

In this chapter we will examine the endocrine system in relation to some common diseases such as diabetes and osteoporosis as well as post-menopausal problems and thyroid disorders. Most people are aware that we have hormones, but what they do may be more of a mystery. Anyway, let's start off with the usual short quiz to find out how much you know before we begin:

1   What is the name of the gland that releases insulin?

 

2   What is the function of insulin?

 

3   Name two hormones produced by the ovaries.

 

4   Does thyroid hormone increase or decrease metabolism?

_____

5   Which pituitary hormone stimulates the development of ovarian follicles?

_____

*Answers are at the end of the chapter on p. 261.*

How did you do? If you haven't studied human biology recently you may have found these questions quite testing. Hormones are rather like vitamins – most people can name them but few could accurately explain their action. If you got them all correct then well done, but if not, don't worry as we will deal with the physiological action of all of the hormones mentioned above later in this chapter.

## 10.1   Principles of endocrine control

The endocrine system complements the nervous system in controlling the body. Both systems can have a major influence on the behaviour of organs and tissues, but generally the nervous system is best suited to spontaneous actions, whereas the endocrine system is most effective in the long-term control of processes. Functions where speed is essential such as sight, speech and movement are best coordinated by the nervous system while processes such as growth, reproduction and the regulation of blood glucose lend themselves to hormonal control. There is, however, close cooperation between the endocrine system and the nervous system and many tissues such as the heart and blood vessels respond to both hormonal and nervous stimulation. An example of both systems working together is the so-called 'fight or flight' response to dangerous situations, where the sympathetic nervous system is reinforced by circulating adrenaline. Some endocrine glands, such as the pituitary, are under the direct control of the nervous system.

The endocrine system is a collection of glands and tissues that secrete hormones into the bloodstream. These hormones circulate around the body until they come into contact with receptor proteins that are found on the cell surface and also inside cells. Many of these hormonal receptors are targets for the drugs discussed in previous chapters. When a hormone binds to its receptor it produces an effect on that cell and that effect will depend on the type of hormone, the class of receptor and the location of the cell. We examined receptors in some detail in Chapter 2 and saw that each tissue expresses its own collection of receptors and, consequently, will only respond to hormones specific to those receptors.

Table 10.1 lists some of the key hormones, especially those that have a pharmacological relevance, either because their receptors form the targets for drugs or drugs interfere with their production.

Table 10.1 Selected hormones released by endocrine glands and their actions

| Gland or tissue | Hormone* | Targets | Effects |
|---|---|---|---|
| Posterior pituitary | Antidiuretic hormone (ADH) – vasopressin | Kidneys and arterioles | Inhibits urine production and so conserves water. Vasoconstriction maintains blood pressure |
| Anterior pituitary | Follicle-stimulating hormone (FSH) | Ovaries (females) Testes (males) | Stimulates ovarian follicles in females and sperm production in males |
| Anterior pituitary | Luteinising hormone (LH) | Ovaries (females) Testes (males) | Causes ovulation in females and testosterone secretion in males |
| Ovaries | Oestrogens | Anterior pituitary Breasts Uterus | Regulates reproductive cycle. Maintains secondary sexual characteristics, etc. |
| Ovaries | Progesterone | Anterior pituitary Uterus | Regulates reproductive cycle. Maintains pregnancy |
| Thyroid | Thyroid hormone | Various tissues | Regulation of metabolic rate and promotion of body growth |
| Adrenal cortex | Aldosterone | Kidneys | Regulates the body's sodium balance (and therefore blood pressure) |
| Adrenal cortex | Cortisol | Various tissues including the liver | Release of glucose, amino acids and fatty acids into the blood |
| Adrenal medulla | Adrenaline (epinephrine) | Various tissues – heart, blood vessels and bronchioles etc. | Increase in blood pressure and blood glucose, bronchodilation, etc. |
| Pancreas | Insulin and glucagon | Various tissues – liver and fat cells | Regulation of blood glucose |

* Note that this is an abbreviated list of hormones, selected because of their pharmacological relevance or because they are key to physiological systems mentioned in other chapters.

Hormones can be divided into three classes . . .

● Peptide (protein) hormones, e.g. insulin

● Steroid hormones, e.g. oestrogen and progesterone

● Amine hormones, e.g. adrenaline and thyroid hormone (thyroxine).

The mechanism of action of these different classes of hormone varies according to the hormone type.

*Peptide hormones* These are hydrophilic (attracted by water) and dissolve in water. From this it follows that they are lipophobic (repelled by lipids) and insoluble

Figure 10.1 Peptide hormones bind to receptors on the surface of cells.

Figure 10.2 Steroid hormones bind to receptors within cells and generally initiate protein synthesis.

in lipids. As cell membranes are essentially lipid in nature, peptide hormones are unable to pass through the cell membrane and exert their influence on the cell by binding to receptors on the cell surface (Figure 10.1).

*Steroid hormones* These are all derived from cholesterol and, being lipid in nature, they are lipophilic (attracted to lipids) and pass through the cell membrane. Inside the cell steroid hormones bind to their receptors and produce an effect within the cell, often the initiation of protein synthesis (Figure 10.2). For example, testosterone stimulates the production of muscle protein (which is why synthetic steroids are sometimes used illegally by some athletes to increase their muscle bulk).

*Amine hormones* These vary in their action. For example, adrenaline behaves as a peptide whereas thyroid hormone behaves as a steroid.

 **A QUICK RECAP on principles of endocrine control**

● The endocrine system comprises various glands and tissues that secrete hormones into the bloodstream.

● Hormones travel in the blood and diffuse into the tissues where they bind to receptors in and on cells.

- The effect of a hormone binding to a tissue depends on the type of hormone, the class of receptor and the location of the cell.

- Hormones can be divided into three types – peptides, steroids and amines.

## 10.2  Disorders of glucose regulation – and associated drugs

### The regulation of blood glucose

Glucose, a *monosaccharide* sugar, is one of the principal fuels used by our body to make energy. In our cells, glucose is broken down to produce adenosine triphosphate (ATP), the energy-providing molecule that powers the millions of biochemical reactions that take place in our body every second.

We obtain glucose from the food we eat, predominantly starch-rich foods such as potatoes, rice, bread and pasta. In the small intestine, glucose is absorbed into the blood and routed to the liver via the hepatic portal vein. The hepatocytes (liver cells) absorb much of the recently acquired glucose and convert it into glycogen, an insoluble polymer of glucose. This is stored in the hepatocytes and can be reconverted to glucose when blood glucose levels fall.

> *Monosaccharide* literally means single sugar. Glucose is a single sugar molecule that can also exist as a disaccharide when two glucoses join to form *maltose*. Glucose molecules can also join together in long chains called polymers to form glycogen.

All cells need to make energy and most can use lipids as fuel as well as sugars. Neurons, however, rely almost exclusively on glucose for their energy, which is why the maintenance of appropriate blood glucose levels is essential for the proper functioning of the nervous system. In hypoglycaemia (low blood glucose levels) neurological processes in the brain can be compromised. At some time, most of us will have missed a meal and experienced the effects of low blood glucose, a feeling of being light-headed along with an inability to concentrate normally. Hyperglycaemia (high blood glucose levels) can also cause neurological disturbance such as blurred vision and headache. Chronic hyperglycaemia, a common feature of diabetes mellitus, can be a contributory factor to atherosclerosis, eye problems and renal failure.

Our blood glucose levels are liable to fluctuation because our food intake can vary greatly over a 24-hour period. After meals, the body absorbs nutrients from the digestive system and, though buffered somewhat by glucose storage in the liver, blood glucose levels rise. When digestion is complete and nutrient absorption

239

tails off, blood glucose levels fall. Despite these fluctuations, the body needs to maintain blood glucose levels within certain limits. The brain is especially sensitive to falls in blood glucose as it relies solely on glucose for its energy and has very little glucose storage capacity of its own. Typical fasting levels of blood glucose lie between 3.3 and 6.1 mmol per litre and results outside this range could indicate a dysfunction in glucose regulation such as occurs in diabetes mellitus.

### IN PRACTICE

Generally a fasting glucose level in excess of 7.0 mmol per litre indicates a strong possibility that the individual is diabetic. For an accurate assessment of a patient's blood glucose levels it is now normal to measure glycated haemoglobin (HbA1c) as this gives an indication of plasma glucose concentrations over previous weeks. HbA1c levels equal or greater than 6.5 per cent generally initiate treatment for diabetes.

## The pancreas

The pancreas is a large gland that nestles under the stomach and plays an important part in glucose regulation. The position of the pancreas relative to adjacent organs is shown in Figure 10.3. The pancreas has a dual role, secreting both digestive enzymes into the duodenum via the pancreatic duct and also releasing insulin and glucagon, the two key hormones in glucose regulation, into the blood. These two hormones are released from small clusters of glandular cells called the *Islets of Langerhans*.

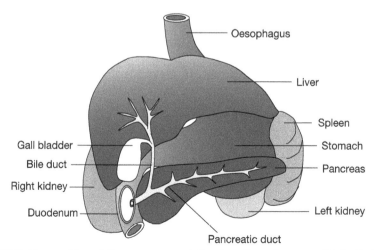

**Figure 10.3** The position of the pancreas relative to adjacent organs. (Note that the pancreas is shown in front of the stomach here for illustrative purposes.)

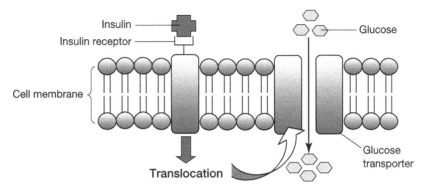

**Figure 10.4** The binding of insulin to insulin receptors causes the translocation of glucose transporters to the cell membrane and this promotes the uptake of glucose from the blood.

## How the body responds to an increase in blood glucose

After a meal the resulting increase in blood glucose is detected by the β (beta) cells of the pancreatic islets, causing them to release more insulin into the blood. Insulin stimulates cells, especially adipose (fat cells) and muscle cells, to take up glucose from the blood. Glucose is a relatively large molecule and to enter cells it requires transmembrane glucose transporters. When insulin binds to insulin receptors, cells are stimulated to increase the numbers of *glucose transporters* in the cell membrane, a process called *translocation* (Figure 10.4). The more transporters that are recruited, the more glucose is transported into cells – with a corresponding drop in blood glucose.

*Translocation* – glucose transporters in the cytoplasm of the cell are moved and inserted into the cell membrane so that glucose can enter through them into the cell.

Insulin also has other effects on the body's cells, all of which contribute to an increase in glucose usage and storage – and therefore a reduction in blood glucose.

**KEY FACT**

When blood glucose levels rise, the body releases more insulin, which allows cells to take up more glucose from the blood.

## How the body responds to a decrease in blood glucose

In the hours after a meal, when digestion is complete and blood glucose and insulin levels fall, this causes the alpha cells of the pancreas to release the hormone glucagon.

Glucagon has the opposite effect to insulin in that it increases blood glucose levels and promotes processes that spare glucose usage. Glucagon works primarily on hepatocytes to convert stored glycogen into glucose and release it into the blood. A summary of the contrasting actions of glucagon and insulin is shown in Figure 10.5.

## Disorders of blood glucose regulation: diabetes mellitus

This very common disease is found in two main forms – Type 1 and Type 2 diabetes, both of which are increasing annually in the UK. Type 2 diabetes is the most common form, accounting for around 90 per cent of all diabetes cases. It is primarily a disease of affluent societies although ironically it is more common among people of lower economic status where obesity, one of the key risk factors for diabetes, is most widespread. A family history of diabetes can also be a pre-disposing factor for diabetes and people of Asian and Afro-Caribbean origin are also at greater risk. Diabetes is fundamentally a disease involving dysfunctions in glucose regulation, but despite it being such a common disease and much research having been undertaken, the mechanisms underlying the problem are by no means fully understood. However, as our knowledge of these diseases improves, so does the possibility for advances in treatment or even a cure.

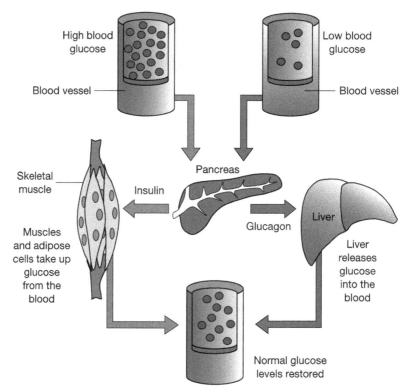

**Figure 10.5** Summary of the actions of insulin and glucagon in the regulation of blood glucose.

Type 1 diabetes is primarily a disease of the young and is the result of an auto-immune destruction of the insulin-producing β cells of the pancreas. Insulin production is severely compromised and regular insulin injections are necessary to regulate blood glucose.

Type 2 diabetes was once a disease of middle age but with an increase in childhood obesity, many younger people are now developing the disease. It is thought that an increase in the consumption of sugar-rich foods is primarily responsible. This causes a long-term elevation of insulin levels and, as a consequence, tissues become resistant to the action of insulin and eventually insulin production itself declines. These two factors result in hyperglycaemia because the mechanism that allows glucose to enter cells has become compromised. Dietary modification may be sufficient to control Type 2 diabetes initially but many sufferers progress to require antidiabetic drugs and insulin injections.

In both forms of diabetes mellitus, abnormally high levels of blood glucose are encountered, typically over 11 mmol per litre. This can overwhelm glucose reabsorption in the kidneys, causing it to appear in the urine, a condition called *glycosuria*. Other symptoms of diabetes include an increase in thirst, an increase in urine production and lethargy.

**DID YOU KNOW ...** that the word *mellitus* has its origin in the Latin word 'mel', meaning honey? Diabetes can result in glucose appearing in the urine, making it sweet, and in days gone by, physicians tested for diabetes by tasting their patient's urine. Be thankful for modern testing methods!

In Type 1 diabetes, *diabetic ketoacidosis* may also be encountered. Ironically, this is caused by cells being starved of glucose. Remember that cells need insulin in order to obtain glucose from the blood so, in the absence of insulin, there is an abundance of glucose in the blood while the cells themselves are starved of this essential energy molecule. In an effort to maintain energy production, cells switch to lipids as their main source of fuel, resulting in the production of *ketones* as a by-product which, being acidic, can cause *ketoacidosis*. Diabetes can be the cause or contributory factor of many other chronic pathologies including nephropathy (disease of the kidneys), retinopathy (disease of the retina) and cardiovascular disease.

**CASE STUDY**

Alison is worried about her 14-year-old daughter Sophie who recently seems tired and listless. Sophie is definitely on the wrong side of slim and, like many girls her age, finds exercise boring. She doesn't go out much, preferring to visit her friends on social network sites. Sophie's aunt developed Type 2 diabetes when she was 25 and Alison is worried that diabetes might be a problem for the family. Should Alison be worried?

*Comment on case study* Sophie is not behaving differently from many other girls her age and her being tired and listless may not necessarily be connected with diabetes. The fact that her aunt developed Type 2 diabetes at a relatively early age may indicate a family predisposition to the disease and these days 14 years old is not particularly young for diabetes to manifest itself. It can be quite difficult for parents to influence the lifestyles of adolescents but Alison can certainly ensure that family meals are regular and healthy with plenty of vegetables and complex carbohydrates. Alison should also do what she can to persuade Sophie to become more active, perhaps paying for dancing or fitness classes. If Sophie continues to cause Alison concern or if she notices changes in behaviour such as drinking more fluids she should discuss her concerns with her GP, who may suggest a precautionary test for diabetes.

## Drugs used in diabetes mellitus – insulins

There are two approaches to the treatment of diabetes. The normal treatment for Type 1 diabetes is insulin given by subcutaneous injection. This is to replace the body's own insulin deficiency where endogenous insulin production is minimal or non-existent. Treatment for Type 2 diabetes is more complex because this form of the disease can vary in its intensity and nature. Oral antidiabetic drugs work by a variety of means, generally either stimulating residual insulin secretion by the β cells of the pancreas, or encouraging muscle and adipose cells to take up glucose from the blood. Supplementary insulin may also be required by some Type 2 diabetics.

> **IN PRACTICE**
> Before Type 2 diabetics are prescribed oral antidiabetic drugs, control of the disease is usually attempted by at least three months of dietary modification and an increase in exercise. Eating moderate amounts of complex carbohydrates that release their sugars slowly can help to maintain stable blood glucose levels. Exercise increases the cellular uptake of glucose.

There are various types of insulin available for injection. All of these are the result of many years of research and development, stretching back to the 1920s when insulin, extracted from the pancreases of cattle, was first used to treat diabetic patients. Modern insulins are from three sources – modified porcine (pig), bovine (cattle) or genetically engineered human insulin. The latter form of human insulin is not extracted from humans but is produced in bacteria and yeast using genetic engineering. The gene that codes for human insulin is inserted into bacteria and yeast, which produce the insulin protein in large quantities. The protein produced in this way requires further purification and modification before it can be used as a medicine. The advantage of human insulin is that it is self-evidently more similar in structure to the patient's own insulin, so there is less chance of it causing an adverse reaction.

Insulin can be further modified to affect the rate at which it is absorbed, thus delaying the time of onset and prolonging the duration of its effect. This modification is effected by attaching zinc or other residues to the insulin molecule or by genetically engineering insulins with a slightly different amino acid sequence. The various insulins currently available are categorised by the rate at which they begin to act and the duration of their action.

- **Short-acting insulins** have a rapid onset (30 to 60 minutes), and a peak action of between 2 to 4 hours with duration up to 8 hours. These insulins include **insulin, insulin aspart, insulin glulisine** and **insulin lispro.**

- **Intermediate and long-lasting insulins** have an onset of between 1 to 2 hours, a peak action of between 4 to 12 hours and duration of 16 to 35 hours. These insulins include **insulin detemir, insulin glargine, insulin zinc suspension, isophane insulin** and **protamine zinc insulin.**

- **Biphasic insulins** are a mixture of intermediate and fast-acting insulins that produce rapid onset but long-lasting effects. These insulins include **biphasic insulin aspart, biphasic insulin lispro** and **biphasic isophane insulin.**

> **DID YOU KNOW ...** the reason that insulin has to be injected is because it is a protein and proteins will not survive digestive enzymes in the gut? Inhaled insulins were introduced a few years ago but subsequently with-drawn following concerns over safety. Modern insulin injection devices resemble fountain pens and make the self-injection of insulin relatively easy and painless.

## Drugs used in diabetes mellitus – antidiabetic drugs

These drugs are used to treat Type 2 diabetes when dietary and exercise changes have failed to control the condition.

1  **Biguanides – metformin** is the only biguanide currently available. It works by reducing hepatic synthesis of glucose and increasing the uptake of glucose by peripheral cells – but only where there is a residual production of insulin by the pancreas. **Metformin** is usually the drug of first choice for the treatment of Type 2 diabetes, especially in overweight patients.

2  **Sulfonylureas** – short-acting sulfonylureas include **gliclazide** and **tolbutamide.** **Glibenclamide, glimepiride** and **glipizide** are longer-acting and may thus have more side-effects such as occasional hypoglycaemia. All of the sulfonylureas work by opening $Ca^{2+}$ channels in the cell membrane of the β cells of the pancreas, stimulating them to release insulin. These drugs are only suitable for use in Type 2 diabetes where the β cells retain some insulin-secreting capacity.

3  **Acarbose** inhibits the *α-glucosidase* enzymes in the gut that have a role in the digestion of starches. This reduces the rate at which starches are broken down and consequently the rate at which glucose is absorbed. This can reduce the

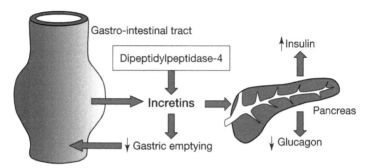

**Figure 10.6** Food in the gastro-intestinal tract stimulates the release of incretins that promote the secretion of insulin while inhibiting both glucagon and gastric emptying. Dipeptidylpeptidase-4 is an enzyme that breaks down incretins.

risk of hyperglycaemia after a meal. Unfortunately, undigested sugars in the gut can feed gas-producing bacteria, resulting in flatulence, a side-effect that (not surprisingly) puts off many patients from continuing with this drug.

4 **Exenatide** and **liraglutide** are relatively recent drugs which increase insulin secretion by the pancreatic beta cells while reducing glucagon release by the alpha cells and also slowing the rate of gastric emptying. They are synthetic forms of *exendin-4*, a hormone first isolated from the saliva of an American desert lizard. Exendin-4 mimics the action of *glucagon-like peptide-1* (GLP-1) of the *incretin* family of peptides, released by the gastro-intestinal tract immediately following a meal (Figure 10.6). These drugs rely on residual activity of the pancreatic beta cells so are only used for the treatment of Type 2 diabetes, generally in combination with **metformin** and a sulfonylurea.

5 **Linagliptin**, **saxagliptin**, **sitagliptin** and **vildagliptin** are recently introduced drugs that work within the same pathways described above for **exenatide**. The 'gliptins', as they are frequently called, are inhibitors of *dipeptidylpeptidase-4*, an enzyme that breaks down the incretins. By blocking dipeptidylpeptidase-4, the 'gliptins' increase natural incretin levels; this increases insulin production and suppresses glucagon production. As with **exenatide** and **liraglutide**, the 'gliptins' are only used for the treatment of Type 2 diabetes, generally in com-bination with **metformin** and a sulfonylurea.

6 **Meglitinides** are currently represented by two drugs, **nateglinide** and **repaglin-ide**. They work by a very similar mechanism to the sulfonylureas, stimulating insulin release by pancreatic β cells in Type 2 diabetes.

7 **Thiazolidinediones** are now represented only by **pioglitazone** and this has recently been issued with a caution about its use in patients at risk from bladder cancer. The mechanism of action of **pioglitazone** is complex and not fully understood but it appears to enhance insulin signalling in adipocytes, and thus the uptake of glucose from the blood.

## Hypoglycaemia

Acute hypoglycaemia can arise from an overdose of insulin and chronic hypogly-caemia from excess endogenous insulin production. Hypoglycaemia is generally treated via the administration of glucose, but if sugar cannot be given by mouth then **glucagon** may be prescribed via injection. This stimulates the liver to convert stores of glycogen into glucose for release into the bloodstream.

**A QUICK RECAP on diabetes, insulins and antidiabetic drugs**

- Glucose levels in the blood need to be regulated to ensure that levels do not fall too low or rise too high.
- When glucose levels rise after a meal, the pancreas releases insulin which encourages muscle and fat cells to take up glucose from the blood.
- When glucose levels fall between meals, the pancreas releases glucagon which stimulates the liver to release glucose to increase blood sugar levels.
- Type 1 diabetes is an auto-immune disease that destroys the insulin-producing cells of the pancreas. Type 1 sufferers cannot produce insulin and require insulin injections.
- Type 2 diabetes usually develops later in life and may be caused by factors such as obesity. Type 2 sufferers may be able to control their diabetes by diet and drugs but sometimes insulin injections are also necessary.
- Injectable insulins are divided into short-acting, intermediate and long-acting, and biphasic, and vary in their time to onset and their duration.
- Antidiabetic drugs are used only for the treatment of Type 2 diabetes.
- By different mechanisms, drugs such as **exenatide**, **sitagliptin**, the sulfony-lureas and the meglitinides stimulate the pancreas to release insulin (where residual capacity remains).
- **Metformin** and **pioglitazone** increase the uptake of glucose by cells.
- **Acarbose** reduces the rate at which glucose is absorbed from the gut.

## 10.3 Hormonal regulation of reproduction – and associated drugs

The introduction of female hormonal contraceptives, 'the pill', in the 1960s, revolu-tionised sexual habits in the UK and probably changed society forever. For the first time it allowed women to take charge of their own fertility and prevented millions of unwanted pregnancies. The contraceptive pill proved to be a safe and (if used correctly) 99 per cent effective method of contraception, and although the formulations have changed somewhat over the last 40 years, the pharmaco-logical action of the drugs is still essentially the same. These drugs have other uses besides contraception, helping to prevent painful periods and alleviating some of the post-menopausal symptoms suffered by many older women.

The 28-day female reproductive cycle produces changes in a woman's body that prepare her for conception. Over the month, the endometrium (the lining of the uterus) develops into a nutrient-rich structure, ready to receive the ovum that is released by the ovaries midway through the cycle. If fertilisation occurs, the fertilised ovum implants itself in the wall of the uterus and the wonderful process of embryological development starts which, in nine months' time, will result in the birth of a new human being. If the woman does not conceive during this time, the endometrium is shed in a flow of menstrual blood – a 'period'. After the period, the process starts all over again. The cycle is controlled by an intricate interplay of two hormones released by the anterior pituitary:

● follicle-stimulating hormone (FSH)
● luteinising hormone (LH)

...and two hormones released by the ovaries:

● *oestrogen*
● *progesterone*.

The cycle can be divided into three phases, as shown in Figure 10.7.

*Oestrogen* and *progesterone* are the common names for the two types of hormones secreted by the ovaries. There are in fact several oestrogens including oestradiol, oestriol and oestrone. Progesterone is the main circulating form of the **progestogen** group.

Figure 10.7 Simplified graph showing changing levels of hormones during the 28-day reproductive cycle (hormone levels are in arbitrary units).

1 **The menstrual phase** – this starts on the first day of menstruation and lasts 4 to 6 days. During this phase the lining of the uterus is shed in a flow of blood.

2 **The follicular phase** – during the next 8 to 10 days, FSH promotes the development of a follicle in one of the ovaries containing the maturing ovum. As the follicle develops it starts to produce oestrogen and the amount of oestrogen steadily increases as the follicle itself enlarges. The increase in oestrogen towards the end of the follicular phase stimulates a surge in luteinising hormone (LH) which causes the follicle to release its ovum in the process, known as *ovulation*. The ovum travels from the ovary to the uterus, along the oviduct where it has the potential to be fertilised by incoming sperm.

3 **The luteal phase** – this final phase can vary considerably depending on whether the ovum is fertilised or not. If fertilisation occurs, the embryo that is implanted in the endometrium sends a hormonal signal to the ovaries. This maintains the high levels of progesterone that occur immediately after ovulation. Progesterone maintains the structural integrity of the endometrium and prevents further menstruation. If fertilisation does not occur, the progesterone levels tail off, removing support from the endometrium which is shed in the menstrual flow.

Control of the reproductive cycle involves a complex interplay between the pituitary and the ovarian hormones. As hormone levels change, this signals the pituitary and ovaries to modify the release of their hormones, which brings about further changes and responses in the intricate hormone balance. Artificially changing hormone levels with synthetic oestrogens and progestogens interferes with the cycle and, as we will see later in this chapter, prevents ovulation and conception.

## Post-menopausal problems and hormone replacement therapy

Around the age of 45 years, most women start to go through a phase of changes called the menopause that marks the end of their reproductive life. For a woman who has kept herself fit and healthy this may seem particularly unfair because while her partner may still be able to father children, she will be unable to conceive them. This seemingly iniquitous situation is generally thought to be an evolutionary adaptation that dates back tens of thousands of years to an era when times were tough and the average human lifespan was less than 40 years. Evolution is ruthless in its economy and will eliminate unnecessary expenditure, so it may well be that there was no selective advantage in the female body storing more ova than necessary for an average lifespan that was less than 40 years. Few women over that age were likely to bring a baby to term or live to look after that baby, so genes for reproductive capacity in what was then 'old age' would not be selected. On the other hand, sperm are relatively cheap on resources, so there was little selective advantage for evolution to limit their production (although sperm production does decline somewhat with age).

Evolutionary history aside, in the twenty-first century many women in their mid-forties are still in excellent physical condition and are looking forward to another 40 or more years of healthy and fruitful life. It is therefore unfortunate for these women that the menopause can be quite distressing because changes in circulating hormone levels can produce some very uncomfortable symptoms.

During the period from menarche (the onset of menstruation) to menopause, oestrogen levels are maintained by the activity of the oestrogen-producing *ovarian follicles*. Menopause occurs because there are a finite number of follicles in the ovaries and when they have all been through the monthly cycle of maturation and ovulation, there comes a point when their supply is exhausted. Without follicles, the supply of oestrogen relies on the adrenal glands which continue to produce some oestrogen but in a form that is less potent. Before menopause, when oestrogen levels are relatively high, these high levels have a suppressive effect on FSH and LH, and when oestrogen levels fall with menopause, FSH and LH levels rise. These changes in hormone levels contribute to the symptoms associated with menopause such as hot flushes, vaginal dryness, loss of sexual drive, mood swings, an increased susceptibility to cardiovascular disease and osteoporosis (thinning of the bones).

*Ovarian follicles* are small, fluid-filled sacs containing the developing ovum that forms each month in the ovaries. Their development is stimulated by the aptly named follicle-stimulating hormone (FSH) and in the middle of the cycle, luteinising hormone (LH) triggers the ovum's release during ovulation.

## Hormone replacement therapy (HRT)

As post-menopausal problems are caused by falling hormone levels, the pharmacological solution is to replace these hormones artificially. Restoring hormones to pre-menopausal levels brings significant relief to many women for whom problems such as hot flushes can cause considerable distress. Many proprietary HRT preparations are available, delivering a combination of oestrogens and progesterone. Low-dose oestrogens in the form of **oestradiol** are usually administered continuously with a synthetic progestogen such as **norethisterone** or **levonorgestrel** added for 12–14 days in the second half of the cycle, mimicking the hormonal environment created in the natural follicular and luteal phases. Because the regime is cyclical in nature, withdrawal bleeding may occur when the progesterone part of the course is completed. Twelve months after the last menstrual period, many women switch to a regime of continuous low-dose combined oestrogen and progesterone which relieves post-menopausal symptoms without the inconvenience of monthly bleeding.

Hormone replacement therapy may be delivered orally or via a transdermal patch, as steroid hormones, oestrogens and progestogens are readily absorbed through the skin. Progesterone itself is not suitable for oral use because it is nearly completely metabolised by first-pass metabolism in the liver (as explained in Chapter 3). This is why synthetic progestogens are used in oral contraceptives.

**Tibolone** acts as a combined synthetic oestrogen and progesterone and is used for the short-term treatment of post-menopausal symptoms.

## Hormone replacement therapy: side-effects and safety

Apart from the usual short-term side-effects with HRT such as nausea and vomiting, there are also symptoms associated with normal cyclical changes in hormonal levels, including bloating, abdominal cramps and tenderness of the breasts – and of course the return of monthly menstruation. Unpleasant though these symptoms may be, there are long-term concerns with extending a woman's exposure to oestrogens. Specifically, there is a small but significant increase in the risk of developing breast, endometrial and ovarian cancers, plus an increase in the risk of stroke and venous thrombosis. The Committee on Safety of Medicines (CSM) has published a series of reports on the safety of HRT based on evidence from clinical trials. In all cases, the increased risk, in particular with combined oestrogen and progesterone HRT, is low and is outweighed by its benefits in the relief of post-menopausal symptoms. The CSM does however recommend that the lowest dose of HRT is used and for the shortest time possible. **Tibolone** also increases the risk of breast cancer but not as much as for combined HRT.

**A QUICK RECAP on the hormonal regulation of reproduction and hormone replacement therapy**

- The 28-day female reproductive cycle is controlled by pituitary and ovarian hormones.

- The pituitary hormone, follicle-stimulating hormone (FSH), promotes the development of the ovarian follicles and luteinising hormone (LH) promotes ovulation.

- The ovarian hormone, oestrogen, plays a part in regulating the follicular phase of the cycle, and progesterone prepares the uterus for pregnancy.

- At menopause, the ovarian production of oestrogen and progesterone is curtailed.

- Falling levels of these hormones produce symptoms such as hot flushes, vaginal dryness, loss of libido and mood swings.

- Hormone replacement therapy, a mixture of oestrogens and progestogens, returns the hormonal profile to its pre-menopausal state.

- There are small additional risks with HRT of developing breast, endometrial and ovarian cancers plus an increase in the risk of stroke and venous thrombosis.

## Osteoporosis

Osteoporosis is primarily a disease of old age that occasionally occurs in men but is most commonly found in post-menopausal women where a reduction in oestrogen is the main cause. Bone density reaches its peak between 20 and 30 years of age, and after that there is a steady, and initially unnoticeable, decline. This is a normal physiological ageing process but when bone density is reduced to the point where the structural integrity of the bone is compromised, it has become osteoporosis. Bone density is maintained by lifestyle as well as hormonal factors. Exercise and a good diet are key factors in keeping bones healthy. Exercise, especially impact exercise such as running, tennis and gymnastics, strengthens bones – as does a diet high in fruit, vegetables and calcium (an important component of both bones and teeth). Unfortunately, most older people do not exercise, relatively few engage in sports, poor nutrition is endemic in our society and all of this adds to their risk of developing osteoporosis.

> **DID YOU KNOW ...** that just walking around can strengthen bones? In the 1970s when humans first started to spend long periods in space, they discovered on their return to earth that the astronauts had lost a lot of their bone density due to months spent at zero gravity. These days, astronauts exercise while in space to stress their bones and keep them healthy.

Besides the acceleration of normal loss of bone density through ageing and menopause, there are diseases such as *hyperparathyroidism* and *thyrotoxicosis* as well as self-inflicted problems such as alcohol abuse that can exacerbate the problem. The long-term use of corticosteroids for diseases such as rheumatoid arthritis can also result in osteoporosis.

> *Hyperparathyroidism* is an excess of parathyroid hormone (PTH) released by the parathyroid glands on the posterior of the thyroid. PTH plays a key role in calcium regulation, so when its levels are elevated it causes calcium to be removed from the bones, which can lead to osteoporosis.

Before we look at the available drugs and their pharmacological action, we need to understand a little more about how bone density is maintained and how this mechanism is compromised in osteoporosis.

Bones are complex living tissue, not, as some may imagine, relatively inert sections of inorganic scaffolding that support the muscles. Various cells are involved in maintaining the bone matrix but of pharmacological relevance are the *osteocytes, osteoblasts* and *osteoclasts*. Unlike most tissues, bone is constantly being remodelled by teams of osteoclast cells that demolish small sections of bone and by teams of osteoblast cells that rebuild it. When this process is finished, osteocyte

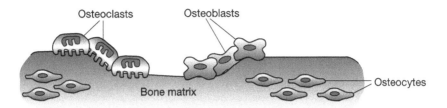

Figure 10.8 Remodelling of the bone matrix by osteoclasts and osteoblasts.

cells are left behind, contained within the bone where their metabolic activity maintains the integrity of the *bone matrix* (Figure 10.8).

## ANOTHER WAY TO PICTURE THIS

Imagine the osteoclasts and osteoblasts as teams of builders whose job it is to replace all the old bricks in a building. Osteoclasts specialise in demolition while the osteoblasts are bricklayers. If the teams follow each other, with the osteoclasts constantly filling in the holes left by the osteoblasts, then eventually the whole building is replaced with new brickwork.

Osteoporosis is primarily a disease of old age and is accelerated in post-menopausal women by lower levels of circulating oestrogen. At a cellular level, the changes observed in osteoporotic bone such as lower density, spongy appearance and fragility are due to changes in the activity of the cells that are involved in maintaining bone density. Essentially, there is an imbalance in activity between the osteoclasts and osteoblasts. Recalling our likening osteoclasts to a demolition team and osteoblasts to bricklayers, you can imagine the situation that would develop if the demolition team carried on working while the bricklayers went on strike. This is effectively what happens in osteoporosis. The post-menopausal fall in oestrogen levels only slightly affects osteoclasts, but it causes osteoblast activity to decline significantly. With the normal balance between these two groups of cells interrupted, bone building fails to keep up with bone demolition and eventually the bone matrix becomes spongy and fragile, leading to an increased risk of fractures – from even minor bumps and falls.

*Bone matrix* is the non-cellular part of the bone that gives bone its strength and rigidity. It comprises inorganic calcium phosphate embedded in a connective tissue called *collagen*. The calcium phosphate gives the bone its hardness and the collagen makes it tough and resistant to breakage.

There are drugs available to help with osteoporosis but ideally it should be prevented by individuals adopting a lifestyle that keeps bones healthy. Women should try to maximise their bone density prior to menopause by regular impact exercise such as aerobics or jogging and adopting a healthy diet with foods con-

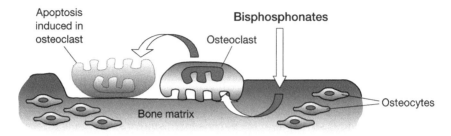

**Figure 10.9** Bisphosphonates absorbed into the bone matrix are taken up by osteoclasts, inducing apoptosis.

taining plenty of calcium and vitamin D – the vitamin essential for the efficient absorption of calcium from food. Going into menopause with strong bones and maintaining a healthy lifestyle after menopause is undoubtedly the best way of delaying the onset of this disease.

Where drug treatment is deemed necessary for osteoporosis, the bisphosphonates are the drugs of choice, in particular, **alendronic acid**, **disodium etidronate** and **risedronate sodium**. **Ibandronic acid** and **strontium ranelate** are also licensed for osteoporosis but are not recommended for general use.

The bisphosphonates have an affinity for calcium and so are naturally absorbed into the bone matrix. During the remodelling process, the osteoclasts absorb the bone and so take up the bisphosphonates. This induces *apoptosis* in the osteoclasts, a form of cell suicide, and so the balance of remodelling shifts back to the bone-builders, the osteoblasts, and this helps to maintain bone density (Figure 10.9).

> *Apoptosis* is programmed cell death, a form of 'cell suicide'. The cell is induced to die in a controlled manner either by external or internal signals. This is very useful in multicellular organisms because cancerous or virally infected cells can be eliminated before the problem spreads.

**IN PRACTICE**

Patients need careful counselling on how to take their bisphosphonate medication. Bisphosphonates can cause irritation and even ulceration of the oesophagus so they need to be taken with plenty of water. The patient then needs to remain standing (or seated upright) for at least 30 minutes to ensure the drug has passed through the oesophagus.

## Other drugs for osteoporosis

Although the bisphosphonates are the main drugs used for the treatment of osteoporosis, another approach is to increase circulating oestrogen levels and so slow the rate of bone loss. Hormone replacement therapy has been discussed above, and although it is effective for helping with post-menopausal symptoms, it is not generally recommended as a first-line treatment for osteoporosis.

**Parathyroid hormone** (PTH) is a hormone licensed for treating osteoporosis. It is involved in calcium balance and is released by the parathyroid gland, found on the posterior of the thyroid gland. Parathyroid hormone is an unlikely candidate to be recommended as an anti-osteoporotic drug because PTH normally promotes bone reabsorption by osteoclasts. This leads to an increase in blood calcium levels at the expense of bone, and chronically high levels of PTH (as found in hyperparathyroidism) can result in osteoporosis. However, the pulsatile release of PTH has the opposite effects and promotes osteoblast activity, which is why daily subcutaneous injections of PTH give the fluctuations in levels that tip the balance towards bone formation and help to increase bone density. **Teriparatide** is a relatively recent recombinant form of PTH that has been licensed to treat osteoporosis.

**Calcitonin** is a hormone responsible for conserving bone by inhibiting osteoclast activity. The drug **salcatonin** (synthetic or recombinant salmon calcitonin) is no longer recommended for the prophylaxis of osteoporosis but can used in patients who may suffer long periods of immobilisation.

**DID YOU KNOW ...** that low body weight is also a risk factor for osteoporosis, and that being overweight can stress the bones and make them stronger? Unfortunately, obesity is also a risk factor for cardiovascular disease and diabetes so, if you want to keep your bones and your heart healthy, reach for your running shoes rather than the cream cakes!

**A QUICK RECAP on osteoporosis**

- Post-menopausal women are particularly susceptible to osteoporosis because of reduced levels of oestrogen, a hormone that supports bone formation.
- Bones are constantly being remodelled by the balanced activity of osteoclasts (bone breakers) and osteoblasts (bone makers).
- In osteoporosis, the balance swings towards the osteoclasts and bones become weaker.
- Bisphosphonates induce apoptosis (cell death) in osteoclasts.
- Calcitonin and parathyroid hormone are used as drugs, mimicking natural hormones to swing the balance of osteoclast and osteoblast activity towards bone formation.

## Oral contraceptives

Oral contraception is a popular method of preventing pregnancy, being easy to use and reliable. There are various types, the most popular of which is the combined oral contraceptive, a mixture of oestrogens and progestogens. However, oestrogen has a pro-thrombotic effect so to lower the risk of venous thromboembolism, it is recommended that combined hormonal contraceptives be discontinued four weeks prior to major elective surgery, surgery to the legs and surgery that involves immobilisation of the lower limbs. Oestrogen also interferes with lactation so combined oral contraceptives are not advised for use after birth when the mother is breast-feeding. In both of these circumstances progestogen-only contraceptives are available which are effective but not quite as reliable as the combined oral contraceptive.

Oral contraceptives work mainly by suppressing the release of the two pituitary hormones, LH and FSH. This inhibits the development of the ovarian follicle and prevents ovulation. Essentially, the body is responding to levels of oestrogens and progestogens that normally equate to pregnancy (where ovulation is suppressed), and if the ovum is not released, fertilisation and conception cannot occur.

**Combined hormonal contraceptives** contain an oestrogen and a progestogen. The oestrogen is commonly **ethinyloestradiol** and the progestogen may be **norethisterone, levonorgestrel, gestodene, norgestimate** or **desogestrel**. There is typically a 5:1 ratio of progestogen to oestrogen. The course of oral contraceptives normally lasts for 21 days and after the final pill in the course, the circulating levels of oestrogen and progesterone fall and withdrawal bleeding occurs, mimicking a menstrual period.

The oestrogen in combined oral contraceptives suppresses FSH release and follicle development is inhibited. The progestogen component of the pill suppresses LH, and ovulation is inhibited. Additionally, the progestogen thickens the cervical mucus, making it inhospitable to sperm, and preventing them from reaching the uterus. The development and maturation of endometrium is also inhibited by the progestogens, discouraging the implantation of any fertilised egg.

Unwanted effects of combined contraceptives include fluid retention, weight gain, nausea, vomiting, headache and breast tenderness.

The use of oral contraceptives may result in a small increase in the risk of thromboembolism, breast cancer and hypertension in certain individuals, depending on age, family history and lifestyle. There is, however, a corresponding protective effect against ovarian and endometrial cancers. Pregnancy itself is also a risk factor that must be weighed against the small risks presented by this relatively secure form of contraception.

There are interactions with other drugs that can reduce the effectiveness of the combined contraceptives. These include **rifampicin, rifabutin, carbamazepine, griseofulvin, phenytoin** and the herbal antidepressant, St John's Wort (see BNF for full list). All of these, but especially **rifampicin** and **rifabutin**, induce hepatic enzyme activity that causes hormonal contraceptives to be metabolised more quickly, lowering their blood concentration levels – with obvious and possibly unfortunate consequences. Broad-spectrum antibiotics, such as **ampicil-lin**, have a similar effect but by a different mechanism.

## Progestogen-only contraceptives

Although this group has a higher failure rate than combined contraceptives, they provide an alternative form of oral contraception when oestrogen is contra-indicated. For example, they are suitable for women undergoing elective surgery because they are less likely to cause clotting than would oestrogen. Those women at risk from cardiovascular disease such as heavy smokers, diabetics and sufferers from hypertension may also be prescribed progestogen-only contraceptives in pre-ference to the oestrogen-containing combined pill. Immediately after childbirth they are useful because, unlike oestrogen, they do not interfere with lactation. Examples include preparations containing **norethisterone, levonorgestrel, des-ogestrel** and **etynodiol diacetate.**

The effect of progestogen-only contraceptives on ovulation is variable and their main contraceptive effect is the thickening of cervical mucus, making it inhospitable to sperm. It may also make the endometrium less susceptible to implantation by the fertilised ovum.

**Parenteral preparations** of progestogen-only contraceptives are available as an effective long-term method of preventing pregnancy in circumstances where daily oral medication may be difficult to maintain. **Norethisterone enantate** and **medroxyprogesterone acetate** are delivered by injection and provide protection for around two and three months respectively. **Etonorgestrel** implants are rods that are inserted subdermally in the upper arm and provide contraceptive protec-tion for up to three years.

## Emergency or post-coital contraception

Emergency contraceptives involve a single dose of **levonorgestrel** or **ulipristal acetate** being taken as soon as possible after unprotected sexual intercourse. The main action of **levonorgestrel** is the inhibition of ovulation and possibly the prevention of implantation. It is effective up to 72 hours after unprotected sexual intercourse. **Ulipristal** is classified as a *selective progesterone receptor modulator* (SPRM) that inhibits ovulation and may delay the maturation of the endometrium. **Ulipristal** is effective up to 120 hours after unprotected sex.

# Drugs for the treatment of erectile dysfunction

Erectile dysfunction is quite a common problem but, before resorting to pharma-cological remedies, it is necessary to eliminate psychological or physiological causes. **Alprostadil** is prostaglandin $E_1$ (PGE1) that is injected into the penis and acts as a vasodilator to produce an erection. Other drugs are *phosphodiesterase type-5* inhibitors and include **sildenafil, tadalafil** and **vardenafil**. These relax smooth muscle cells in the blood vessels of the spongy tissue of the penis, pro-moting blood flow and erection.

**A QUICK RECAP on oral contraceptives and drugs for erectile dysfunction**

● Combined hormonal contraceptives contain an oestrogen and a progestogen that raise hormone levels, similar to those in pregnancy.

● This suppresses LH and FSH release, therefore follicle development and ovulation are both inhibited. As the ovum is not released, fertilisation cannot take place.

● Many drugs such as **rifampicin** and **rifabutin** interact with combined contraceptives and reduce their effectiveness.

● Progestogen-only contraceptives are useful after childbirth and before elective surgery. Their primary action is the thickening of cervical mucus.

● Emergency contraception involves a single dose of either **levonorgestrel** or **ulipristal**, both of which inhibit ovulation.

● Drugs for erectile dysfunction promote vasodilation in the spongy tissue of the penis.

## 10.4 The thyroid gland: physiology, pathology and associated drugs

The thyroid is quite a large gland situated in the neck, in front of the trachea and just below the thyroid cartilage, a protuberance in men known as the 'Adam's apple'. In shape the thyroid consists of two lobes and looks rather like a butterfly (Figure 10.10).

**Figure 10.10** Location of the thyroid gland.

The thyroid releases various hormones, the most pharmacologically important ones being thyroxine ($T_4$) and the more active triiodothyronine ($T_3$). Thyroxine $T_4$ has a much longer half-life than $T_3$ and is the main circulating thyroid hormone. However, $T_4$ has relatively weak activity and is effectively a *pro-hormone* because before it becomes active it has to be converted to $T_3$ inside the cells of the body. Iodine is an essential component of both of these hormones and over 99.9 per cent of the body's iodine is concentrated in the thyroid gland. The release of the thyroid hormones is controlled by *thyroid-stimulating hormone* (TSH) released by the anterior pituitary gland under control of the nearby hypothalamus.

The thyroid hormones are important regulators of metabolism. They increase the body's usage of carbohydrates and lipids to make energy and this maintains body temperature. Thyroid hormones are important promoters of protein synthesis, which is why they are essential for normal growth in children.

## Disorders of thyroid function

These can basically be divided into two groups, those that increase and those that inhibit thyroid hormone production.

**Hyperthyroidism** is a condition where the thyroid gland releases abnormally high quantities of thyroid hormones into the blood. There are various types, the most common being *Grave's disease*, an auto-immune condition, and also benign *adenomas*, non-cancerous growths within the thyroid. Both of these conditions can result in a visible enlargement of the thyroid gland called *goitre*, and in some cases *exophthalmia* (protruding eyeballs). Patients with hyperthyroidism have elevated temperatures, nervousness and an increase in appetite, linked paradoxically with a reduction in body weight.

Severe hyperthyroidism is referred to as thyrotoxicosis, which can lead to a *thyrotoxic crisis* or 'thyroid storm'. Treatment here is of a specialist nature involving IV fluids and corticosteroids – as well as some of the anti-thyroid drugs.

**Hypothyroidism** is another auto-immune problem of the thyroid that causes a reduction in the release of thyroid hormones. In extreme cases this can cause a condition called *myxoedema*. Patients have a reduced metabolism, are lethargic and often speak very slowly. Hypothyroidism can also be caused by a diet severely deficient in iodine, but this is rarely seen in the UK.

## Drugs used to treat disorders of thyroid function

There are two drugs used in the treatment of long-term hyperthyroidism, **carbimazole** and **propylthiouracil**. These drugs inhibit the release of thyroid hormones and can return levels to near normal in around four to eight weeks. Their mechanism is not fully understood, but they are believed to inhibit an enzyme in the thyroid gland involved in the production of thyroid hormones.

**Iodine/iodide**, also known as **Lugol's solution**, is another drug available for the treatment of thyrotoxicosis. It is also used prior to elective surgery for partial *thyroidectomy* (removal of part of the thyroid gland). In the body, iodine is converted to its ionic form, iodide, and high levels of iodide appear to interfere with the regulatory mechanism of the thyroid gland, resulting in a reduction in the release of thyroid hormones.

Hypothyroidism is treated with synthetic thyroid hormone in the form of **levothyroxine sodium** (thyroxine $T_4$) and **liothyronine sodium** (triiodothyronine $T_3$). There are currently no drugs available that stimulate the body to increase its own production of thyroid hormones. **Liothyronine** has a faster action than **levothyroxine** and can be used for emergency cases of severe hypothyroidism.

**A QUICK RECAP on the thyroid gland, disorders and associated drugs**

● Thyroid hormones $T_3$ and $T_4$ are important regulators of the body's metabolic rate.

- In Grave's disease, which is the most common form of hyperthyroidism, elevated thyroid hormone levels can result in goitre, exophthalmus, nervousness and weight loss.

- **Carbimazole** and **propylthiouracil** inhibit the release of thyroid hormones by the thyroid gland.

- In hypothyroidism, the metabolic rate is much reduced, resulting in lethargy. Treatment is mainly by **levothyroxine**, effectively thyroxine ($T_4$).

### FURTHER RECOMMENDED READING

All recommended websites are open access (but free registration is sometimes required).

The Committee on Safety of Medicines (CSM) – http://www.mhra.gov.uk/

NHS website – diabetes, contraception and thyroid disorders – http://www.nhs.uk/Conditions/

Diabetes UK – http://www.diabetes.org.uk/

NICE Guidelines on Diabetes – http://www.nice.org.uk/Guidance/CG66/

National Osteoporosis Society – https://www.nos.org.uk/

NICE Guidelines – Type 2 Diabetes – newer agents (partial update of CG66) (2009) – http://guidance.nice.org.uk/CG87

Medscape – endocrinology – http://emedicine.medscape.com/endocrinology

## Test yourself

Now you have finished reading through this chapter try answering these questions to see how much you have learned.

*The answers to these questions are at the end of the book (see p. 317).*

1   How do peptide hormones communicate with cells?

2   Which class of hormones binds to intracellular receptors?

3   How does the liver store glucose?

4   What is the role of *glucagon* in glucose regulation?

5   What are the key differences between Type 1 and Type 2 diabetes?

6   Ketoacidosis is a problem when cells are starved of sugar, and can occur in diabetics whose blood sugar levels are high. Explain this apparent anomaly.

7   Why can drugs such as **gliclazide**, **tolbutamide** and **metformin** not be used in Type 1 diabetes?

8   Which ovarian hormones are dominant in the follicular and luteal phases of the female reproductive cycle?

9   What symptoms are common in post-menopausal women?

10 What are the roles of osteoblasts and osteoclasts in osteoporosis?

11 How do the bisphosphonates attenuate osteoporosis?

12 How do combined oral contraceptives prevent conception?

13 Why are combined oral contraceptives not recommended immediately after childbirth?

14 What potential problems are there in prescribing antibacterial drugs to a woman taking combined oral contraceptives?

15 Name two observable symptoms that may occur in hyperthyroidism.

Answers to the questions on pp. 235-6.

1 The pancreas.
2 Reduces blood sugar levels.
3 Oestrogen and progesterone.
4 Increases metabolism.
5 Follicle-stimulating hormone.

# Chapter 11

# Mental health and neurological disorders

This chapter examines the physiological basis of mental health problems and neurological disorders and the action of the major drug groups used in the treatment of these problems.

## CONTENTS

The chapter contains some brief case studies and ends with self-test questions to help you to ensure you have understood the neurophysiological nature of mental health problems, neurological disorders and the pharmacology of drugs used to treat those disorders.

**IN PRACTICE**

Mental health problems are more common among the population than many would think. The UK Office for National Statistics in its most recent survey estimated that around one in six people at any one time are suffering from mental health problems. These will vary from mild anxiety to serious problems such as schizophrenia and bipolar disorders (popularly termed *manic depression*). Eating disorders and post-natal depression can also be included under the umbrella of mental health problems. Another closely related group of illnesses that have a physiological effect on the brain (and often a psychological effect) are the dementias such as Parkinson's and Alzheimer's disease, which are becoming increasingly common with our ageing population. Epilepsy is another common disorder that affects the brain, resulting in periodic seizures.

Regardless of your area of clinical practice, it is highly likely that some of your patients or their close relatives will have some form of mental health or neurological problem and may well be on medication for that problem. Although the treatment of people with mental health problems involves many different therapies such as counselling and psychotherapy, psychoactive drugs are used extensively. Drugs that are used to treat neurological disorders of the brain have many similarities with those used to treat mental health disorders (which is why they have been included in the same chapter). This is why it is important that all clinical practitioners have a working knowledge of the various groups of drugs used to treat people with mental health and neurological problems, and especially how those drugs can cause their many side-effects and interactions.

## Introduction

Since before recorded history, humans have used psychoactive drugs to induce changes in their mental state. These drugs were mostly obtained from plants and fungi found growing in the locality and were often imbued with sacred powers and used in rituals and ceremonies. This ability of organic substances to bring about changes in our perception has continued through the ages to the present day. Some of these ancient drugs such as opium and cocaine are now classed as illegal narcotics and heavy penalties await those who deal in them. However, this is a fairly recent phenomenon and in the early part of the twentieth century, both opium and cocaine were sold over the counter in vast numbers of patent medicines. Cocaine was even part of the original formula of a popular American non-alcoholic carbonated drink that still bears the remnants of the drug's name (although cocaine as an ingredient was withdrawn long ago).

The therapeutic use of these drugs for mental health problems also stretches back into history. In eighteenth-century Britain, laudanum, a mixture of opium and alcohol, was recommended for melancholy and the Austrian psychoanalyst Sigmund Freud used cocaine for depression. One would hope that modern synthetic mental health drugs would be far removed from narcotic derivatives, but despite them being much more specific in their action, many such as barbiturates and amphetamines continue to be used illegally for recreational purposes.

Mental health problems range from mild depression to serious psychoses and there are a wide range of drugs available to help. As we will see in this chapter, our understanding of the psychophysiological action of most of these drugs is fairly limited because our understanding of the workings of the brain is fairly limited. There are many factors that contribute to an individual's psychological health and, in these more enlightened times, no one would argue that pharmaceuticals are the best and only way to help people with mental health problems. However, the drugs we are about to discuss do have a role in therapy and many people depend on these therapeutic psychoactive drugs to help them to live a reasonably normal and productive life.

## WHERE ARE WE STARTING FROM?

In this chapter we will examine the physiological basis of mental health disorders, neurological disorders affecting the brain, and their associated drugs. Most problems that affect the brain are poorly understood, as is the mechanism of the drugs used to treat them. However, let's start with the usual short quiz to find out how much you know before we begin:

1   Name the outer layer of the brain responsible for advanced thought processes.

   _____

2   Do emotions such as fear originate in the inner or outer sections of the brain?

   _____

3   What type of chemicals are noradrenaline and dopamine?

   _____

4   5-Hydroxytryptamine is another name for . . . ?

   _____

5   What is the name of the structure that transmits signals between neurons?

   _____

*Answers are at the end of the chapter on p. 286.*

*Answers are at the end of the chapter on p. 286.*

How did you do? Don't worry if you found these questions a bit tough. The brain is a particularly complex structure, perhaps *the* most complex structure, so the associated neurophysiology is equally complex. However, we need to understand the basics in order to have some inkling of how mental health and associated drugs work, and we will cover those basics in the forthcoming chapter.

## 11.1 The neurophysiological basis of mental health and neurological disorders

The origins and mechanisms of most mental health problems are poorly understood. Some neurological disorders such as Alzheimer's and Parkinson's disease do have an identifiable pathology involving the formation of abnormal proteins or the degeneration of neurons in specific areas of the brain. Most mental health disorders, however, have no apparent physiological manifestation and a tissue sample from the brain of a sufferer would in most cases be no different from the tissue sample of an individual without that problem. Sometimes there is the suggestion that a particular receptor is either over- or under-expressed, or there may be some slight difference in the density of neural tissue in a particular region of the brain, but the relevance of these small differences is as yet poorly understood. Genetics, life experiences, relationships, even illegal drugs can all have an influence on our mental health, but the precise nature and consequence of that influence will vary between individuals and it is almost impossible to predict how these factors may result in a mental problem.

### ANOTHER WAY TO PICTURE THIS

The brain is like the central processing chip in your computer. Sometimes programs seem to crash for no apparent reason. Turn the computer off and frequently the problem will have righted itself when you turn it on again. The chip is in some ways like the brain – there may be no identifiable damage but sometimes the software malfunctions.

While the mechanisms behind most mental health disorders are as yet poorly characterised, we do know that chemical imbalance is a contributory factor in some disorders because most of the drugs used to treat mental illness alter the balance of chemicals in the brain. In some disorders, the influence of drugs may be to override processes rather than to correct imbalances, but either way, changing the chemical balance of the brain is a therapeutic strategy that can sometimes produce beneficial results.

Many mental health drugs seem to exert their effects on the sections of the brain that control emotions and feelings. These are generally areas deep within the brain, centred around the *basal ganglia* (Figure 11.1). Changing the chemical balance within these areas can have a profound effect on an individual's sense of well-being.

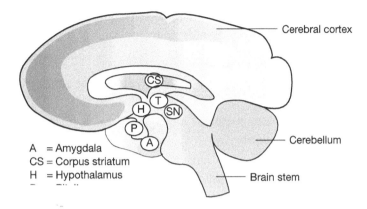

Cerebral cortex

Cerebellum

Brain stem

A   = Amygdala
CS = Corpus striatum
H   = Hypothalamus

showing some of the basal ganglia.

deep within the brain that control basic
s system, the endocrine system, move-

re generally referring to the neurotrans-
iined synapses in Chapter 6 where we
:h other by releasing neurotransmitters
eurons called the synaptic cleft. These
· inhibit activity in neighbouring neurons.
brain, vast complex systems of neuronal
es stimulating and sometimes inhibiting,
ctivity. It is here that our mental health
:he emphasis of stimulation or inhibition
e emotional brain, making the individual
to mood swings, etc. Precisely how this
ito a change in mood or behaviour is at

iin

ansmitter found in the brain. Some neuro-
tylcholine excite adjacent neurons while
id glycine inhibit them. Noradrenaline and
dopamine can be excitatory or inhibitory.

The receiving neurons will thus be targeted by a variety of signals, some
excitatory and some inhibitory, and it is the balance of excitation and inhibition

---

[1] GABA = gamma-aminobutyric acid.
[2] 5-HT = 5-hydroxytryptamine or serotonin.

that determines whether the receiving neuron is excited or inhibited. Imagine this happening in millions of interconnected neurons and you will understand why the brain is still relatively poorly understood.

**A QUICK RECAP on the neurophysiological basis of mental health disorders**

- Mental health problems seem to originate in the emotional centres, deep within the brain.

- Except perhaps for neurodegenerative diseases such as Alzheimer's and Parkinson's, for most mental health problems there is as yet no identifiable physical pathology.

- Mental health problems are poorly understood but neurotransmitter imbalance may be a contributory factor because psychoactive drugs change the chemical balance in the synapses of the brain and produce a therapeutic effect.

- Neurotransmitters can be either excitatory or inhibitory and it is the sum of excitatory and inhibitory signals on an individual neuron that determines whether it is excited or inhibited.

## 11.2 The principles of drug treatment for mental health and neurological disorders

Drugs used in mental health operate in or around the synapses deep within the brain. Before we examine their action in more detail, let us remind ourselves of the mechanisms taking place in the synapse. Figure 11.2 shows a typical synapse that might be excitatory or inhibitory – depending on the neurotransmitter that is being released. As a nervous impulse reaches the neuron terminal it causes the release of neurotransmitters from their pre-packed vesicles. These neurotransmitters diffuse across the synaptic cleft and bind to receptors on the post-synaptic membrane of an adjacent neuron. When the receptors are activated they cause associated ion channels to open and (depending on the ion) the adjacent cell is either stimulated or inhibited. Whether the adjacent cell is stimulated enough to generate its own nervous impulse depends on the sum of excitation and inhibition from all of the adjacent neurons.

Neurotransmitters quickly uncouple from their receptors and are either re-cycled back into the releasing neuron terminal through re-uptake transporters or de-activated by enzymes in the synapse. *Presynaptic receptors* on the neuron terminal respond to a variety of *neuromodulators*, chemicals that play a part in limiting the release of the neurotransmitters.

Drugs acting on the synapses of the brain do so in a variety of ways that we will discuss shortly but, essentially, by various means they tend either to *potentiate* or to *attenuate* the action of a particular neurotransmitter.

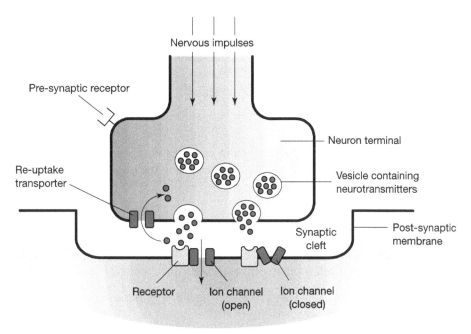

**Figure 11.2** Synapse showing neurotransmitters binding to receptors and opening ion channels.

> To *potentiate* is to increase or amplify the activity of something and is the opposite of *attenuate*, which is to decrease its activity.

If the neurotransmitter is excitatory then potentiating its action shifts the synapse even more towards excitation, whereas attenuating its action shifts the synapse away from excitation – towards inhibition. If the neurotransmitter is inhibitory then potentiating its action shifts the synapse even more towards inhibition, whereas attenuating its action shifts the synapse away from inhibition – towards excitation. If that sounds rather complicated, Table 11.1 may explain it better.

## ANOTHER WAY TO PICTURE THIS

Excitatory neurotransmitters are like the accelerator pedal on your car. If you potentiated the action of the accelerator (more acceleration) the car would go

**Table 11.1** The effect on synapses of potentiating or attenuating the action of excitatory and inhibitory neurotransmitters

|  | Excitatory neurotransmitter | Inhibitory neurotransmitter |
|---|---|---|
| Action of neurotransmitter is potentiated | Increase in excitation | Increase in inhibition |
| Action of neurotransmitter is attenuated | Decrease in excitation | Decrease in inhibition |

faster. Conversely, if you attenuated the action of the accelerator (less acceleration) the car would slow down. Now compare inhibitory neurotransmitters to your
car's braking system. If you potentiated the action of the brakes (more braking)
the car would slow down. Conversely, if you attenuated the action of the brakes
(less braking) the car would speed up.

### KEY FACT

Drugs used in mental health alter the balance of neurotransmitters in the
brain, either potentiating or attenuating their activity.

Yes, this idea of drugs potentiating or attenuating inhibitory and excitatory neurotransmitters can appear rather puzzling at first, but it is an important principle in
the action of mental health drugs. Sit down with a piece of scrap paper and work
through it a few times – you will soon get the idea.

We will explain the action of the various drugs shortly but to demonstrate
how central synapses are to their action, take a moment to examine Figure 11.3.
This shows the site of action of the main groups of drugs used in mental health.
You will see that all of the drugs interfere in some way with the workings of the
synapse, either enhancing or inhibiting its action. It is important to note that
the drugs highlighted in the figure will not all act on exactly the same synapse
because many different classes of synapses are located in many different areas

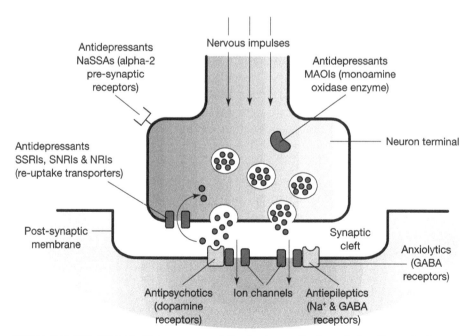

Figure 11.3 Structures in the synapses of the brain are the targets for the main drug
groups used for mental health problems.

of the brain. However, it should help you to appreciate just how important a target the synapses are to mental health drugs.

We now arrive at the main problem in explaining the action of drugs used in the treatment of mental health disorders – namely, we do not fully understand how any of the drugs work! The reason for this is that we do not fully understand how the brain itself works. Neuroscientists have discovered much about the workings of the brain but there is much that remains a mystery. The brain is composed of billions of neurons interconnected by trillions of synapses that makes the most complex computer ever made look like a child's toy in comparison. We may know that a particular drug increases the concentration of a particular neurotransmitter in a particular area of the brain, but why it should relieve a feeling of depression is a matter of conjecture. Undoubtedly, techniques such as PET and CAT scans will enable us to explore more about the workings of the living brain. In the meantime, however, we have to admit that there is a large gap in our understanding between a drug's action in the synapse and its psychological effect on the patient.

> **KEY FACT**
>
> Our knowledge of the action of drugs used in mental health is by no means complete and we can only speculate on how most may produce their psychological effect.

PET and CAT scans are nothing to do with vets, dogs and moggies but are acronyms for *Positron Emission Tomography* and *Computer Aided Tomography*. These non-invasive, high-tech imaging devices enable neurologists to examine the workings of the brain.

## Mental health drugs and dependence

Most drugs that are used in mental health can cause dependence, similar in many aspects to the dependence some people develop on legal and non-legal drugs such as alcohol, nicotine and cocaine. The administration of a therapeutic drug may not produce a particularly pleasurable effect (as might illegal drugs) but withdrawal from it often causes discomfort or distress – especially if the individual has been taking the drug for a long time. The mechanisms that cause dependence are poorly understood. There may certainly be a biochemical basis for dependence, probably connected with the *limbic* system, an area of the brain concerned with emotions, mood and reward, but there is often a psychological element as well. Some drugs, especially the antipsychotic drugs, can produce acute withdrawal symptoms such as convulsions and confusion if the drug is discontinued suddenly. Hypnotics, anxiolytics and antidepressants can all cause dependence and are generally advised to be used for as short a period as possible to avoid this problem.

The *limbic system* incorporates various basal ganglia and has a major but poorly understood role in the coordination of mood and emotions.

**IN PRACTICE**

Mental health drugs have the possibility of producing many side-effects and can cause dependence. As a general principle, mental health drugs should be prescribed cautiously, especially where an alternative, non-pharmacological treatment is available. If drugs are prescribed, it should be for as short a period as possible.

**A QUICK RECAP on the principles of drug treatment for mental health disorders**

- Almost all drugs used for mental health disorders are targeted at synapses deep within the emotional centres of the brain.
- Drugs change the excitatory or inhibitory neurotransmitter balance in the synapses.
- Beyond their effect on the neurotransmitter balance in the synapses, we have relatively little understanding of how most psychoactive drugs produce their psychological action.
- Many drugs used for mental health disorders can create dependence – both biochemical and psychological.

## 11.3 Drugs used in the treatment of mental health disorders

### Mental health drug group 1: anxiolytics

Anxiety is not necessarily an abnormal state of mind and if you are in a stressful situation, such as a job interview, then it is perfectly normal to be anxious. These stressful situations result in a programmed series of physiological and psychological responses that include an increase in sympathetic activity, the release of stress hormones and an increase in alertness. This response is common to all mammals and prepares them for potential danger, and while a job interview is not particularly dangerous, it is still stressful and will provoke a stress response. Some people, however, suffer from anxiety brought about by situations that for most people would neither be stressful nor present a cause for concern or apprehension. This is unnatural anxiety, which can often be helped by anxiolytics that relieve anxiety and help those with stress-related problems. They are not, however, appropriate for use in cases of depression, although some antidepressants such as **trazodone** are also licensed for anxiety.

The benzodiazepines are the main group of drugs used for the relief of short-term anxiety. They include **diazepam, alprazolam, chlordiazepoxide, lorazepam** and **oxazepam**. These drugs bind to a site on gamma-aminobutyric acid (GABA) receptors and enhance the inhibitory action of GABA. Because GABA receptors are widely distributed in the brain, the site of their action and the mechanism whereby they relieve anxiety is poorly understood. **Buspirone** is an anxiolytic not in the benzodiazepine group. It is a partial agonist for 5-HT (serotonin) receptors. Beta-blockers such as **propranolol** are also licensed for use in anxiety but their action is predominantly physiological rather than psychological. However, reducing physical symptoms such as tremor and palpitations (disturbances in heart rhythm) can be reassuring for the patient and help to allay anxiety.

Side-effects for the anxiolytics are similar to those of the hypnotics (sleep inducers), drowsiness being the chief problem, which is why there is a caution for those driving or operating machinery.

> **DID YOU KNOW ...** that beta-blockers such as **propranolol** and **atenolol** are banned in target sports such as archery and shooting as they steady the aim by reducing tremor and give the participants an unfair advantage?

## Mental health drug group 2: hypnotics

Hypnotics are prescribed for those suffering regularly from insomnia (lack of sleep). Drugs in this category include the benzodiazepines such as **nitrazepam, flurazepam, loprazolam, lormetazepam** and **temazepam. Zaleplon, zolpidem** and **zopiclone** are a closely related group of hypnotics that work in a similar manner to the benzodiazepines. If anxiety is a cause of the patient's insomnia then the anxiolytic benzodiazepine **diazepam** is sometimes used to treat both symptoms. The mechanism of action for the hypnotic benzodiazepines is the same as those used for anxiety alone. Also licensed for use in acute alcohol withdrawal, **clomethiazole** can be used for severe insomnia in elderly patients. It has a similar pharmacological effect to the benzodiazepines, enhancing the inhibitory action of the neurotransmitter GABA.

Hypnotics are recommended for short-term use only for those with persistent insomnia.

As might be expected with drugs that send you off to sleep, drowsiness is one of the chief side-effects. Of course, this is a desirable action if the patient has retired to bed, but if the symptoms last over into the next day then this can present problems. **Nitrazepam** and **flurazepam** tend to have a longer duration of action compared to the other hypnotics mentioned above, so would be avoided in patients who may be driving or operating machinery the following morning.

**CASE STUDY**

Zaheer is a successful businessman but recently he has been involved in stressful negotiations for an important contract. He is also worried about his son, who is ill. He presents at your clinic with anxiety that he says is keeping him awake at night. What would you suggest?

*Comment on case study* Being anxious when your children are ill is perfectly normal and quite likely to cause insomnia, and Zaheer's sleep problems are likely to be compounded by his stressful work life. Before hypnotics or anxiolytics are prescribed, you might try to find out more about his home circumstances and the nature of his son's illness. Some men can find it quite difficult to discuss their problems but talking in confidence to a practitioner may help to allay Zaheer's anxieties. Find out what his evening routine is: does he allow himself time to unwind after work? If his problems appear to be short-term, then a hypnotic for a week or two might help him to get a good night's sleep, but preferably choose one that has a shorter duration of action so as not to interfere with his daytime activities. His anxiety is not a clinical problem because it is a normal response to a stressful situation, so you would be reluctant to prescribe an anxiolytic drug at this stage.

## Mental health drug group 3: antidepressants

Depression is relatively common in our society and around 15 per cent of us will suffer from this problem at some time. Depression is more than being sad such as when a loved one dies: it is a clinical syndrome that can produce feelings of apathy, bleakness and lack of self-esteem – even when the individual may, to all intents and purposes, have no appreciable problems in their domestic, social and financial circumstances. Psychological symptoms can also be accompanied by physical symptoms such as loss of appetite, tiredness and digestive problems. Post-natal depression is quite common in mothers of newly-born children.

As with all mental health problems, the pathophysiology of depression is poorly understood. We do know, however, that pharmacological interference in brain chemistry can, in many cases, improve the symptoms and often allows people afflicted with depression to live a relatively normal life. There are three main groups of antidepressants – **tricyclic antidepressants** (TCAs), **selective serotonin re-uptake inhibitors** (SSRIs) and **monoamine oxidase inhibitors** (MAOIs). There are also antidepressants, some of them recently introduced, that do not fit into a neat group so we will refer to them as 'other antidepressant drugs'.

Activity of the first three groups centres on serotonin (5-HT) and noradrenaline-releasing neurons in the brain. Both of these neurotransmitters are of the same monoamine chemical group and share the same re-uptake transporter. They are released from their neuron terminals and bind to receptors on the post-synaptic membrane where they have an inhibitory effect on that cell. The neurotransmitter then decouples from the receptor and is taken back via a re-uptake transporter protein in the pre-synaptic terminal. Here some of the neurotransmitters are degraded by the enzyme *monoamine oxidase* as part of the terminal's regulatory mechanism (Figure 11.4).

Tricyclic antidepressants (TCAs) are non-selective monoamine re-uptake inhibitors that block the re-uptake transporters for 5-HT (serotonin) and noradrenaline so the neurotransmitters remain in the synaptic cleft; in other words, their concentration there is effectively increased. With more neurotransmitter molecules to bind to the receptors, the effect of the neurotransmitter is enhanced. Some TCAs such as **amitriptyline, clomipramine, dosulepin, doxepin, nortriptyline, mianserin** and **trazodone** have a sedative action so are more suitable for the agitated patient. Others such as **imipramine** and **lofepramine** are less sedating.

## IN PRACTICE

**Amitriptyline** used to be a popular drug for the treatment of depression but is no longer recommended as it is dangerous in overdose, causing hypotension convulsions and arrhythmias. The potential for self-harm is greater in depressed patients so it is sensible not to prescribe such a potentially toxic drug. **Dosulepin** is also no longer recommended for the same reason.

Figure 11.4 Synapse of noradrenaline/serotonin releasing neurons.

Selective serotonin re-uptake inhibitors (SSRIs), such as **fluoxetine, citalopram, escitalopram, fluvoxamine, paroxetine** and **sertraline** are more specific for the re-uptake transporters of 5-HT and tend to exert their effects predominantly in 5-HT synapses.

Monoamine oxidase inhibitors, such as **phenelzine, isocarboxazid** and **tranylcypromine**, irreversibly inhibit the intracellular enzyme monoamine oxidase. This enzyme breaks down monoamines such as noradrenaline, dopamine and 5-HT. Inhibition of the enzyme therefore increases the concentration of these neurotransmitters in the synapse. These drugs are less frequently used these days because of their potential side-effects and interactions (see below). Another member of the group, **moclobemide**, is a reversible inhibitor of the MAO enzyme and is claimed to have fewer side-effects.

## Other antidepressant drugs

There are some drugs that do not easily fit into the main classes of antidepressants. Included in this 'group' are **agomelatine, duloxetine, flupentixol, mirtazapine, reboxetine, tryptophan** and **venlafaxine**.

- **Agomelatine** is a relatively recent drug, used in the treatment of major depression, that has an agonist action on *melatonin* receptors and an antagonist action on 5-HT serotonin receptors. Melatonin has a bewildering number of functions including the regulation of biorhythms, mood and sleep. It is closely related to 5-HT serotonin, being part of the same synthesis pathway (Figure 11.5).

- **Duloxetine** and **venlafaxine** are used in the treatment of major depression. Both inhibit the re-uptake of serotonin and noradrenaline and are therefore referred to as serotonin and noradrenaline re-uptake inhibitors (SNRIs).

- **Reboxetine** is used in the treatment of major depression. It is a selective inhibitor of the re-uptake of noradrenaline and is therefore referred to as a noradrenaline re-uptake inhibitor (NRI).

- **Flupentixol** is a dopamine receptor antagonist that can also be used as an antipsychotic drug. It blockades dopamine receptors in the mid-brain but can also affect motor neuron relays in the substantia nigra, which may explain the Parkinson-like problems of muscle control experienced by some patients.

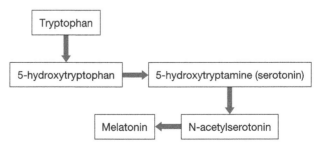

**Figure 11.5** The synthesis of melatonin and 5-hydroxytryptamine from tryptophan.

- **Mirtazapine** is used in the treatment of major depression. It is an alpha-2 adrenergic receptor antagonist, classified pharmacologically as a noradrenergic and selective serotonin antidepressant (NaSSA). This drug is believed to work by blocking presynaptic alpha-2 adrenergic receptors that normally inhibit the release of noradrenaline and serotonin. This increases the availability of these two neurotransmitters in the synapse and so has an effect similar to that of the SNRIs, **duloxetine** and **venlafaxine**.

- **Tryptophan** is an amino acid that is converted via 5-hydroxytryptophan into 5-hydroxytryptamine (serotonin) – Figure 11.5. Not the drug of first choice for depression, tryptophan works by increasing the production of serotonin. **Tryptophan** has been linked to eosinophilia–myalgia syndrome, a debilitating muscle problem caused by abnormally high levels of circulating white blood cells called eosinophils.

Yes indeed, all these acronyms can get somewhat confusing so let's list them again . . .

- **SSRI** – Selective Serotonin Re-uptake Inhibitor
- **SNRI** – Serotonin/Noradrenaline Re-uptake Inhibitor
- **NRI** – Noradrenaline Re-uptake Inhibitor
- **NaSSA** – Noradrenergic and Selective Serotonin Antidepressant.

### St John's Wort ( *Hypericum perforatum* )

Up to this point we have resisted the inclusion of any unlicensed drug that does not appear in the *British National Formulary*. We are making an exception for St John's Wort, first because there is good evidence that it relieves mild to moderate depression and second, although unlicensed, it does get a mention in the BNF (albeit for its interactions). A third reason for its inclusion here is because it is very popular with the public who see it as a safe, natural alternative to conventional antidepressant drugs. *Hypericum perforatum* is a small, rather scruffy, yellow-flowered plant that is common on uncultivated open ground. It gets its species name from the leaves, which that can be seen to have small perforations when held against the light. The leaves and flowers contain a myriad of organic chemicals including hypericin, hyperforin, various *flavonoids*, tannins and essential oils. It appears to exert its antidepressant effect mainly by inhibiting serotonin re-uptake transporters, in a similar way to **fluoxetine** and **paroxetine**. However, side-effects from this herb are claimed to be fewer than with conventional SSRIs – although whether side-effects are dose-related is difficult to determine as the chemical composition of the raw herb can vary considerably between batches.

*Flavonoids* are plant chemicals that have antioxidant properties and so are believed to be beneficial to human health, helping to prevent cancer and cardiovascular disease. *Tannins* give tea and wine their astringent flavour.

## Side-effects of antidepressants

Each patient may react differently with regard to side-effects. The tricyclic anti-depressants are less selective, binding to both noradrenaline and 5-HT re-uptake transporters, so tend to have a greater potential for side-effects than do the SSRIs. Antimuscarinic side-effects include dry mouth, sedation, blurred vision, constipation, nausea, etc. TCAs also have the potential to cause arrhythmias, tachycardia and postural hypotension and their use is contra-indicated in patients with arrhythmias and those who have suffered a recent heart attack. TCAs are dangerous in overdose and it is recommended for safety reasons that they are only prescribed in limited quantities.

SSRIs are less sedating and less likely to cause cardiovascular problems, their main side-effects being on the gastro-intestinal system, where they can cause diarrhoea, nausea, dyspepsia, etc.

Like all substances that have a genuine pharmacological effect, *Hypericum perforatum* has side-effects and interactions. This herb can induce P450 enzymes in the liver and increases the metabolism (and so reduces the plasma concentration) of various drugs, for example, anti-epileptics such as **carbamazepine**, cardiac glycosides such as **digoxin**, anticoagulants such as **warfarin**, oral contraceptives (both oestrogens and progestogens) and many more.

Monoamine oxidase inhibitors have their own range of unwanted effects such as dizziness and postural hypotension (especially in the elderly). A significant problem with MAOIs is that they interact with many other drugs and also some foods. The monoamine oxidase enzyme is distributed widely in the body where it breaks down a wide variety of nitrogenous molecules, including those ingested with food. Inhibiting monoamine oxidase with a MAOI drug can result in a build-up of **tyramine**, an amine that is found in foods such as mature cheese, soy sauce, game meats such as pheasant, as well as those perennial and uniquely British favourites, Bovril®, Oxo® and Marmite®. Tyramine can cause the release of noradrenaline from storage vesicles in sympathetic neurons resulting in vasoconstriction and tachycardia, which together can cause a dramatic increase in blood pressure, the so-called *'tyramine pressor response'*.

Drugs such as **flupentixol** that blockade dopamine receptors have their own set of problems, associated with motor neuron relays in the basal ganglia that can result in problems with motor coordination.

## Mental health drug group 4: antipsychotics

Antipsychotic drugs have a tranquilising and sedative effect on the mind and are used selectively for serious problems such as schizophrenia, severe anxiety and violent or unpredictably impulsive behaviour. Their use requires specialist knowledge in the field of mental health prescribing, so we will discuss them only briefly here. They can be divided into two groups, the typical and the newer atypical antipsychotics.

Most of the first-generation (typical) antipsychotics are of the **phenothiazine** group and include **chlorpromazine, flupentixol, haloperidol, levomepromazine,** pericyazine, perphenazine, pimozide, prochlorperazine, sulpiride, trifluoperazine and zuclopenthixol. All of these drugs are dopamine antagonists that block $D_2$ dopamine receptors in the CNS, but precisely how this produces the effect of stabilising mood and feelings is poorly understood. Second-generation (atypical) anti-psychotics form a sub-group that includes amisulpride, aripiprazole, clozapine, olanzapine, quetiapine, paliperidone and risperidone. These include some of the more recently introduced antipsychotics which are considered to be better tolerated than the older drugs. As with the typical antipsychotics, these drugs act by binding to synaptic dopamine receptors but may have less affinity for the motor neuron relays in the *substantia nigra*, which explains why some produce fewer side-effects related to motor coordination. Some in the group also appear to have an affinity for 5-HT (serotonin) receptors as well as alpha-2 adrenergic receptors, perhaps explaining other effects on mood.

Although most of these drugs are available in tablet form, in slow-release formulations, some can be given by *depot injections*. Drugs such as flupentixol decanoate, fluphenazine decanoate, haloperidol (as decanoate), olanzapine embonate, paliperidone, pipotiazine palmitate, risperidone and zuclopenthixol decanoate may be administered every two to four weeks, which may help with patients whose compliance with oral medication is poor.

> *Depot injections* are given to patients for whom compliance may be a problem. The special formulations allow the drug to be released slowly from its site of injection (usually the buttocks) over a period of several weeks.

## Side-effects of antipsychotics

Any drug that interferes with the normal working of the brain can be expected to have profound side-effects and the antipsychotics are no exception. Dopamine is an important neurotransmitter in areas of the brain, such as the substantia nigra, that are involved in control of movement and muscles. Blocking the action of dopaminergic relays with antipsychotic drugs can cause problems such as involuntary movements and symptoms similar to those in Parkinson's disease. Here, the degeneration of dopaminergic neurons in the substantia nigra produces *dyskinesia* (lack of motor coordination), difficulty walking, tremor, loss of facial expression, etc. Another cause of the many side-effects produced by this group of drugs is their tendency to bind to 5-HT, acetylcholine and noradrenaline receptors, causing problems such as hypotension, dizziness, drowsiness, headache, confusion, etc.

## Mental health drug group 5: anti-manic drugs

Mania is a state of psychosis where an individual experiences an extreme state of excitement and elevation, sometimes with delusions and often with great physical energy. It is often a facet of bipolar disorder where the mood of the individual can swing from mania to depression, which is why it used to be called *manic depression*.

**Lithium** is the main drug that is used both in the prophylaxis and treatment of mania. It can also be used for the prophylaxis of bipolar disorder and recurrent depression. Its mechanism of action has yet to be elucidated. Lithium levels need to be carefully monitored to avoid toxicity that may cause convulsions and damage the kidneys. **Valproic acid** is also available for the treatment of mania. It appears to enhance the activity of the inhibitory neurotransmitter GABA as well as inhibiting sodium channels in certain CNS neurons, giving it an anti-convulsant action.

**A QUICK RECAP on drugs used in the treatment of mental health disorders**

- Anxiolytics such as **diazepam** and **lorazepam** relieve anxiety by enhancing the action of GABA receptors.

- Hypnotics induce sleep and include benzodiazepines such as **nitrazepam** and **temazepam**. Closely related to the anxiolytics, they have a similar mechanism of action.

- Antidepressants are divided into three main groups – tricyclic antidepressants (TCAs), selective serotonin re-uptake inhibitors (SSRIs) and monoamine oxidase inhibitors (MAOIs). They relieve depression by enhancing the action of 5-HT (serotonin) and noradrenaline.

- Other antidepressants include **duloxetine, flupentixol, mirtazapine, reboxetine, tryptophan** and **venlafaxine**. They have a variety of selectivity for 5-HT (serotonin), noradrenaline and dopamine activity.

- Antipsychotic drugs are divided into typical and atypical antipsychotics and have a tranquilising and sedative effect on the mind, mainly through the action of dopamine blockade. They tend to interfere with other receptors and have many side-effects.

- **Lithium** and **valproic acid** are the main drugs used in the prevention and treatment of mania.

## 11.4 Drugs used in the treatment of neurological disorders

So far we have examined disorders and drugs for mental health problems and we have broadly defined these as problems of the mind that affect people's mood and behaviour, but may not have an easily identifiable physiological origin. This section relates to physiological pathologies that affect the brain and often result in psychological disorders that may edge them towards the category of mental health problems. There are many different types of disorder that affect the brain, but we will concentrate on the three that are most common and have drugs associated with their treatment. Epilepsy results in periodic seizures while Parkinson's disease and Alzheimer's disease are termed dementias, a form of neurological deterioration that mostly affects the elderly.

## Drugs used in the control of epilepsy

Epilepsy is a neurological disorder affecting over 450 000 people in the UK which results in recurrent seizures (previously called fits). Some cases of epilepsy may have had an identifiable origin such as a motor accident, a difficult birth or an infection such as meningitis, but for the majority of people the cause of their epilepsy is unknown. In reality, epilepsy is not one disease but various complex pathologies affecting different areas of the brain in different ways – but all resulting in some form of seizure. Some of these seizures are apparently minor, resulting in confusion and an inability to speak, while others can result in unconsciousness and convulsions. Sometimes the seizures arise for no apparent reason, but others have specific triggers such as flashing lights. Many people with epilepsy have few other symptoms beside their seizures and otherwise may live a normal life.

DID YOU KNOW ... that some very famous people in history have suffered from epileptic seizures, including Julius Caesar, Napoleon Bonaparte, Leo Tolstoy, Lenin and Vincent van Gogh?

   Epilepsy appears to be caused by uncontrolled discharges in the thalamic – cortical neurons that connect the thalamus and areas of the cerebral motor cortex (Figure 11.6). Generally the excitation of neurons is controlled by regulatory mechanisms in neural circuits that attenuate (damp down) neuronal activity

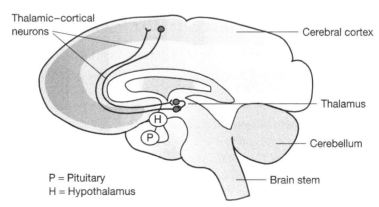

**Figure 11.6** Uncontrolled discharges in the thalamic–cortical pathways are involved in epilepsy.

and keep it confined to the immediate area. In epilepsy, however, this attenuation somehow malfunctions and neurons fire in a random and uncontrolled manner, affecting both the thalamus and cerebral cortex resulting in seizures, jerky muscle contractions and loss of consciousness.

All anti-epileptic drugs reduce excess neuronal activity in the brain, especially in the thalamic – cortical relays between the thalamus and the cerebral motor cortex. Drugs such as **carbamazepine, lamotrigine** and **phenytoin** block Na⁺ channels in high-frequency discharge neurons. **Ethosuximide** inhibits calcium ion channels in the relay of neurons between the thalamus and the cortex. Calcium ions entering neurons stimulate activity, therefore the blocking of $Ca^{2+}$ channels damps down excessive neuronal activity in these areas.

Various anti-epileptic drugs centre their activity on GABA synapses in the thalamus. As GABA is an inhibitory neurotransmitter, enhancing its action will increase inhibition in the adjacent neurons, which is beneficial when they are over-excited, as in epilepsy.

**Sodium valproate** and **phenobarbital** (phenobarbitone) interact with GABA receptors, enhancing the opening of associated chloride channels which increases levels of inhibition in the thalamus. **Clonazepam** is a benzodiazepine that also enhances GABA activity. **Gabapentin**, despite its name, has relatively little affinity for GABA receptors and is thought to act on presynaptic $Ca^{2+}$ channels, possibly inhibiting the release of excitatory neurotransmitters such as glutamate and noradrenaline. **Vigabatrin** inhibits the GABA-metabolising enzyme *GABA transaminase* and thus increases the availability of GABA. **Tiagabine** decreases GABA re-uptake into cells and thus more GABA is available to bind to GABA receptors.

The side-effects of the drugs used to control epilepsy are, as one might imagine, extensive. They include nausea, vomiting, drowsiness, dizziness, impaired co-ordination, depression, constipation, dry mouth, etc. Often given in combination, anti-epileptics have a distinct tendency to interact, often via induction or inhibition of hepatic P450 enzymes. Given the narrow therapeutic window of many of these drugs, special care is needed when prescribing in this complex area.

## Drugs used in the control of Parkinson's disease

Parkinson's disease is a form of chronic neurological deterioration that affects around 120 000 people in the UK. It is generally a disease of old age that affects the substantia nigra, a region of the basal ganglia that has a role in the coordination of movement. For reasons unknown, the dopamine-releasing neurons in this area start to degenerate and this causes progressive deterioration, resulting in symptoms such as tremor, rigidity and slow movement (bradykinesia). The problem can also result in loss of facial expression and everyday tasks such as speaking and writing may become difficult. Drugs used in the treatment of Parkinson's can help with the symptoms associated with the disease but do not halt its progression.

Because lack of dopamine is the major cause of problems in patients with Parkinson's disease, many drugs aim to increase dopamine levels in the brain.

Although providing relief of symptoms on most individuals, the effectiveness of these drugs tends to decline after a year or two.

Dopamine itself is unsuitable for use as a drug but its precursor **levodopa** is widely used in the treatment of Parkinson's disease. However, before it reaches the central nervous system **levodopa** is quickly converted into dopamine by the enzyme *dopa-decarboxylase*, resulting in dopamine-associated side-effects, including nausea and cardiovascular problems (Figure 11.7a). In order to over-come this problem, dopa-decarboxylase inhibiting drugs such as **benserazide** or **carbidopa** are combined with **levodopa** and this allows **levodopa** to enter the central nervous system where it is finally converted into dopamine and can exert its therapeutic effect (Figure 11.7b). **Benserazide** or **carbidopa** themselves are unable to cross the blood–brain barrier and so have no effect on the conversion of **levodopa** into dopamine in the central nervous system. **Co-beneldopa** is a combination of **benserazide** and **levodopa**. **Co-careldopa** is a combination of **carbidopa** and **levodopa**.

Catechol-*O*-methyltransferase (COMT) is an enzyme that degrades **levodopa** in the periphery (Figure 11.7a). **Entacapone** and **tolcapone** inhibit the action of COMT, thus conserving levodopa, allowing it reach the CNS and be converted into dopamine (Figure 11.7b).

Figure 11.7a Outside the central nervous system levodopa is converted into dopamine by the enzyme dopa-decarboxylase, causing dopamine-induced side-effects. Levodopa is also converted to an inactive metabolite by the enzyme COMT (catechol-*O*-methyltransferase).

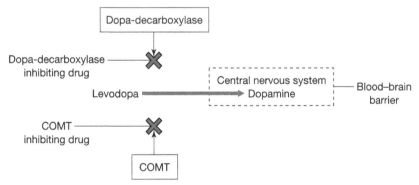

Figure 11.7b Dopa-decarboxylase inhibiting drugs such as **benserazide** or **carbidopa** allow **levodopa** to enter the CNS where it is converted to dopamine. COMT inhibiting drugs such as **entacapone** and **tolcapone** prevent the degradation of **levodopa**.

Dopamine receptor agonists include drugs such as **apomorphine hydrochloride, bromocriptine, cabergoline, pergolide, pramipexole, ropinirole** and **rotigotine**. These drugs mimic the action of dopamine in the motor relays of the central nervous system and restore some of the function caused by loss of dopaminergic neurons. These drugs have fewer long-term complications with regard to motor coordination compared to **levodopa** but may produce more psychological side-effects such as confusion and hallucinations – especially those *ergot-derived* drugs such as **bromocriptine, cabergoline** and **pergolide**. Another dopamine receptor agonist is **amantadine**, which may also enhance the release of dopamine in the CNS.

In Parkinson's, a reduction in dopamine is also associated with an increase in acetylcholine (ACh) in the corpus striatum, an area in the basal ganglia, adjacent to the substantia nigra. Elevated acetylcholine levels in this region can increase tremor and rigidity so drugs such as **orphenadrine, procyclidine** and **trihexyphenidyl** that inhibit muscarinic ACh receptors can help with these symptoms. As with most antimuscarinics, these drugs have constipation, dry mouth and nausea as common side effects.

The enzyme, monoamine-oxidase-B (MAO-B) degrades dopamine in the brain so MAO-B inhibitors such as **selegiline** and **rasagiline** prolong the action of dopamine.

*Ergot-derived* drugs are extracted from the *Claviceps* fungus that infects cereals and contains the alkaloid ergotamine that is used to synthesise the hallucinogenic drug LSD (which may possibly explain some of the side-effects).

## Drugs used in the control of Alzheimer's disease

Alzheimer's disease is the most common form of dementia, affecting around 450 000 people in the UK, most of them over the age of 65. It is a progressive condition that starts with forgetfulness and difficulty remembering the right words. As the disease progresses the individual is subject to mood swings and confusion and eventually major changes in personality and behaviour can occur. The pathology of Alzheimer's disease is not well understood but it is known that there is a gradual loss of neurons and synapses, especially in the cerebral cortex. This is compounded by a build-up of abnormal proteins around the neurons and fibril tangles within the neurons. The production of the neurotransmitter acetylcholine is also affected.

There is no cure for Alzheimer's disease but drugs such as **donepezil, galantamine, memantine** and **rivastigmine** can slow the development of symptoms. **Donepezil, galantamine** and **rivastigmine** are inhibitors of the enzyme *acetylcholinesterase* that breaks down synaptic acetylcholine. Inhibiting this enzyme therefore reduces the rate of degradation of acetylcholine and thus synaptic levels of this neurotransmitter increase, partially compensating for a reduction in cholinergic activity. **Memantine** is an antagonist of the NMDA (*N-methyl d-aspartate*) glutamate receptors. Excessive amounts of this excitatory neurotransmitter are believed to overstimulate neurons, causing damage through a process called excitotoxicity that can result in cell death. By shielding the NMDA receptor from the effects of glutamate, **memantine** reduces excitoxicity, along with cell death. These drugs may delay the progression or alleviate the symptoms of Alzheimer's disease but it inevitably results in steady neurological deterioration and death.

### A QUICK RECAP on drugs used in the treatment of neurological disorders

- Drugs used in the treatment of epilepsy have a variety of actions, most of which delay neural transmission in the thalamic–cortical pathways. **Carbamazepine** and **phenytoin** block Na⁺ channels in high-frequency discharge neurons. **Valproate, vigabatrin, phenobarbital** and **tiagabine** increase the inhibitory effects of GABA.
- Drugs used to treat Parkinson's disease such as **apomorphine** and **bromocriptine** are dopamine agonists that increase dopamine activity in the basal ganglia and restore some motor coordination.
- Dopa-decarboxylase inhibiting drugs such as **benserazide** or **carbidopa** allow more **levodopa** to enter the CNS where it is converted to dopamine.
- COMT inhibiting drugs such as **entacapone** and **tolcapone** prevent the degradation of **levodopa** outside the CNS.
- Alzheimer's disease is an irreversible form of dementia whose pathology is not fully understood. Drugs such as **donepezil, galantamine** and **rivastigmine** increase the activity of acetylcholine activity in the brain and help with symptoms. **Memantine** reduces damage from excitotoxicity and helps to prevent the loss of neurons.

### REFERENCES AND FURTHER RECOMMENDED READING

Books

Healy, D. (2008) *Psychiatric Drugs – Explained* (5th edn). Churchill Livingstone

Linde, K., Mulrow, C.D., Berner, M. and Egger, M. (2005) *St John's Wort for Depression*. The Cochrane Collaboration.

Office for National Statistics (2000) *Psychiatric Morbidity Among Adults Living in Private Households in Great Britain*.

Websites

All recommended websites are open access (but free registration is sometimes required).

MIND (mental health charity) – http://www.mind.org.uk

Mental Health Foundation – http://www.mentalhealth.org.uk

NHS website – http://www.nhs.uk/Conditions

National Society for Epilepsy – http://www.epilepsynse.org.uk

The Parkinson's Disease Society – http://www.parkinsons.org.uk

The Alzheimer's Society – http://www.alzheimers.org.uk/

## Test yourself

Now you have finished reading through this chapter try answering these questions to see how much you have learned.

*The answers to these questions are at the end of the book (see p. 317).*

1 What is the name of the clusters of nerve cells deep within the brain that form the target for most mental health drugs?

2 GABA is short for . . . ?

3 Are GABA, 5-HT and glycine inhibitory or excitatory neurotransmitters?

4 What is a re-uptake transporter and where is it situated?

5 What is the effect of potentiating the effect of an inhibitory neurotransmitter?

6 What is the effect of attenuating the effect of an excitatory neurotransmitter?

7 Which receptors are the main targets for anxiolytics such as the benzodiazepines?

8 What is the main side-effect of hypnotic drugs?

9 What is the main side-effect of drugs that block dopamine receptors?

10 Tricyclic antidepressants increase the concentration of which two neurotransmitters in the synaptic cleft?

11 Which group of drugs might be incompatible with Marmite® on toast?

12 What is the main concern taking *Hypericum perforatum* with conventional drugs?

13 What are the main group of receptor targets for antipsychotic drugs?

14 Lithium is prescribed for which disorder?

15 Which neural pathways are targeted by anti-epileptic drugs?

Answers to the questions on p. 265.

1 The cerebral cortex.
2 The inner section of the brain.
3 Neurotransmitters (catecholamines, to be precise).
4 Serotonin.
5 The synapse.

# Chapter 12

# Cancer and anti-cancer drugs

This chapter explains the cellular origins and pathophysiology of common cancers and the pharmacological action of anti-cancer drugs.

## CONTENTS

The chapter contains some brief case studies and finishes with some self-test questions to enable you to be certain that you have understood the physiology, pathology and pharmacology of this important area.

## Introduction

Above all other diseases, cancer is perhaps the one that people fear most. Even in the second half of the twentieth century, a diagnosis of cancer was regarded as a prediction of an early demise. Treatments, where available, were often ineffective or as dangerous as the disease itself. Over the last thirty or so years, things have changed dramatically. New methods of screening, diagnosis and treatment have been developed that offer genuine hope to cancer patients. Whilst not all cancers have a good chance of cure, there are many that do respond well to treatment and these days a diagnosis of cancer is by no means the 'death warrant' it was forty or fifty years ago.

Cancer is a disease that has been with humankind since our earliest days. References to cancer-like diseases have been found in the Ancient Egyptian hieroglyphs and some mummified remains have shown signs of cancerous growths. The word 'cancer' derives from a description of the disease by Hippocrates, a Greek physician who lived around 2400 years ago. He used the term 'carcinos', as the finger-like projections emanating from some tumours reminded him of a crab. The Greek word was later translated into the Latin word 'cancer'.

For the next 2350 years not much happened to help those unfortunate enough to contract cancer. The diagnosis and treatment of the disease were mostly based on the writings of the Roman physician Galen, who surmised that cancer was caused by an 'excess of black bile'. This theory showed imagination but was somewhat wide of the mark so it's not surprising that treatments such as purgatives and poultices based on Galen's ideas were ineffective. With the advent of anaesthetics and aseptic techniques in the nineteenth century, there were a few successful operations for the removal of tumours but, generally, a positive outcome was rare.

Successes in the pharmacological treatment of cancer did not really emerge until after the middle of the twentieth century. Before then, there were virtually no drugs that could be used with confidence. Mercury and lead compounds were used but these were extremely toxic and not particularly effective. The first successful drugs, introduced soon after the end of World War II, were the nitrogen mustards, still in use today, which had some success with lymphomas (cancer of lymphocytes – white blood cells). Since those early days, continuous research into the disease itself and the development of new medicines has introduced a vast number of effective pharmaceutical weapons that can treat and often cure what is still our most feared disease.

**WHERE ARE WE STARTING FROM?**

In this chapter we will be down among the molecular and cellular structures where the problem of cancer originates. Not familiar territory to most people, so let's start off with the usual short quiz to find out how much you know before we begin:

1 Some cancers result from DNA mutations. What is 'DNA' short for?

_____

2 Is DNA a single, double or triple helix?

_____

3 Is cancerous cell division mitosis or meiosis?

_____

4 What are genes?

_____

5 What is apoptosis?

_____

*Answers are at the end of the chapter on p. 309.*

How did you do? DNA and genetics can be quite challenging but this is where cancer starts and also where the anti-cancer drugs work. If you found the questions a bit tough then start at the beginning of the chapter and work through the background bioscience that explains the origins of cancer. Once you understand this then the action of the anti-cancer drugs will be relatively straightforward.

## 12.1 The physiology behind cancer – cell division

There is no one disease called cancer – it is a collection of diseases with one common feature – the uncontrolled proliferation of cells. Most anti-cancer drugs inhibit cell division so we need to understand the process of cell division in order to understand how these drugs work.

In the healthy individual, trillions of cells work cooperatively to maintain the proper functioning of the body. Heart cells do their job as heart cells, nerve cells do their job as nerve cells, skin cells do their job, immune cells do their job and so on . . . You can compare the body to a large industrial company where individuals working at their own job in their own departments, collectively ensure the smooth running of the organisation. With trillions of 'worker' cells, there obviously needs to be a degree of control that determines which cells do what task, where they do it and at what rate they work. Much of this control is at a cellular level with adjacent cells exchanging chemical signals to regulate their activity.

Figure 12.1 Cell division; a cell replicates its DNA and organelles, then divides into two new identical cells.

There also needs to be control over cell division. In children there's lots of cell division because new tissue needs to be made as each child grows toward adulthood. In the adult body, however, the majority of cells do not need to reproduce themselves and signals from adjacent cells instruct them that further cell division is unnecessary – except to replace old cells that have been lost, worn out or damaged. There are some tissues where, even in adulthood, new cells are constantly being produced. For example, epithelial tissue such as the skin and digestive tract is constantly being replaced as old cells are lost. Blood cells have a finite lifespan and these are recycled by the spleen and replaced by cell division in the bone marrow.

Cells reproduce by cell division. A cell copies its DNA, replicates its internal organelles then pinches in the middle and finally splits into two daughter cells (Figure 12.1).

Normal cell division takes place under tight control from circulating hormones and chemical mediators released from adjacent cells. Take, for example, the production of skin cells. New cells are constantly being produced at the base of the epidermis to replace old skin cells that are constantly being lost from the surface of the skin. If production and loss are in balance then we have healthy skin. If, however, we produced too few new cells or too many new cells then our skin would lose its normal character, becoming either too thin or too thick. This is a rather simplistic example but it illustrates the body's need for the regulation of cell division. Now consider what would happen if one rogue cell totally ignored all restraint signals and started reproducing in an uncontrollable manner. We would soon have a mass of rogue cells and this is precisely what happens in cancer, with a subtle twist that the rogue cells can migrate to other parts of the body.

## DNA (deoxyribose nucleic acid) and protein synthesis

We discussed DNA and protein synthesis briefly in Chapter 1 but now we need to consider the process in a little more depth in order to understand how cancer develops and ultimately how drugs work to arrest the growth of cancerous cells.

Each of the body's cells contains a full set of instructions to make the 20 000 or so different proteins required for the body to function properly. Each cell or tissue will only produce a small selection of proteins, specific to its own requirements, but nevertheless it has the instructions for all 20 000. The code for our proteins is contained within DNA (deoxyribose nucleic acid), a thin ribbon-like molecule found in the nucleus of each cell. The DNA is divided into 46 separate sections, called chromosomes. There are 46 chromosomes in all cells except the sperm and egg which both have 23 chromosomes. Humans are *diploid*, meaning our chromosomes are arranged in pairs. We have a set of 23 chromosomes from our mother and a matching set of 23 chromosomes from our father. Each chromosome codes for many hundreds of proteins which are constructed of one or more chains of amino acids. The length of DNA that codes for a single chain of amino acids is called a *gene*.

**KEY FACT**

The code for the body's proteins is contained in each cell's DNA. The length of DNA that codes for a protein is called a gene.

**DID YOU KNOW...** human genetics are relatively simple – compared to many plants. Humans are *diploid* with just two of each chromosome while oats *(Avena sativa)* are *hexaploid* – six of each chromosome! The amount of DNA in the plants is also surprising. Lilies such as *Lilium davidii* have *seven* times our DNA packed into their 24 chromosomes. So, as you sit down to eat your porridge, consider for a moment that the cereal in your breakfast bowl and the flowers on the table might be genetically more complex than you are...!

## DNA (deoxyribose nucleic acid)

DNA is a long chain of nucleotide units. A nucleotide comprises of a nitrogenous base, a ribose sugar and a phosphate. There are four types of nitrogenous base, **adenine** (A), **guanine** (G), **thymine** (T) and **cytosine** (C). The ribose sugar found in DNA nucleotides lacks an oxygen atom found in normal ribose so is called deoxyribose. The four bases form the coded instructions for the 20 000 or so proteins that are made in cells. The nucleotides are joined in two long ribbons arranged in a double helix (Figure 12.2).

**Figure 12.2** DNA – two ribbons of nucleotides arranged in a double helix.

Figure 12.3 The DNA code for a protein is transcribed into mRNA which is then translated by ribosomes into a chain of amino acids that form a protein.

## Protein synthesis

When a cell needs to make a particular protein it first locates the appropriate gene, i.e. the section of DNA that codes for the protein. The gene is copied into mRNA (messenger ribose nucleic acid) in a process called *transcription* and the mRNA is then translated into the protein by ribosomes in a process called *translation* (Figure 12.3). Proteins are made of long chains of amino acids and the DNA code is essentially an instruction to the ribosomes as to the sequence of amino acids that are to be assembled into the protein.

**DID YOU KNOW ...** the structure of DNA was first determined by Francis Crick and James Watson working at the Cavendish Laboratories in Cambridge in 1953? Together with Maurice Wilkins they received the Nobel Prize for Chemistry in 1962. Rosalind Franklin, who made a major contribution to the work of Watson and Crick, should have been honoured with them but sadly died of cancer in 1958, and the Nobel Prize is not awarded posthumously.

## DNA replication

When a cell divides, the two new cells need to be identical to the original cell. Each needs to have the full complement of organelles and each needs to have a full set of 46 chromosomes. This means that the DNA in the original cell has to be copied exactly into 46 new chromosomes. The original cell now has 92 chromosomes and these need to be distributed equally between the two new cells so each new cell has a full complement of 46 chromosomes.

The copying of DNA during replication is done by a group of enzymes that form a *replication complex*. This consists of *topoisomerase* and *helicase* enzymes that configure the original DNA to allow *polymerases* to assemble the new DNA strands (Figure 12.4). You need to know about these enzymes because some of them are targeted by anti-cancer drugs.

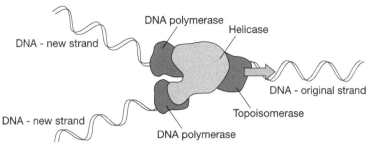

Figure 12.4 In cell division the replication complex copies the original strand of DNA and produces two identical copies. Helicase and topoisomerase enzymes configure the original DNA strand and DNA polymerases assemble the new DNA strands.

## ANOTHER WAY TO PICTURE IT

Imagine a thick piece of rope made of twisted strands of fibre. Now imagine pulling the strands apart – it would end in a tangled knot. This is what would happen when DNA is copied, were it not for the action of the helicase and topoisomerase enzymes. These clever enzymes pull the DNA apart, untwisting the two strands as they go.

## The cell cycle

Generally, most of the cells in the body are in a resting phase but when stimulated they move into the *cell cycle*. The control of cell division is complex, involving a bewildering array of internal regulatory proteins and signal mediators from adjacent cells. Any breakdown in the regulation of the cell cycle can result in uncontrolled cell proliferation, and eventually cancerous tissue growth.

The cell cycle can broadly be divided into two parts, *interphase* and *mitosis* (Figure 12.5). Interphase is when the cell prepares for cell division and mitosis is when the division actually takes place. In interphase the chromosomes double in number so that when the cell divides each new cell will have a full complement of chromosomes. During mitosis half the (doubled) chromosomes migrate into each

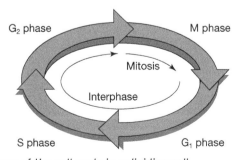

Figure 12.5 The phases of the cell cycle in a dividing cell.

new cell. At the conclusion of mitosis the cell divides into two new daughter cells in a process called *cytokinesis*. The time taken for these phases can vary but on average lasts around twenty-four hours.

The cell cycle is divided into discrete sections:

- $G_0$ phase – the cell's resting phase.
- $G_1$ phase – the cell grows and prepares for division.
- S phase – the cell synthesises new DNA.
- $G_2$ phase – further growth prior to mitosis.
- M phase – mitosis, where the chromosomes migrate into their new cells.

**A QUICK RECAP on the physiology behind cancer**

- Cancer is uncontrolled cell division.
- Cell division is normal in certain tissues – skin, gut, bone marrow, etc.
- Cell division first requires the copying of a cell's DNA.
- DNA codes for the body's 20 000 or so proteins.
- The length of DNA that codes for a protein is called a gene.
- The copying of DNA is complex, involving helicase and topoisomerase enzymes.
- In cell division, cells pass through a series of phases called the cell cycle.

## 12.2  The pathophysiology of cancer

### The epidemiology of cancer

Although there have been major advances in the treatment of cancer over the past few years, it is second only to coronary heart disease as the most common cause of death in the UK. Although all cancers involve the uncontrolled proliferation of aberrant cells, individual cancers vary in their origin and cause. Table 12.1 shows the mortality rates for the most common cancers in the UK.

**Table 12.1 Mortality rates of common cancers in the UK by gender 2007/09\***

|  | Lung (%) | Breast (%) | Colorectal (%) | Prostate (%) | Lymphomas & leukaemias (%) |
|---|---|---|---|---|---|
| Female | 32 | 26 | 14 | n/a | 10 |
| Male | 51 | n/a\*\* | 22 | 24 | 17 |

\*UK Office for National Statistics (2012).
\*\* Note: males can develop breast cancer but relatively rarely.

There is for some cancers, however, a significant difference between incidence and mortality. For example, in men, prostate cancer is easily the most common type but treatment can slow its progression. Lung cancer is actually not as common as prostate cancer but it responds less well to treatment. In women, breast cancer is the most common type but again it responds to treatment better than lung cancer.

There is also a difference in incidence between social classes for some cancers. According to the UK Office for National Statistics (UK ONS), manual workers are twice as likely to contract lung cancer compared to professionals – and this difference in risk is similar for circulatory and respiratory diseases. The reason for this is probably mainly due to lifestyle and environment. We also know from UK ONS data that professionals are much less likely to smoke than manual workers and that over 80 per cent of lung cancers are attributable to cigarette smoking. Colorectal cancer has been linked to diets low in fibre and high in red and processed meat, and the gender difference here may be due to women being more health-conscious with regard to food.

Not all cancers have an environmental or lifestyle origin. The incidence of breast cancer, for example, has been increasing steadily over the years, partly due to women having fewer children, although obesity and smoking add to the risk. This is also a cancer that has a heritable component, parents passing the susceptibility to cancer on to their daughter. Prostate cancer has also been increasing but this may well reflect higher detection rates due to more readily available tests.

**CASE STUDY**

Sharon is 32 and visits her Practice Nurse to discuss 'family planning'. She has a steady boyfriend and wants to continue using combined oral contraceptives – until she is ready to start a family. Sharon is obviously overweight and you can smell cigarette smoke on her clothes. You are aware that her mother has recently been treated for breast cancer. How would you assess Sharon's risk of breast cancer?

*Comment on case study* Sharon's risk of breast cancer is likely to be higher than average. If she smokes and is overweight then it's unlikely she exercises overmuch. These are all known risk factors. Being childless and long-term oral contraceptive use are also risk factors. Her mother having had breast cancer indicates a possible genetic predisposition to the disease. Sharon needs to be made aware of the risks and the changes in lifestyle that may reduce her risk, including possibly non-hormonal methods of contraception. Regular breast screening in the UK does not start until later in life but Sharon can be advised on breast awareness that can help a woman spot the early signs of cancer.

## The development of cancer

What is it that turns a normal cell, living in harmony with other cells, into a rogue cell that seems intent on dividing to the extent that it can cause the death of its host? To answer this we need to look at how the body regulates cell division.

Earlier in the chapter we saw how cells use the DNA code to produce proteins. Provided the code is correct then the protein produced from the code will function normally. However, what happens if a mutation occurs in the DNA, causing an error in the code – how might this affect the finished protein? Will it function normally, abnormally or not at all?

## ANOTHER WAY TO PICTURE IT

Imagine the DNA as a knitting pattern that has a single printing error. What will be the effect on the finished jumper? Well, it depends on the error. The final jumper might be fine except for a small flaw on the back that no one would notice. Perhaps one sleeve may be slightly shorter but the jumper is still wearable. Catastrophically, the error may cause the sleeve to fall off.

Mutations happen regularly in DNA as a consequence of exposure to environmental carcinogens – chemicals that can cause cancer. Obvious carcinogens include asbestos, ionising radiation, tobacco smoke and some pesticides which are all known to damage DNA by various mechanisms. Less obvious carcinogens include viruses such as *hepatitis B and C* and *human papillomavirus* (HPV), the latter linked to genital cancers. Sunlight can damage DNA in skin cells, leading to *melanomas*. Red, processed and barbecued meats have been implicated in bowel cancer. Conversely, some foods are considered anti-carcinogenic. We are constantly encouraged to consume plenty of fruit and vegetables because they contain anti-oxidant vitamins that neutralise toxic metabolites produced by carcinogens.

Whatever the source, mutations happen regularly in DNA and most of them are inconsequential as they either cause no problem or are rectified by the cell's repair mechanisms. One mutation may not cause a cell to become cancerous but an accumulation of mutations can. This is demonstrated by the fact that the incidence of most cancers increases with age. As the body's cells get older they build up more and more mutations and a cell may eventually develop into the one that is the source of a cancer.

Why some cells become cancerous and others do not is not fully understood but we do know that these cells exhibit specific behaviours different from normal cells.

- They divide and ignore the STOP signals from adjacent cells.
- They invade adjacent tissues.
- They fail to respond to self-destruct signals.
- They release signal chemicals that promote the growth of new blood vessels.
- They become immortal (normal cells stop dividing after 50 cycles of division).
- They can spread in the blood or lymph to other parts of the body (metastasis).

Normal cells have genes for groups of proteins that regulate cell division. These fall into two categories – *tumour suppressor genes* that suppress cell division and *proto-oncogenes* that promote cell division. If mutations occur in these genes then the resulting proteins may malfunction, causing uncontrolled cell division. If a tumour suppressor protein malfunctions, this removes restraint on cell division. Conversely, if a proto-oncogene mutates into an *oncogene* and the resulting protein becomes over-active then this may push the cell into uncontrolled cell division.

### ANOTHER WAY TO PICTURE IT

Imagine the tumour suppressor protein as the brake on your car and the onco-gene protein as your accelerator. If your brakes fail then your car won't stop. A similar fate befalls you if your accelerator sticks full on. In either situation, you are in danger from an uncontrollable car that is going too fast. It's unfortunate (but less dangerous) if your brake won't release and your accelerator cable snaps. Better to keep your car serviced so none of these problems happen . . . !

When a cell's DNA is so damaged that the cell becomes abnormal then it under-goes a form of programmed suicide called *apoptosis*. With the death of the cell the problem is normally resolved but cancer cells ignore these signals and refuse to self-destruct.

All cells need a good supply of blood for oxygen and nutrients but cancer cells quickly outgrow their blood supply. To resolve the problem they release signal molecules such as *vascular endothelial growth factor* (*VEGF*) that promotes the growth of new blood vessels, a process called *angiogenesis*.

Cells that are accustomed to reproducing, such as epithelial cells, have a built-in limiting mechanism that prevents them from reproducing more than fifty or so replication cycles. Cancer cells have found a way round this problem that allows them to become immortal and keep dividing indefinitely.

> **DID YOU KNOW . . .** immortal cancer cells are very useful to scientists as they can be kept alive indefinitely in the laboratory? The oldest line of cells are designated HeLa after Henrietta Lacks, who died of cancer in 1951 in Maryland, USA. These cells have been extensively used for biomedical research for over half a century but unfortunately, no one ever thought to ask Henrietta's permission . . . !

A tumour that divides and grows but remains at its point of origin is said to be benign, as in most cases it can be removed surgically. Unfortunately, many cancers migrate to other parts of the body in a process called *metastasis*. Cancer cells move into the lymphatic system and spread to other tissues of the body where again they ignore signals from their new neighbouring cells and continue to grow, forming secondary tumours.

### A QUICK RECAP on the pathophysiology of cancer

- Cancer is the second most common cause of death in the UK.
- The most common cancers are breast cancer in women and prostate cancer in men.

- Lung cancer is the cancer with the highest mortality – in women and men.
- Environmental and genetic factors influence the development of cancer.
- Cancers start with cumulative mutations in the DNA of a single cell.
- Cancer cells ignore the stop signals from adjacent cells and invade adjacent tissues.
- They ignore signals to self-destruct and become immortal.
- Cancer can spread to other parts of the body, a process called metastasis.

## 12.3   Anti-cancer drugs – chemotherapy

Cancer is not a single disease but a collective term for over a hundred similar diseases. Each cancer has a different genetic and cellular origin which is why there is unlikely to be a universal 'cure for cancer'.

### General principles of anti-cancer chemotherapy

There are three therapeutic tactics used against cancer – surgery, radiotherapy and drugs – chemotherapy and targeted biotherapy that utilises genetically engineered proteins. Surgery and radiotherapy play an important role in the treatment of cancer but, this being a pharmacology book, we shall consider only chemotherapy and targeted biotherapy.

An ideal anti-cancer drug would kill all cancer cells while leaving normal, healthy cells untouched but targeting cancerous cells is difficult because differences from other body cells are small. They may behave very differently from normal cells but the usual protein targets for drugs – receptors, enzymes ion channels, etc. – are mostly the same on cancer cells as they are on normal, non-cancerous cells.

The chief difference between cancer cells and normal cells is that cancer cells divide rapidly, so most anti-cancer drugs target processes and structures associated with cell division.

### Fraction-kill hypothesis

An ideal anti-cancer drug would target and kill all of the cancer cells in a single treatment. However, some tumours have a poor blood supply and not all of the drug can reach all of the cells, so only a percentage of the cancer cells are killed. With the second round of treatment, the same percentage of cells will be killed, and so on. For example, if a tumour contains 1 000 000 000 cancer cells and a drug kills 90 per cent of them then after the first round of treatment there will still be 100 000 000 left. The second round will kill a further 90 per cent of the remaining cells but still leave 10 000 000 cells. Eventually, after six or so cycles, nearly all of the cells in the tumour should have been killed, leaving any remaining cancerous cells to be mopped up by the body's immune system.

## Combination therapy

Many anti-cancer drugs are effective for a specific phase of the cell cycle. If only a single drug is used then it may well kill most of the cells in a particular phase of a cell cycle but what about cells in other phases – or cancer cells resting in $G_0$ phase? To resolve this problem, cell-cycle specific drugs can be used in combination. An example of this is the R-CHOP regime used for *non-Hodgkin's lymphomas*. This is a combination of five drugs: **rituximab, cyclophosphamide, hydroxydaunorubicin (doxorubicin), oncovin (vincristine)** and **prednisolone**. Each of these drugs will target specific phases of the cell cycle, ensuring the maximum number of cancer cells are killed with each round of treatment. **Prednisolone** is not an anti-cancer drug but it recruits resting cancer cells from $G_0$ phase into $G_1$ phase of the active cell cycle where they are targeted by other drugs in the R-CHOP regime.

## Side-effects of anti-cancer drugs

No one pretends that anti-cancer drugs do not produce unpleasant side-effects. It is widely recognised that these drugs have some of the most unpleasant side-effects in the pharmacopoeia. One might wonder why anyone would subject themselves to drugs that have such unpleasant side-effects but for many patients the alternative would be a steady progression of the disease, a worsening of symptoms or even death.

Anti-cancer drugs target cells that are dividing rapidly, with the intention of either stopping cell division or damaging the cell to the extent that it either self-destructs or is destroyed by the body's own immune cells. Unfortunately, cell division is not restricted to cancer cells. Skin, gut, blood, hair and sperm cells are all engaged in legitimate replication so any drug that inhibits cell division in cancer cells is also likely to affect these tissues and cells.

The gut is constantly replacing cells that have been shed in the digestive process. Anti-cancer drugs inhibit the replacement of cells in the gut epithelium leading to malabsorption and other disturbances of digestion. Sperm production can be severely affected and some drugs may result in permanent sterility. Men of reproductive age are often encouraged to store sperm for use after treatment. Alopecia (hair loss) is a common side-effect but hair usually returns after treatment is finished.

Most anti-cancer drugs cause *myelosuppression* – suppression of activity in the bone marrow where most blood cells are made. This can cause a reduction in numbers of red blood cells, neutrophils and platelets. The risk of anaemia, infection and haemorrhage are increased and it is often low levels of blood cells that limit the frequency of drug administration. Blood samples may need to be taken regularly to monitor the patient's blood cell count.

Probably the most common and possibly the most unpleasant side-effects are nausea and vomiting. Some drugs such as **cisplatin** are particularly unpleasant in this respect while others are less so, but susceptibility to nausea and vomiting varies between patients. Pre-treatment with anti-emetics such as **domperidone** or **metoclopramide** can help with this problem. Other drugs used to prevent nausea and vomiting associated with cytotoxic therapy include the 5-HT$_3$ (serotonin) receptor antagonists: **granisetron**, **ondansetron** and **palonosetron**. Two relatively recent drugs are the *neurokinin-1 receptor* antagonists, **aprepitant** and its injectable pro-drug version **fosaprepitant**.

### IN PRACTICE

**Extravasation,** the leakage of intravenous drugs from the cannulated vein into the surrounding tissue, can be a significant problem in cancer chemotherapy, especially if impaired circulation in a limb reduces venous flow, allowing IV drug solutions to pool and leak around the site of cannulation. Most anti-cancer drugs are cytotoxic and if they leak out of the vein they can cause necrosis to tissues in the area surrounding the *cannulation*. Drugs such as **doxorubicin** are especially likely to cause tissue necrosis. Children can be at risk because they have immature skin but elderly patients with fragile skin can also present a problem. Often a *central line* is used to ensure the safe delivery of the drug into the bloodstream. Cytotoxic drugs are dangerous which is why they are prepared and administered only by clinical staff with appropriate training.

## Anti-cancer drugs during pregnancy

Ideally no drugs should be taken in pregnancy because of the risk of harming the developing foetus. Drugs that cause foetal abnormalities are termed *teratogenic* and should not be used if a woman is pregnant, especially during the first trimester (three months) of pregnancy. Anti-cancer drugs damage cells and inhibit cell division, a process necessary for the normal development of a baby in the womb. This is why anti-cancer drugs should not be administered during pregnancy. Women who are of child-bearing age are usually counselled before treatment begins and contraceptive advice given to prevent conception. A woman with cancer who subsequently becomes pregnant presents a treatment dilemma for the physician and may limit treatment options. Anti-cancer drugs can also damage sperm so men undergoing treatment may be advised to use condoms.

### CASE STUDY

Jenny is four months into her pregnancy. It was progressing normally when a pap smear revealed abnormal cells. Further tests revealed early-stage cervical cancer. What is the best treatment?

*Comment on case study* Jenny's consultant will probably recommend that treatment is reserved until after the baby is born. Even though Jenny is into her second trimester of pregnancy, no surgical procedure or drug would be without risk to her baby. A caesarean section may allow the hospital to ensure the prompt delivery of the baby so that treatment of Jenny's cancer can be started as soon as possible.

## Pharmacology of anti-cancer drug groups

Having briefly outlined the principles for the use of anti-cancer drugs, we can now examine the main groups of drugs in detail and explore their mechanism of action.

### Alkylating agents

This group of drugs includes the nitrogen mustards – **bendamustine, chlorambucil, cyclophosphamide, estramustine, ifosfamide** and **melphalan**, and the nitrosoureas – **carmustine** and **lomustine. Busulfan, thiotepa** and **treosulfan** are also alkylating agents. They are used to treat a wide range of cancers but especially leukaemias and lymphomas. **Cyclophosphamide** is also widely used to treat some solid tumours. Platinum-based drugs such as **cisplatin, carboplatin** and **oxaliplatin** treat various cancers and have a mechanism of action similar to the alkylating agents.

Without delving into the biochemistry of alkylation, essentially these drugs cross-link adjacent guanine bases (Figure 12.6). This has the effect of sticking together the two adjacent strands of DNA, making it difficult for the replication complex to copy and synthesise new DNA. The resulting damage can cause programmed self-destruction (apoptosis).

**ANOTHER WAY TO PICTURE THIS**

Have you ever got a zip jammed by fluff or some other unwanted material? Tug as you might, you can't separate the two halves of the zipper. Alkylating agents are the fluff in the DNA helix, preventing the strands being separated in transcription.

### Anti-metabolites

This group of drugs includes **methotrexate, fluorouracil, azacitidine, capecitabine, cladribine, clofarabine, cytarabine, fludarabine, gemcitabine, mercaptopurine, nelarabine, pemetrexed, raltitrexed, tegafur** (with uracil) and **tioguanine**. Rapidly dividing cells need to synthesise new DNA so require a good supply of the nitrogenous bases: adenine, guanine, thymine and cytosine. These bases are synthesised in the dividing cell using amino acids as their raw materials. Some antimetabolite drugs inhibit key enzymes in the biosynthesis pathways and so prevent cells making new bases and new DNA.

**Figure 12.6** Alkylating agents such as **cyclophosphamide** cross-link guanine bases, impeding DNA replication.

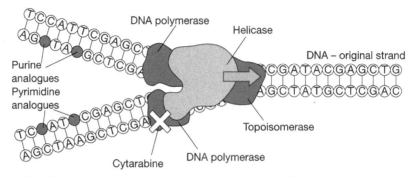

**Figure 12.7** Purine and pyrimidine analogues such as **cladribine** and **gemcitabine** replace authentic nitrogenous bases in newly synthesised DNA, causing it to malfunction. **Cytarabine** inhibits DNA polymerase.

Some of these drugs are so similar in molecular structure to the nitrogenous bases that they are mistakenly inserted into the new DNA strands during replication. The insertion of these synthetic analogues causes the DNA assembly to malfunction (Figure 12.7). The cell cycle is halted in S (synthesis) phase (see Figure 12.5 above), potentially triggering apoptosis of the cell. Cancer cells have an exceptionally high demand for new nitrogenous bases and it is believed that this renders them particularly susceptible to antimetabolite drugs.

The DNA bases are divided into two chemically similar groups. Adenine and guanine belong to the *purine* group while cytosine and thymine belong to the *pyrimidine* group. *Uracil*, a nitrogenous base found only in RNA is also a pyrimidine. Purine analogues include **cladribine, fludarabine, mercaptopurine, nelarabine, clofarabine** and **azacitidine**. Pyrimidine analogues include **gemcitabine** and **tioguanine**. **Tegafur** works synergistically with uracil to inhibit pyrimidine synthesis. **Cytarabine** directly inhibits DNA polymerase, the enzyme that assembles the nucleotides.

Both **cladribine** and **fludarabine** are potent immunosuppressive agents and patients receiving these drugs are at risk from opportunistic microbial infection.

Uracil, a nitrogenous base found in mRNA, is converted to the nitrogenous DNA base thymine via the enzyme thymidylate synthetase. **Fluorouracil** and **capecitabine** directly inhibit thymidylate synthetase. *Folic acid* (vitamin B9) or *folate* is essential to the pathway that synthesises pyrimidines. **Methotrexate, pemetrexed** and **raltitrexed** are folate antagonists that inhibit *dihydrofolate reductase*, another enzyme crucial to the conversion of uracil to thymine (Figure 12.8).

**DID YOU KNOW ...** that folic acid (or vitamin B9), is essential for DNA synthesis and the healthy development of cells and tissues? A shortage of folic acid can cause a baby to be born with congenital problems such as *spina bifida*. The UK Food Standards Agency has recommended 'mandatory fortification' of bread or flour with folic acid. Naturally, folate antagonists such as **methotrexate** are contra-indicated during pregnancy.

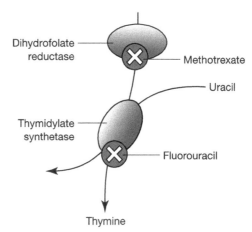

**Figure 12.8** Simplified diagram showing how **methotrexate** and **fluorouracil** inhibit key enzymes in the pathway that synthesises the DNA base thymine.

## Cytotoxic antibiotics

This group of anti-cancer drugs include the anthracycline antibiotics: **daunorubicin, doxorubicin, epirubicin** and **idarubicin. Mitoxantrone** is an anthracycline derivative. Other cytotoxic antibiotics include **bleomycin, dactinomycin** and **mitomycin.** They are used to treat various cancers including breast cancer, leukaemias and lymphomas.

They are mainly produced by species of *Streptomyces*, a genus of Gram-positive, soil bacteria. These organisms produce metabolites that inhibit competition from other soil organisms and these metabolites have antibiotic characteristics. They are however, far too toxic to be used as antibacterial drugs but their cytotoxicity makes them very useful in the treatment of cancer.

The mechanism of action of this group is varied but most of them bind to DNA and prevent its transcription into mRNA and its replication during cell division. **Doxorubicin** and **bleomycin** also appear to inhibit the action of topoisomerase II, an enzyme in the replication complex (see Figure 12.7). **Bleomycin,** used in the treatment of lung cancer, also produces free radicals that fragment DNA.

The anthracycline antibiotics such as **doxorubicin** are renowned for their potential to cause *cardiomyopathy*, damage to the heart – and their use can even result in heart failure. **Dexrazoxane** is a drug used to counteract doxorubicin-induced cardiomyopathy. Ironically, it has its own side-effect profile including the usual nausea and vomiting as well as myelosuppression.

## Cytotoxic plant alkaloids

Anti-cancer plant alkaloid drugs include derivatives of the Madagascar periwinkle *Catharanthus roseus* (formerly *Vinca rosea*), **vincristine, vinblastine, vindesine, vinflunine** and the semi-synthetic derivative **vinorelbine.** From the Pacific yew *Taxus brevifolia* we derive **docetaxel, paclitaxel carlizataxel.** These drugs are

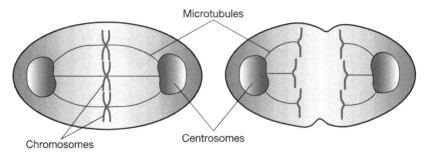

**Figure 12.9** During mitosis, chromosomes are pulled apart from their pairs as the microtubules shorten. Drugs such as **paclitaxel** and **vincristine** incapacitate microtubules, thus inhibiting mitosis.

used for a variety of cancers: lymphomas, leukaemias and some solid tumours, e.g. breast, ovarian, lung cancers and sarcomas.

The plant alkaloids work by inhibiting the activity of cellular microtubules that are crucial to cell division. Earlier in this chapter we learned that during mitosis half the (doubled) chromosomes migrate into each new cell. This means that a full set of 46 chromosomes has to migrate to one end of the dividing cell and a corresponding set of 46 chromosomes migrates to the opposite end. The mechanism whereby this happens is quite ingenious. When each chromosome is copied, they are joined together as a pair of identical chromosomes. Attached to each chromosome is a microtubule, a thin, thread-like strand which is anchored to structures called *centrosomes* at the far end of each newly-forming cell. As mitosis progresses, the microtubules contract, pulling the pairs of chromosomes apart so that each new cell receives one of the pair of chromosomes (Figure 12.9). By inhibiting the action of the microtubules, mitosis is halted, triggering apoptosis in the dividing cell. Vinca alkaloids inhibit the assembly of microtubules while the taxanes prevent the microtubules from shortening and so separating the chromosomes.

## Topoisomerase inhibitors

During DNA replication, topoisomerase enzymes in the replication complex configure the DNA strand being copied to prevent it becoming irrevocably twisted and tangled (see Figure 12.7 above). Various drugs inhibit topoisomerase enzymes, thus halting the process of DNA replication in rapidly dividing cancer cells. Topoisomerase 1 inhibitors include **irinotecan** and **topotecan.** Extracted from the root of *Mandragora officinarum* (the mandrake plant), **etoposide** is a Topoisomerase II inhibitor – as are **doxorubicin** and **bleomycin**, discussed above under 'cytotoxic antibiotics'.

DID YOU KNOW ... in the Middle Ages there was a superstition that anyone pulling up a mandrake plant would drop dead instantly? To get around this problem, a dog was tied to the plant so that it would pull up the mandrake (and presumably die instead). It was unlikely that any dog ever died (unless it ate the plant it had just pulled up) so it is surprising no one noticed this myth had no factual basis.

### Protein kinase inhibitors

This is a large group of relatively recent drugs used to treat a wide range of cancers including myeloid leukaemia, pancreatic cancer, lung cancer, renal cancer, metastatic breast and colorectal cancers. Drugs in this group include **dasatinib, erlotinib, everolimus, gefitinib, imatinib, lapatinib, nilotinib, pazopanib, sorafenib, sunitinib temsirolimus vendetanib** and **vemurfenib**. Their mechanism of action is complex but essentially they suppress cell division by inhibiting the signalling pathways that promote cell division in cancer.

Protein kinases are enzymes involved in signalling pathways in cells. Some are complexed with cell-surface receptors that respond to growth-stimulating messengers such as epithelial and epidermal growth factors. Binding of the messenger to the receptor triggers intracellular signalling cascades that regulate cell division. Other kinases are found within the cell and are part of the mechanism that regulates the transcription of genes. Some of these genes, such as the oncogenes and tumour suppressor genes, mediate the over-proliferation of cells in cancer. Protein kinase inhibitors act on a variety of these kinases to suppress cell division (Figure 12.10).

In some cancers there is an over-expression of a particular receptor involved in promoting cell division. In non-small cell lung cancer, for example, it is the over-expression of a protein kinase receptor to epidermal growth factor. **Gefitinib**

**Figure 12.10 Protein kinase inhibitors block signalling pathways that promote cell division.**

binds to the kinase domain of the receptor, so blocking its normal signalling pathway and inhibiting the growth of cancerous cells in the lungs.

## Hormone antagonists

*Aromatase Inhibitors* Prolonged exposure to oestrogen can increase the likelihood of breast cancer. This is a contributory factor to the increase in the incidence of breast cancer in Western countries where women are having fewer children and so prolonging their exposure to oestrogen. In pre-menopausal women oestrogen is produced by the ovaries but after menopause it is converted from adrenal androgens such as testosterone by aromatase enzymes. Aromatase inhibitors such as **anastrazole**, **exemestane**, and **letrozole** block the aromatase enzyme thus reducing the production of oestrogen. These drugs are only used in women who have oestrogen receptor-positive breast cancer.

These drugs are not suitable for use in pre-menopausal women as a reduction in oestrogen would stimulate the hypothalamus to release hormones that stimulate the release of oestrogen – which would be self-defeating.

*Selective oestrogen receptor modulators (SERMs)* These drugs include **tamoxifen** and **toremifene** and are used in women who have oestrogen receptor-positive breast cancer. They block receptors on breast tissue from the influence of oestrogen while sparing oestrogen receptors on tissues such as bone where the hormone has a beneficial function of maintaining bone integrity and preventing osteoporosis.

*Androgen receptor antagonists* **Bicalutamide**, **cyproterone** and **flutamide** are for use in men, blocking androgen receptors and reducing the stimulating effects of testosterone on prostate cancer. As expected from drugs that block testosterone, they can have a feminising action on the male body including gynaecomastia (breast development).

## Targeted biotherapy – monoclonal antibodies

Antibodies (immunoglobulins) are small immune proteins produced by B lymphocytes. These cells respond to microbial infection by releasing millions of antibodies into the bloodstream. Here they home in on the microbes, binding tightly and promoting their destruction by other immune cells such as macrophages. A key characteristic of the antibodies is that they are produced by one group or clone of B cells – hence the term 'monoclonal antibodies'. They are also specific for one protein – usually that present on the microbe causing the infection. This specificity is very useful because antibodies can be genetically engineered to respond not to bacteria but to proteins on cancer cells.

An antibody drug you will no doubt be familiar with is **trastuzumab** (Herceptin®) used in the treatment of early breast cancer. This drug binds to and blocks HER2 receptors, so reducing the rate of proliferation of cancerous breast cells.

Rituximab and ofatumumab are engineered antibodies used in the treatment of B-cell lymphoma. B lymphocytes have CD20 protein on their cell surface and these drugs are specific for this protein, binding and preventing the B cells reproducing. Alemtuzumab targets CD52 protein found on B and T cells in lymphocytic leukaemia.

Other monoclonal antibody drugs include panitumumab, bevacizumab and cetuximab, all used for metastatic colorectal cancer and targeting growth factor receptors.

The exquisite specificity of monoclonal antibodies presents some of the most exciting opportunities for the development of new drugs. Several monoclonal antibodies are currently undergoing clinical trials that deliver anti-cancer drugs exclusively to cancerous cells. Compounds such as cytotoxic antibiotics and radioactive isotopes too toxic to be delivered systemically can be attached to antibodies that deliver them directly to cancer cells without damaging other tissues.

DID YOU KNOW ... that the ending of monoclonal antibody names gives a clue to their origin? Drugs ending in 'umab' such as trastuzumab are fully humanised antibodies while those ending in 'ximab' such as cetuximab are chimeric, i.e. half human, half mouse.

A QUICK RECAP on drugs used in the management of cancer

- Alkylating agents include the nitrogen mustards such as cyclophosphamide, the nitrosoureas and platinum-based drugs such as cisplatin. They all cross-link DNA, hindering DNA replication in cancer cells.

- Antimetabolites such as methotrexate and 5-fluorouracil interfere with the process of DNA synthesis. If cells do not have the components to make new DNA then they cannot replicate.

- Drugs that incapacitate microtubules include the plant alkaloids vincristine and paclitaxel. If chromosomes can't segregate properly then cells cannot replicate.

- Drugs such as tamoxifen block receptors to growth-stimulating mediators which inhibits the stimulus for cell replication.

- Topoisomerase inhibitors such as doxorubicin, irinotecan and etoposide inhibit enzymes that prevent DNA strands becoming irrevocably twisted and tangled during replication.

- Protein kinase inhibitors such as gefitinib inhibit signalling pathways in cell division.

- Aromatase inhibitors such as anastrazole and letrozole block aromatase enzymes, reducing the production of oestrogen in post-menopausal women.

- Monoclonal antibodies such as rituximab and trastuzumab are engineered immunoglobulins, highly specific for cancer cells.

## REFERENCES AND FURTHER RECOMMENDED READING

Books

Brown, M. & Cutler, T. (Eds) (2012) *Haematology Nursing*. Wiley-Blackwell.

Wilkes, G.M. and Barton-Burke, M. (2012) *Oncology Nursing Drug Handbook*. Jones and Bartlett Publishers International.

Websites

All recommended websites are open access (but free registration is sometimes required).

Medscape – oncology – http://emedicine.medscape.com/oncology

National Cancer Institute – http://www.cancer.gov/

National Institute of Health and Clinical Excellence (NICE) – http://www.nice.org.uk/

Office for National Statistics – http://www.ons.gov.uk/

## Test yourself

Now you have finished reading this chapter it is worthwhile finding out how much you have learned and remembered. Cancer is a very common disease so it is important that you understand the action of the various anti-cancer drugs.

*The answers to these questions are at the end of the book on p. 318.*

1 Name three tissues where cell division continues in the adult body.

2 Name the four nitrogenous bases found in DNA.

3 How many chromosomes would you find in most adult cells?

4 Outline the function of topoisomerase and helicase enzymes in DNA replication.

5 Name the two main phases in the cell cycle.

6 What is happening to the cell in $G_0$ phase?

7 What is combination therapy?

8 Name five side-effects common to many anti-cancer drugs.

9 How do alkylating agents such as **cyclophosphamide** interfere with DNA replication?

10 Drugs such as **fludarabine** and **gemcitabine** are synthetic analogues of nitrogenous bases. How does this inhibit DNA replication?

11 How does the inhibition of thymidylate synthetase by **fluorouracil** inhibit DNA replication?

12 What is a common and serious side-effect of **doxorubicin**?

13 How do vinca alkaloids and taxanes prevent mitosis?

14 What group of anti-cancer drugs inhibits enzymes involved in signalling pathways?

15 Why are aromatase inhibitors not used in pre-menopausal women?

Answers to the questions on p. 289.

1 DNA is short for deoxyribose nucleic acid.
2 DNA is a double helix.
3 Cancerous cell division is mitosis.
4 Genes are sections of DNA that code for proteins.
5 Apoptosis is the programmed self-destruction of a cell.

# General resources: books and websites

## Useful reference books

Some of these books focus primarily on the use and administration of drugs in clinical practice rather than on pharmacological mechanisms, but as they all add to the reader's understanding of the subject they are worthy of mention.

**Adams, M.P.** *et al.* (2010) *Pharmacology for Nurses – A Pathophysiologic Approach* (3rd edn). Prentice Hall.

**Coleman, M.** (2010) *Drug Metabolism* (2nd edn). Wiley–Blackwell.

**Galbraith, A.** *et al.* (2007) *Fundamentals of Pharmacology* (2nd edn). Pearson Education.

**Golan, D.E.** *et al.* (20011) *Principles of Pharmacology* (3rd edn). Lippincott, Williams & Wilkins.

**Greenstein, B. and Gould, D.** (2009) *Trounce's Clinical Pharmacology* (18th edn). Churchill Livingstone.

**McGavock, H.** (2010) *How Drugs Work* (3rd edn). Radcliffe Publishing Ltd.

**Rang, H.P.** *et al.* (20011) *Rang and Dale's Pharmacology* (7th edn). Churchill Livingstone.

## Useful websites

There is plenty of information on the web but not all of it is reliable. Here are a few useful websites run by more reputable organisations – and with free access.

**NHS Direct: Health encyclopaedia** – This site contains some useful information on the symptoms, causes, diagnosis and treatment of a wide range of diseases – http://www.nhsdirect.nhs.uk/

**Bandolier** – UK website assessing the evidence base for the use of drugs and other treatments. Hosted by Oxford University – http://www.medicine.ox.ac.uk/bandolier/

**The Cochrane Collaboration** – Independent, non-profit-making organisation that evaluates clinical trials and publishes systematic reviews on drugs and other treatments – http://www.cochrane.org/

**Student BMJ** – Website maintained by the *British Medical Journal*. Primarily aimed at medical students, it contains useful articles on various aspects of medicine including diagnosis and treatment – http://student.bmj.com/

**eMedicine** – An open-access US-based website that provides extensive information on the nature and treatment of a wide range of diseases. Written by health professionals, the information is evidence-based, but note that information may not be in concordance with UK clinical protocols – http://emedicine.medscape.com/

**RxList** – An open-access US-based website that provides extensive information on therapeutic drugs. Information on generic drugs will be useful to UK practitioners but note that US dosages, prescribing protocols and the formulations of proprietary drugs may be different from those in the UK – http://www.rxlist.com/

**Merck manuals** – An online medical library maintained by the US pharmaceutical company, Merck & Co. Inc. This is an extensive database that provides detailed information on a wide range of conditions and their treatment. Note that information may not be in concordance with UK clinical protocols – http://www.merck.com/mmpe/index.html

# Answers to 'Test yourself'

## Chapter 1, p. 20

1  (a) Nucleus – contains the DNA that codes for proteins.
   (b) Ribosomes – assemble amino acids into proteins.
   (c) Mitochondria – produce ATP.
   (d) Cell membrane – controls the passage of materials in and out of the cell.
2  Lipid.
3  Receptors, ion channels, enzymes and carrier proteins.
4  A gene.
5  Amino acids.
6  An oil is liquid at room temperature whereas a fat is solid.
7  Cholesterol.
8  Starch
9  Fuel (glucose or lipids) and oxygen.
10  $CO_2$ is transported in the blood from the cells to the lungs where it is breathed out.

## Chapter 2, p. 40

1  Approximately 20 000 proteins in the human body.
2  (1) There are many different types of protein.
   (2) Proteins have important roles in physiological processes.
   (3) Each organ and tissue has protein distinctive to that organ and tissue.
3  Hormones, neurotransmitters and mediators.
4  They are the appropriate shape for that receptor (right key for lock).
5  It is a similar shape/molecular structure to adrenaline.
6  An agonist drug binds to a receptor and has the same effect as the natural chemical messenger binding to that receptor. An antagonist drug binds to and blocks a receptor from its natural chemical messenger.
7  A sympathomimetic drug has an adrenergic effect, i.e. the same effect as stimulation by the sympathetic nervous system.
8  Acetylcholine.
9  Cations are *positively* charged ions.
10  Voltage-controlled ion channel.
11  Stops the transmission of nervous impulses (action potentials) along the pain neurons.
12  The enzyme's active site.
13  The cholesterol synthesis pathway (in the liver).
14  A carrier protein requires energy in the form of ATP to transport ions (and other molecules) across membranes.

## Chapter 3, p. 69

1  Antihypertensives that result in hypotension, anticlotting drugs such as warfarin and heparin that can cause haemorrhage, laxatives that can cause diarrhoea, etc.
2  Increases the heart rate.
3  **Salbutamol** targets $\beta_2$ receptors in the bronchioles but may also bind to $\beta_1$ receptors on the heart and produce the same effects as adrenaline – tachycardia.

4 Kininases degrade bradykinin but if their action is blocked the bradykinin levels build up and irritate the lining of the lungs.

5 Calcium channel blockers inhibit the contraction of smooth muscle, including that found in the walls of the digestive tract. A reduction in peristalsis can result in constipation.

6 Enteral, parenteral and topical.

7 Drugs pass from the gut into the hepatic portal vein and into the liver from where they are released into the circulatory system via the hepatic vein.

8 **Insulin** is a protein so is broken down by digestive enzymes (proteases).

9 GTN is almost completely metabolised during its initial passage through the liver and not enough emerges into the blood to be of therapeutic value.

10 The initial metabolism of an orally ingested drug as it passes through the liver.

11 Most likely to increase in their bioavailability as P450 enzymes generally inactivate drugs so their inhibition will slow the rate of inactivation – and so increase bioavailability.

12 An increase in vitamin K competes with **warfarin** and promotes coagulation.

13 The level of drug in the blood that is greater than the minimum effective concentration but less than the maximum safe concentration.

14 The time it takes a drug to fall from 100 per cent of its concentration in the blood by one half, to 50 per cent concentration.

15 Hepatic and renal insufficiency may delay metabolism and elimination of drugs and their metabolites.

## Chapter 4, p. 108

1 Transport of nutrients, gases, wastes, metabolites and hormones plus repair, thermoregulation and immunity.

2 Capillaries.

3 Coronary arteries.

4 Cholesterol.

5 Blood supply is reduced so insufficient oxygen is available to heart muscle cells. These cells start to produce lactic acid and this stimulates pain receptors.

6 More blood and oxygen is supplied to the heart muscle cells so they do not produce lactic acid.

7 A thrombus forming, possibly leading to a heart attack.

8 A slower heart rate reduces the workload of the heart and so reduces angina pain.

9 Low-density lipoprotein (LDL).

10 The hepatocytes of the liver synthesise cholesterol to make good the shortfall.

11 HMG CoA reductase is an enzyme involved in the production of cholesterol in the liver. Inhibiting HMG CoA reduces cholesterol production, so the liver pulls in LDL cholesterol from the blood, thus lowering circulating levels of LDL.

12 Platelets, fibrin and red blood cells.

13 **Aspirin** inhibits the enzyme COX-1 in platelets and so reduces the production of thromboxane-A2, a mediator that increases the expression of GPIIb/IIIa receptors on platelets. These receptors bind with fibrin to form the mesh-like structure that makes up a blood clot.

14 **Warfarin** inhibits the process that produces the proteins involved in the clotting cascade. Heparins block the clotting cascade itself.

15 To break up a clot that has formed in the coronary arteries and is causing a heart attack.

## Chapter 5, p. 137

1 Yes, heart rate and pulse are the same.

2 Systole is the higher pressure.

3 Blood pressure falls.
4 Angiotensin-II, ADH-vasopressin and adrenaline.
5 Noradrenaline.
6 Heart rate would increase via the baroreceptor response.
7 BP falls because SVR has fallen.
8 Vasoconstriction, stimulation of ADH-vasopressin release, increase in blood sodium levels (and therefore blood volume and stroke volume).
9 With lower aldosterone levels, the kidneys recycle less sodium so blood sodium levels fall. This reduces blood volume, stroke volume, cardiac output and so blood pressure.
10 Diuretics decrease the water reabsorbed so more urine is produced.
11 Hyponatraemia – more sodium is lost in the urine.
12 Contraction of the smooth muscle is reduced and this causes vasodilation of the arterioles.
13 CCBs also block calcium channels in the smooth muscle of the gut wall, inhibiting their contraction so causing a general reduction of gut motility.
14 Reduce heart rate, increase peripheral vasodilation and reduce sympathetic stimulation. Reduction in renin release so RA system is inhibited.
15 Beta-blockers may block $\beta_2$ receptors in the lungs – the targets for bronchodilators such as **salbutamol**.

## Chapter 6, p. 166

1 'Pain is whatever the patient informs you that they are experiencing'.
2 Neuropathic.
3 Chronic.
4 Painful stimuli such as heat, mechanical pressure and chemical stimulation.
5 The painful stimulus detected by nociceptors and nervous impulses is sent along nociceptive neurons in the arm to the spinal cord. Impulses arrive via the dorsal horn and synapse with ascending neurons that synapse with corticothalamic neurons in the thalamus. From here they travel to the cerebral cortex.
6 Opioid-like peptides are released during injury and block transmission between nociceptive neurons, so inhibiting the experience of pain.
7 Inflammation manifests itself by the following symptoms – redness, heat, swelling, pain and alteration of function.
8 Phospholipids – arachidonic acid – cyclic endoperoxides – prostaglandins and thromboxanes.
9 Cyclo-oxygenase 2.
10 $PGE_2$ causes vasodilation and (along with histamine) increases the permeability of small blood vessels, resulting in swelling and pain. $PGE_2$ also sensitises nociceptive neurons to the painful stimulation of bradykinin.
11 NSAIDs target COX-2 produced in inflammation but may also bind to and inhibit COX-1, an enzyme involved in the synthesis of non-inflammatory prostaglandins that maintain and protect the gastric mucosa (the lining of the stomach).
12 Because it can damage the liver at only 2–3 times the standard dose.
13 Nausea, vomiting, respiratory depression, drowsiness and constipation.
14 Local anaesthetics block sodium ion channels in nociceptive neurons that are involved in the transmission of nervous impulses. If the nervous impulse is blocked from travelling to the brain, there will be no awareness of pain from the surgical procedure.
15 Intravenous anaesthetics and the inhalational anaesthetics.

## Chapter 7, p. 184

1 Duodenum, jejunum and ileum.
2 Amino acids.
3 Amylase.
4 Gastro-oesophageal and pyloric sphincters.
5 Pepsin.
6 Acetylcholine, histamine and gastrin.
7 Pancreas.
8 Gastro-oesophageal reflux disease (GORD).
9 *Helicobacter pylori*.
10 Constipation – increased passage time allows more time for reabsorption of water.
11 They form a raft that floats on top of the acidic stomach contents, protecting the oesophagus.
12 Histamine $H_2$ receptors.
13 PPIs block the pumping of $H^+$ (protons) into the lumen of the stomach. There $H^+$ normally combines with $Cl^-$ to form hydrochloric acid.
14 Opiates.
15 They pull water into the large intestine by osmosis, thus softening the stools and making their evacuation easier.

## Chapter 8, p. 210

1 Bacteria, viruses, fungi and protozoa.
2 Bacteria.
3 Bacteria are prokaryotes, meaning they do not have a true nucleus. All other organisms such as plants, animals and fungi are eukaryotic with true nuclei.
4 Cell wall, shape and oxygen requirement.
5 Peptidoglycan.
6 They inhibit the enzyme transpeptidase that produces peptidoglycan. This weakens the cell wall and the organism lyses.
7 They produce beta-lactamase enzymes that attack and denature the drugs.
8 It acts as a substrate for beta-lactamase, blocking its action so allowing the antibacterial drugs to kill the bacteria.
9 A bactericidal drug kills bacteria while a bacteriostatic drug prevents the bacteria from dividing.
10 Bacterial ribosomes.
11 They bind to calcium so may interfere with calcium supplies to the growing foetus.
12 Ergosterol, a sterol found in fungal cell membranes.
13 They have little in the way of structure to target and reproduce inside human cells, which makes it difficult for drugs to reach them.
14 Vaccination.
15 **Metronidazole** is indicated for trichomoniasis and anaerobic bacterial infections.

## Chapter 9, p. 231

1 Mouth, trachea, bronchi, bronchioles, alveoli.
2 Around 80 $m^2$ or the area of half a tennis court.
3 The rate and depth of breathing increase.
4 In the medulla in the brain stem.
5 Long-term COPD patients switch from carbon dioxide to oxygen as the main driver of breathing.

6  Mucus traps bacteria and detritus and moves them out of the lungs.

7  Dust mites, pet hair, pollen, exercise, cold weather.

8  Shortness of breath.

9  In emphysema the walls of the alveoli break down, and in bronchitis excess mucus is trapped in the lungs, leading to infections.

10 Smoking.

11 Smooth muscle cells surrounding the bronchioles.

12 Acetylcholine muscarinic receptors.

13 They suppress the activity of mast cells which release inflammatory mediators and eosinophils that damage the bronchial epithelium.

14 Corticosteroids inhibit protein synthesis and thus stunt growth.

15 Constipation.

## Chapter 10, p. 261

1  They bind to and stimulate receptors on the cell surface.

2  Steroid hormones.

3  As glycogen, a polymer of glucose.

4  It stimulates the liver to break down glycogen into glucose which it releases into the bloodstream.

5  Type 1 diabetes is an autoimmune disease that destroys the beta islet cells of the pancreas so they cannot produce insulin. Type 2 diabetes usually occurs later in life and cells of the body become less sensitive to insulin, so their uptake of glucose falls. With time, insulin production may also be affected.

6  Diabetes is a disease caused either by lack of insulin or the cells' inability to take up glucose from the blood. This means that blood glucose levels can be abnormally high while intracellular glucose levels can be abnormally low. This can result in the cells switching to lipids for their fuel and producing acid ketones as a by-product.

7  These drugs rely on the beta cells of the pancreas having some residual insulin-producing capacity. In Type 1 diabetes these cells are destroyed, so cannot produce any insulin (which is why patients rely on insulin injections).

8  Oestrogen is the dominant ovarian hormone in the follicular phase and progesterone in the luteal phase.

9  Hot flushes, vaginal dryness, loss of sexual drive and mood swings.

10 Over-activity of the osteoclasts increases bone reabsorption and under-activity of the osteoblasts reduces bone reconstruction. This results in a net shift towards bone reabsorption, so bones become weaker.

11 Bisphosphonates are incorporated into the bone matrix from where they are taken up by osteoclasts as they reabsorb bone. The bisphosphonates cause apoptosis (programmed cell death) in the osteoclasts, so shifting the balance towards bone-building.

12 They mimic the hormonal environment of pregnancy which inhibits ovulation.

13 They interfere with lactation so are unsuitable if the woman is breast-feeding.

14 Some antibacterial drugs can interact with combined oral contraceptives, reducing their blood concentration and so reducing their effectiveness.

15 Goitre (swelling of the thyroid gland), exophthalmus (bulging eyeballs), nervousness and loss of weight.

## Chapter 11, p. 286

1  Basal ganglia.

2  Gamma-aminobutyric acid.

3 All inhibitory neurotransmitters.
4 Re-uptake transporters are situated in the presynaptic membrane. They are responsible for removing neurotransmitters from the synaptic cleft.
5 Greater inhibition.
6 Less excitation.
7 GABA receptors.
8 Drowsiness.
9 Problems with motor coordination, i.e. Parkinson-like symptoms.
10 5-HT and noradrenaline.
11 Monoamine oxidase inhibitors.
12 It can interact with conventional drugs such as warfarin to reduce their serum concentrations.
13 Dopamine (specifically $D_2$) receptors.
14 Mania and bipolar disorders.
15 Thalamic–cortical pathways.

## Chapter 12, p. 309

1 Bone marrow (blood cells), skin, digestive tract and hair.
2 Adenine (A), guanine (G), thymine (T) and cytosine (C).
3 46 chromosomes (23 in sperm and 23 in egg).
4 Topoisomerase and helicase enzymes prevent DNA tangling during replication.
5 Interphase and mitosis.
6 In $G_0$ phase the cell is resting, i.e. not dividing.
7 Several drugs are given at the same time in order to target the cell in all phases of the cell cycle.
8 Myelosuppression, nausea and vomiting, malabsorption of nutrients and hair loss.
9 Alkylating agents bind strands of DNA together so they cannot be copied during replication.
10 Synthetic analogues of nitrogenous bases are inserted into DNA strands during DNA synthesis which interferes with replication.
11 Thymidylate synthetase is essential for the conversion of uracil into thymine.
12 Cardiomyopathy – heart disease.
13 Vinca alkaloids and taxanes inhibit microtubules.
14 Protein kinase inhibitors.
15 In pre-menopausal women aromatase inhibitors would stimulate the production of oestrogen.

# Glossary of biomedical terms

Acetylcholine  A neurotransmitter of the parasympathetic system.

Acetylcholinesterase  A synaptic enzyme that metabolises the neurotransmitter acetylcholine.

Action potential  A nervous impulse, the chemo-electrical signal that travels along neurons.

Active site  The region of an enzyme where it binds to and modifies its substrate.

Adenoma  A benign localised tumour that has not spread to other tissues.

Adenosine diphosphate (ADP)  The cells' energy molecule in its low-energy state.

Adenosine triphosphate (ATP)  The cells' energy molecule in its fully charged state.

ADH-vasopressin  A hormone released by the posterior gland that opposes the production of urine and increases peripheral vasoconstriction.

Adrenergic receptor (also known as an adrenoceptor)  A receptor for adrenaline or noradrenaline.

Adrenoceptor (also known as an adrenergic receptor)  A receptor for adrenaline or noradrenaline.

Aerobes  Bacteria that have a requirement for oxygen.

Agonists  Drugs that are similar is shape to a natural chemical messenger, bind to its receptor and produce the same cellular response as the messenger.

Allergens  Normally non-toxic substances that stimulate the immune system and initiate an allergic response.

Alpha-glucosidase  An enzyme in the gut that breaks down starch into monosaccharides such as glucose.

Alveolar macrophages  Amoeba-like immune cells that patrol alveoli and destroy bacteria.

Amylase  An enzyme that catalyses the breakdown of starch into sugars and is present in human saliva.

Anaerobes  Bacteria that require an oxygen-free environment.

Angiogenesis  The development of new blood vessels.

Angiotensinogen, angiotensin-I and angiotensin-II  A sequence of proteins activated by an increase in renin production in response to a fall in BP. Angiotensin II promotes vasoconstriction and indirectly increases $Na^+$ retention in order to maintain BP.

Anions  Negatively charged ions.

Antagonists  Drugs that are similar in shape to a natural chemical messenger, bind to and block its receptor without producing a cellular response.

Antibiotic-associated colitis  An infection of the bowel caused by *Clostridium difficile* that proliferate when antibacterial drugs have killed off more susceptible gut bacteria.

Anticholinergic  A drug that opposes the action of the parasympathetic system.

Antithrombin  An anticlotting protein that inactivates the clotting cascade. Antithrombin itself is activated by heparin.

Apoptosis  The programmed self-destruction of a cell.

Arachidonic acid  A precursor in the synthesis pathway of prostaglandins, thromboxanes and leukotrienes.

Arterioles  Small arteries that can constrict under sympathetic stimulation.

Atheromata  Plaques that form in the subendothelium of arteries.

β-endorphin, dynorphin and enkephalins  Naturally occurring opioid-like peptides that inhibit the transmission of pain.

β-haemolytic streptococci  A genus of Gram positive bacteria responsible for diseases such as meningitis, rheumatic and scarlet fever and necrotising fasciitis.

Bacilli  Rod-shaped bacteria.

Baroreceptor reflex  A sympathetic response that attempts to restore blood pressure by increasing vasoconstriction and cardiac output.

Beta-lactam ring  The ring-like structure found in the molecular skeleton of penicillins, cephalosporins and carbapenems.

Beta-lactamases  Enzymes produced by bacteria that break the B-lactam ring of penicillins, cephalosporins and carbapenems.

Biochemical pathways  A series of biochemical reactions where each reaction is catalysed by an enzyme.

Blind therapy  The prescribing of a broad-spectrum antibiotic when it is not possible to identify precisely the type of bacterium responsible for an infection.

Blood-brain barrier  A layer of cells that separates neural tissue from the blood vessels supplying the central nervous system.

Bowman's capsule  The structure that encapsulates the glomerulus at the head of each nephron.

Bradykinin  A small peptide involved in pain modulation.

Caecum  The first section of the large intestine, separated from the ileum by the ileocaecal valve.

Cannulation  The insertion of a hollow needle into (usually) a vein for the administration of medicines or extraction of blood samples.

Cardiac sphincter  Another name for the gastro-oesophageal sphincter.

Cardiomyopathy  A disease of the heart.

Catalysis  In biochemistry, an enzyme-assisted biochemical reaction. The enzyme participates in the reaction but is itself unchanged.

Cations  Positively charged ions.

Cell cycle  Stages in cell division.

Cell organelles  Small structures within cells that perform various functions, mostly associated with energy production and protein synthesis.

Cellular respiration  The process inside cells that breaks down glucose and lipids in the presence of oxygen to convert ADP into ATP.

Central line  A catheter inserted into a major vein, often for the delivery of drugs.

Centrosomes Cellular structures that organise microtubules during mitosis.

Cephalosporinases B-lactamases that specifically attack the B-lactam ring of cephalosporins.

Cerebral cortex The outer layer of the brain, sometimes referred to as 'grey matter'. Responsible for processing conscious thought and reasoning.

Cerebrospinal fluid The fluid that surrounds the brain and spinal cord.

Chelating In organic chemistry, the binding of an organic molecule to a metallic ion.

Cholinergic A drug that mimics the action of the parasympathetic system.

Cocci Bacteria that are spherical in shape.

Coeliac disease A disorder affecting the small intestine caused by intolerance to the gluten in wheat; symptoms include diarrhoea, bloating and pain.

Collagen A tough filamentous protein molecule found in connective tissue such as tendons.

Collateral circulation The blood supply to a tissue bed from more than one artery.

Compliance The ability of the lungs to stretch and expand.

Congenital analgesia A neurological condition present from birth that renders an individual insensitive to pain.

Contra-indicated Circumstances under which a drug should not be prescribed or administered.

Crohn's disease An inflammatory disease affecting sections of the small or large bowel.

Cryptococcosis A fungal infection, frequently from *Cryptococcus neoformans*, especially serious in immunocompromised patients.

Cyclic endoperoxide A chemical in the biochemical pathway that produces prostaglandins, thromboxanes and leukotrienes.

Cyclo-oxygenase 1 (COX-1) A key enzyme in the synthesis of prostaglandins, thromboxanes and leukotrienes.

Cysteinyl leukotriene receptors Receptors to leukotrienes, members of the inflammatory eicosanoid pathway that includes prostaglandins.

Cytochrome p450 enzymes Hepatic enzymes involved in the metabolism of exogenous compounds including drugs.

Cytokines Chemicals that relay signals between cells, especially immune cells.

Cytokinesis The process whereby a cell divides into two new cells after having replicated DNA and organelles.

Defecation reflex An automatic reflex that promotes defecation as faecal pressure builds up in the sigmoid colon. The social requirement of overriding this reflex is learned in childhood.

Depot injections Deep injections of (usually) anti-psychotic drugs that are released slowly, giving a prolonged therapeutic action.

Diabetic ketoacidosis (DKA) A condition of Type 1 diabetes where lack of insulin causes the production of excessive quantities of acidic ketones.

Diastole The period of falling pressure in the ventricle or arteries.

Dihydrofolate reductase An enzyme in the thymine production pathway.

**Dihydropyridines** A group of calcium channel blockers defined by their chemical relatedness and including **amlodipine** and **nifedipine**.

**Dipeptidylpeptidase-4** An enzyme that breaks down glucagon-like peptide-1.

**Diplococci** Bacteria that are often found co-joined in pairs.

**Diploid** Organisms (including humans) which have two of each chromosome.

**Diverticula** Out-swellings in the wall of the colon that can cause diverticular disease.

**Diverticular disease** Pain or discomfort caused by diverticula (out-swellings in the wall of the colon).

**Diverticulitis** Inflammation of diverticula in the colon wall.

**Dopa-decarboxylase** A peripheral enzyme that converts **levodopa** into dopamine.

**Dose-related** A close correlation between the dose and the therapeutic effect (or side-effect) of a drug.

**Duodenum** The section of the digestive tract after the stomach.

**Dyskinesia** Motor coordination disorder, resulting in involuntary movements such as tics and tremors.

**Dyspepsia** Upper abdominal discomfort (often called indigestion).

**Electrocardiogram (ECG)** A medical device that measures electrical activity in the heart and displays it on a graph. Used to detect heart problems such as MI.

**Endogenous ligands** Chemical messengers (ligands) produced within the body (endogenous).

**Endoplasmic reticulum** An organelle involved in the folding of proteins and the synthesis of lipids.

**Endospores** The hard, impervious coats formed by bacteria such as *Clostridia*, allowing them to survive in a form of hibernation when conditions become unfavourable.

**Eosinophils** White blood cells that act as mediators in the inflammatory response.

**Epidural** The introduction of a local anaesthetic such as **bupivacaine** into the spinal cord to produce anaesthesia for surgical procedures.

**Ergosterol** The fungal equivalent of cholesterol. Essential for the stability of fungal membranes.

**Exendin-4** A hormone found in the saliva of the Mexican gila monster lizard (*Heloderma suspectum*) that has a similar structure and action to glucagon-like peptide-1.

**Exophthalmia** Protruding eyeballs, a symptom of hyperthyroidism.

**Expiration** The movement of air out of the lungs.

**Facultative anaerobes** Bacteria that prefer aerobic conditions but can survive without oxygen.

**Filtrate** The fluid filtered from the blood by the glomerulus.

**Fimbriae** Adhesion filaments found on certain bacteria.

**First-pass metabolism** The metabolism of a drug by hepatic enzymes during its first passage through the liver from the digestive system.

**Flagella (singular flagellum)** The whip-like tails that provide motility for certain bacteria.

**Folate** Folic acid as found in the body.

**Folic acid** Vitamin B9 – essential for the synthesis of pyrimidines.

Fusion proteins  High-tech drugs produced by recombinant technology. Two genes are fused and inserted into a bacterium that produces a novel protein with a therapeutic action.

GABA transaminase  An enzyme that removes the neurotransmitter GABA. Inhibiting GABA transaminase with drugs such as vigabatrin increases levels of GABA.

Gastric mucosa  The epithelial lining of the stomach, containing glands that secrete mucus, hydrochloric acid and pepsin.

Gastrin  A hormone secreted by the stomach in response to the ingestion of protein, stimulating the production of HCl by the parietal cells of the gastric mucosa.

Gastro-oesophageal reflux disease  Pain caused by stomach acid flowing into the oesophagus; commonly called heartburn.

Gastro-oesophageal sphincter (also known as the cardiac sphincter)  The ring of muscle between the stomach and oesophagus; usually prevents reflux of stomach contents.

Ginkgolides  Organic molecules found in *Ginkgo biloba* with anticoagulant action.

Glomerulus  Small filtration units at the head of nephrons in the kidney.

Glucagon-like peptide-1 (GLP-1)  A hormone produced by the gut in response to the presence of food. GLP-1 increases insulin production by the pancreas.

Glucose transporters  Transporter proteins that allow glucose to enter cells.

Glycosuria  The presence of glucose in the urine caused by abnormally high levels of glucose in the blood (as found in diabetes).

Goblet cells  Cells in epithelial mucous membranes that produce mucus.

Goitre  A swelling of the thyroid gland. May be caused by either hyperthyroidism or hypothyroidism.

Golgi apparatus  An organelle that packages newly synthesised proteins for dispatch.

Gram negative  A bacterial classification relating to the ability of a microbe to hold a stain for microscopy. Gram negative bacteria do not hold the Gram stain.

Gram positive  A bacterial classification relating to the ability of a microbe to hold a stain for microscopy. Gram positive bacteria hold the Gram stain.

Grave's disease  An auto-immune disease causing hyperthyroidism resulting in exophthalmia, goitre, insomnia, hyperactivity, etc.

Haemoglobin  A protein found in red blood cells that transports oxygen.

Half-life  The time it takes for the concentration of a drug in the body to fall by 50 per cent.

Helicase  An enzyme in the replication complex that, along with topoisomerases, configures DNA during replication and prevents DNA tangling.

Hepatic portal vein  The large vein that carries blood from the mesenteric (digestive) system into the liver.

Hepatic vein  The vein that transports blood from the liver to the vena cava.

Hexaploid  Organisms (mainly plants) which have six of each chromosome.

High-density lipoprotein (HDL)  Beneficial lipoproteins that help remove cholesterol from tissues.

Hippocampus and amygdala  Regions of the limbic system in the brain associated with memory.

Histamine  A locally acting mediator involved in many functions including inflammation.

**Human papillomavirus (HPV)** A virus that is a common cause of cervical cancer.

**Hydrogen bonds** Tiny forces of attraction between a hydrogen atom and an electronegative atom such as oxygen.

**Hypertrophy** An over-growth of muscle tissue.

**Hypoxic drive** A condition induced in COPD patients where the prime drive for breathing switches from carbon dioxide to oxygen.

**Idiopathic** A term used to indicate that the cause of an illness is unknown.

**Ileum** The final section of the small intestine after the jejunum.

**Incretin** A member of a family of peptide hormones released by the gut that include glucagon-like peptide-1.

**Inflammatory bowel disease** A serious condition involving ulceration and inflammation of the colon.

**Inspiration** The movement of air into the lungs.

**Interleukins** Chemical signals between white blood cells.

**Interleukin-6 (IL-6)** A cytokine secreted by T cells that stimulates the immune response in inflammation.

**Interphase** A phase in the cell cycle where cells copy their organelles and DNA in preparation for division.

**Invasive systemic candidiasis** A serious *Candida albicans* infection invading organs and tissues.

**Irritable bowel syndrome (IBS)** A mild problem with symptoms of abdominal pain and constipation or diarrhoea.

**Islets of Langerhans** Clusters of cells in the pancreas that release the hormones insulin (beta cells) and glucagon (alpha cells).

**Jejunum** The middle section of the small intestine between the duodenum and the ileum.

**Ketoacidosis** Acidosis resulting from low insulin in Type 1 diabetes. Cells starved of glucose switch to lipids as a fuel, producing acid ketones as a by-product.

**Ketones** By-products of fatty-acid metabolism. Most can be used as a fuel by certain tissues.

**Kininases** Enzymes that inactivate kinins.

**Late-phase response** An exacerbation of asthma symptoms that occurs several hours after the initial attack.

**Leukotrienes** Chemical mediators related to the prostaglandin group. Implicated in the exacerbation of asthma.

**Ligands** Chemical messengers such as hormones that bind to (usually) a receptor.

**Lipase** Enzyme secreted by the pancreas that breaks down fats into more simple components such as fatty acid.

**Lipoproteins** Small spheres that carry lipids in the blood.

**Loop of Henle** Part of the nephron tubule.

**Low-density lipoprotein (LDL)** Lipoproteins transport cholesterol to tissues where they can contribute to the formation of atheromata.

**Manic depression** The popular term for bipolar disorder where a patient experiences mood swings ranging from mania to depression.

**Melanomas** Skin cancers originating in the melanocytes of the skin.

**Melatonin** A hormone released by the pineal gland that has many functions including the regulation of body rhythms.

**Meningitis** Inflammation of the meninges, the membranes surrounding the brain, often caused by bacterial infection.

**Mesenteric artery** The blood vessel supplying blood to the mesenteric (digestive) system.

**Metastasis** The spread of a cancer from its site of origin to another tissue.

**Metered dose inhaler** A small patient-controlled device that delivers a precise dose of a bronchodilator to asthmatics.

**Mitochondria** The powerhouses of the cell. Organelles that produce ATP.

**Mitosis** The segregation of chromosomes during cell division that ensures each of the two new cells has a complete set of (in humans) 46 chromosomes.

**Modulators** The word 'modulate' simply means 'to change' so a modulator changes the way that something functions.

**Monoamine oxidase** A common enzyme that metabolises monoamines such as adrenaline, dopamine, serotonin, etc.

**Myelosuppression** The suppression of blood cell production in the bone marrow.

**Myxoedema** A condition caused by low thyroid levels, evidenced by slowness, lethargy and fatigue.

**N-acetyl-para-benzoquinoneimine** A toxic metabolite of paracetamol that can cause liver damage in overdose.

**Nebuliser** A face mask adapted to deliver (usually) bronchodilators to patients.

**Nephron** A microscopic structure in the kidney. Collectively, millions of nephrons filter waste from blood and produce urine.

**Neurokinin-1 (NK-1) receptor** A receptor for the neuromodulatory peptide, substance P.

**Neuromodulators** Locally acting signal molecules that influence the operation of synapses.

**Neutrophils** White blood cells that migrate to inflamed tissues and destroy bacteria.

**NMDA (N-methyl d-aspartate) receptors** Glutamate receptors in the brain that control the movement of cations such as $Na^+$ and $Ca^{2+}$ across synaptic membranes.

**Non-dihydropyridines** A group of calcium channel blockers defined by their chemical relatedness and including **verapamil** and **diltiazem**.

**Non-Hodgkin lymphomas** All blood cancers excluding Hodgkin's lymphoma.

**Noradrenaline** (also known as **norepinephrine**) A neurotransmitter in the sympathetic system.

**Nucleus** The largest of the cell's organelles. It contains the chromosomes made of DNA that code for our proteins.

**Oncogenes** Genes that can cause the uncontrolled cell division seen in cancer. Often mutations in proto-oncogenes result in them becoming oncogenes.

**Opportunistic pathogen** A microbe that generally acts as a commensal but can cause disease when conditions favour it.

**Osteoblasts** Bone cells that construct new bone.

**Osteoclasts** Bone cells that absorb the bone matrix in the process of remodelling.

**Osteocytes** Resident bone cells that help maintain healthy bone structure.

**Ovulation** The release of an ovum by the ovaries.

**Parietal** Cells of the gastric mucosa that secrete hydrochloric acid.

**Penicillinases** B-lactamases that specifically attack the B-lactam ring of penicillins.

**Pepsin** An enzyme produced by the gastric mucosa that breaks down ingested proteins.

**Peptic ulcers** Ulceration of the gastric mucosa, frequently caused by *Helicobacter pylori* infection.

**Peptidoglycan** A structural molecule only found in bacteria.

**Phosphodiesterase type-5** An enzyme involved in intracellular signalling in smooth muscle cells. Inhibition of the enzyme results in relaxation of muscle cells and vasodilation.

**Phospholipid bilayer** A double layer of mainly lipid molecules that forms the cell membrane of human cells.

**Plaques** Fatty deposits in the subendothelium of arteries.

**Plasma** The non-cellular part of the blood.

**Polymerases** Enzymes that produce polymers – e.g. DNA and mRNA.

**Polypharmacy** The situation where a patient (who is often elderly) is taking many drugs at the same time.

**Preload** The pressure exerted on the ventricle prior to systolic contraction. The more blood present in the ventricle, the greater the preload.

**Presynaptic receptors** Receptors on the presynaptic membrane; they respond to various neuromodulators in the control of synaptic transmission.

**Primary/essential hypertension** High blood pressure where the cause is unknown. Around 90 per cent of cases of hypertension fall into this category.

**Pro-drugs** Drugs that do not have pharmacological action until transformed by hepatic enzymes.

**Pro-hormone** The precursor of a fully active hormone.

**Prostaglandins thromboxanes** and **leukotrienes** A group of chemical mediators released by mast cells and macrophages that play a key part in the inflammatory response.

**Proteases** Enzymes secreted by the stomach and pancreas that break down proteins into component amino acids.

**Protoctista** A diverse group of single and multiple-celled eukaryotic organisms. Most do not cause disease, but some (such as *Trichomonas vaginalis*) do.

**Proto-oncogenes** Genes that code for proteins that promote cell division.

**Pulmonary system** A section of the circulatory system that carries deoxygenated blood from the right side of the heart to the lungs and then to the left side of the heart.

**Purine** Adenine and guanine nitrogenous bases found in DNA.

Pyloric sphincter  A ring of muscle between the stomach and the duodenum, which controls the release of stomach contents into the small intestine.

Pyrimidine  Thymine and cytosine nitrogenous bases found in DNA.

Recombinant technology  A bioengineering technique that involves the production of proteins by transferring a gene from one organism (usually a bacterium) to another.

Re-entrant rhythm  An aberrant heart rhythm caused by electrical signals in the myocardium travelling in the wrong direction.

Referred pain  Pain that appears to emanate from an area different from the actual source of the pain.

Renin  A circulating enzyme that converts angiotensinogen into angiotensin II in the renin–angiotensin pathway.

Replication complex  A cluster of enzymes that configures and copies DNA during replication.

Respiratory membrane  The epithelial cells of the alveoli and the endothelial cells of the pulmonary capillaries, across which oxygen and carbon dioxide diffuse.

Retrovirus  An RNA virus that copies itself into DNA in the host cell. The DNA provides the code for new viral particles.

Rheumatoid arthritis  A chronic inflammatory disease of the joints.

Ribosomes  Small organelles that assemble amino acids into proteins.

Secondary hypertension  Hypertension with an identifiable cause, such as renal failure.

Selective progesterone receptor modulator (SPRM)  A ligand that interacts with progesterone receptors, producing different effects in different tissues.

Selective toxicity  The ability of an antibacterial drug to kill a bacterium while leaving the host's cells unharmed.

Sino-atrial (SA) node  A group of cells in the myocardium that sets the heart's own rhythm.

Sinus rhythm  The normal rhythm of the heart as set by the sino-atrial node.

Specificity  How well a ligand or drug binds to its target rather than other proteins.

Spina bifida  Congenital spinal malformation. Prevention is aided by folic acid supplements.

Staphylococci  Bacteria that tend to aggregate into grape-like bunches.

Starling's law  Simply put, this law states that the more the heart's ventricles are stretched (the bigger the preload), the more forcefully they contract. This explains the increase in stroke volume during exercise.

Streptococci  Bacteria that tend to form into chains.

Substantia nigra  One of the basal ganglia responsible for the coordination of movement. Its degeneration causes Parkinson's disease.

Substrate  The substance converted by an enzyme into another substance.

Suppositories  Small rectally inserted capsules (usually) of glycerine containing drugs that are absorbed through the rectal membranes.

Swallowing reflex  An automatic response to food being positioned at the rear of the mouth.

Sympathetic nervous system  A division of the autonomic nervous system that is dominant during stress and exercise.

**Sympathomimetic** A drug that mimics the action of the sympathetic system.

**Systemic system** A section of circulatory system that carries oxygenated blood from the left side of the heart to the tissues of the body and then returns to the right side of the heart.

**Systole** The period of rising pressure in the ventricle or arteries.

**Thalamic–cortical neurons** Relay neurons between the thalamus and *cerebral cortex* that exhibit excess excitability in epilepsy.

**Thalamus** The region of the basal ganglia in the brain involved in relaying signals relating to movement to and from the cerebral cortex.

**Therapeutic index** The serum concentration of a drug in the range above minimum effective concentration but below maximum safe concentration.

**Thrombocytopenia** A low level of circulating platelets that can result in haemorrhage.

**Thromboxane A2** A member of the prostaglandin family. Induces the expression of GPIIb/IIIa receptors in platelets.

**Thrombus** A blood clot.

**Thymidylate synthetase** A key enzyme in the synthesis of DNA.

**Thyroidectomy** A surgical operation that involves the removal of part or all of the thyroid gland, often to correct hyperthyroidism.

**Thyroid-stimulating hormone** A hormone released by the anterior pituitary that stimulates the thyroid gland to produce thyroid hormones.

**Thyrotoxic crisis** A complication of hyperthyroidism resulting in high temperature, tachycardia and other symptoms associated with elevated levels of thyroid hormone.

**Thyrotoxicosis** Hyperthyroidism, manifested by nervousness, irritability, tachycardia, etc.

**Tissue plasminogen activator (t-pa)** A protein that converts plasminogen into its active form, plasmin, an enzyme that attacks fibrin.

**Topoisomerase** An enzyme in the replication complex that, along with helicases, configures DNA during replication and prevents DNA tangling.

**Transcription** The copying of a gene from DNA into mRNA.

**Translation** The production of a protein by ribosomes using the code contained in mRNA.

**Transpeptidase** A bacterial enzyme responsible for the synthesis of peptidoglycan. The main target for beta-lactam antibacterial drugs.

**Tumour necrosis factor alpha (TNF$\alpha$)** A pro-inflammatory cytokine released by T cells and macrophages.

**Tumour suppressor genes** Genes that code for proteins that inhibit cell division.

**Tyramine pressor response** A sudden rise in blood pressure caused by the release of noradrenaline in response to a rise in tyramine levels.

**Ulcerative colitis** Severe inflammation of the lining of the colon with ulceration.

**Ulcerative oesophagitis** Severe inflammation of the lining of the oesophagus with ulceration.

**Uracil** Nitrogenous bases found in RNA (instead of thymine).

**Vaccination** Exposing the body to a viral and bacterial antigen that stimulates an immunological memory, protecting the body against future infection.

Van der Waals forces  Tiny forces of attraction between molecules.

Vascular endothelial growth factor (VEGF)  A signal protein that promotes the growth of blood vessels.

Ventilation  The mechanical movement of air into and out of the lungs.

Venules  Small veins that emerge from the capillary bed to form veins.

Vitamin K reductase  An enzyme with vitamin K as its substrate, key in the production of various clotting factors.

Voltage-controlled ion channels  Ion channels that open or close in response to changes in the voltage across cell membranes (membrane potential).

White coat syndrome  A rise in blood pressure caused by anxiety when a doctor or nurse measures an individual's blood pressure.

# Index